SCHIZOPHRENIA

SCHIZOPHRENIA
Origins, Processes, Treatment, and Outcome

Edited by

Rue L. Cromwell
C. R. Snyder

New York   Oxford
OXFORD UNIVERSITY PRESS
1993

Oxford University Press

Oxford   New York   Toronto
Delhi   Bombay   Calcutta   Madras   Karachi
Kuala Lumpur   Singapore   Hong Kong   Tokyo
Nairobi   Dar es Salaam   Cape Town
Melbourne   Auckland   Madrid

and associated companies in
Berlin   Ibadan

Library of Congress Cataloging-in-Publication Data
Schizophrenia : origins, processes, treatment, and outcome /
edited by Rue L. Cromwell and C. R. Snyder
p.   cm   . Includes bibliographical references and index.
ISBN 0-19-506922-6
1. Schizophrenia.   I. Cromwell, Rue L., 1928–
II. Snyder, C. R. [DNLM: 1. Schizophrenia.
WM 203S337945]   RC514.533625   1993
616.89′82—dc20
DNLM/DLC   for Library of Congress   92-48996

9 8 7 6 5 4 3 2 1

Printed in the United States of America
on acid-free paper

Preface

Many advances have occurred recently both in the molecular sciences concerning schizophrenia and in the precise clinical effects when the disorder is treated. At the same time, often in separate and parallel development, advances have occurred in the behavioral science investigations of the disorder. The need seemed both increasing and timely for a book that could illustrate how such variables and findings could interrelate. In some instances the variables of behavioral science could be the glue by which to organize and bridge the disparate gap between the molecules, topical metabolism, and structure, on the one hand, and the travails of a clinician searching for the best possible care for a given person with disordered functioning. In other instances it appeared that the variables of other disciplines were necessary in order to understand fully the phenomena of the behavioral laboratory. For the scientist or clinician outside behavioral science would come the message in this book that different levels of construction and integration of variables are needed—not just an isolated molecular reductionism or just a humanistic or mentalistic expansionism. For the behavioral scientist would come the increased recognition of how other disciplines contribute to and profit from this cross-disciplinary journey.

Consequently, this book is a product of many converging forces; it spans professions and disciplines. The contributors are those who not only have separate areas of research and clinical expertise, but they also think flexibly enough to "break from the pack" and reach for ideas that may make a difference in advancing knowledge and amelioration. In this respect, a special thanks is offered Prof. dr. med. Manfred Bleuler, who shared personal stories about his father as he broke from the pack and created the schizophrenia construct.

The setting within which the book has developed is the Clinical Psychology Graduate Training Program of the University of Kansas. With its Psychology Clinic and research laboratories, this program has maintained a balanced focus in research and practitioner skills. With its recently endowed M. Erik Wright Distinguished Professorship in Clinical Psychology, a major focus has been placed upon psychopathology. The "crew" of graduate students devoted to psychopathology issues has been a rich source for inspired questions and inquiry during the development of this book. Work on the book was first initiated with a conference in the Kansas Series in Clinical Psychology (KSCP), which was sponsored by the Clinical Psychology Graduate Training Program, the Psychological Clinic, and the Continuing Education Division of the University of Kansas.

In the production of the final manuscript, much appreciation is owed to Joan Bossert and to Berta Steiner for their professional assistance and patient support. Many hours have been spent by Sharon Vaughn in proofing, detecting unclear passages, and preparing some of the artwork. Thanks also are extended to Jennifer Snyder and J. Jeffrey Crowson who have assisted in the indexing of the volume.

Finally, thanks are offered to the people with schizophrenia and to their relatives as they have separately borne the burdens of the disorder and yet have cooperated and worked with us in the various studies.

June 1993   R. L. C.
Lawrence, Kansas   C. R. S.

Contents

Contributors

Ralph N. Adams
Department of Chemistry
University of Kansas
Lawrence, Kansas

Lawrence E. Adler
Department of Psychiatry
University of Colorado Health Sciences
*   Center*
Denver, Colorado

Alvin S. Bernstein
Department of Psychiatry
State University of New York
Health Sciences Center at Brooklyn
Brooklyn, New York

Paula Bickford-Wimer
Department of Psychiatry
University of Colorado Health Sciences
*   Center*
Denver, Colorado

Larry A. Carver
Department of Psychiatry and
*   Neuroscience*
School of Medicine
Louisiana State University
New Orleans, Louisiana

Ellen Cawthra
Department of Psychiatry
University of Colorado Health Sciences
*   Center*
Denver, Colorado

Rue L. Cromwell
Department of Psychology
University of Kansas
Lawrence, Kansas

Terrence S. Early
Department of Psychiatry
Washington University School of
*   Medicine*
St. Louis, Missouri

Robert Freedman
Department of Psychiatry
University of Colorado Health Sciences
*   Center*
Denver, Colorado

Michael J. Goldstein
Department of Psychology
University of California, Los Angeles
Los Angeles, California

Martin Harrow
Department of Psychiatry
University of Illinois College of Medicine
Michael Reese Medical Center
Chicago, Illinois

David R. Hemsley
Department of Psychology
Institute of Psychiatry
De Crespigny Park, Denmark Hill
London University
London, United Kingdom

Shara Highgate
Department of Psychology
University of Western Ontario
London, Ontario, Canada

Lee Hoffer
Department of Psychiatry
University of Colorado Health Sciences
*   Center*
Denver, Colorado

William G. Iacono
Department of Psychology
University of Minnesota
Minneapolis, Minnesota

Raymond A. Knight
Department of Psychology
Brandeis University
Waltham, Massachusetts

Alice Madison
Department of Psychiatry
University of Colorado Health Sciences
    Center
Denver, Colorado

Peter McGuffin
Department of Psychological Medicine
University of Wales College of Medicine
Heath Park, Cardiff, Wales

David J. Miklowitz
Department of Psychology
University of Colorado, Boulder
Boulder, Colorado

Herbert Nagamoto
Department of Psychiatry
University of Colorado Health Science
    Center
Denver, Colorado

Richard W. J. Neufeld
Department of Psychology
University of Western Ontario
London, Ontario, Canada

Michael C. O'Donovan
Department of Psychological Medicine
University of Wales College of Medicine
Heath Park, Cardiff, Wales

Arvin F. Oke
Department of Chemistry
University of Kansas
Lawrence, Kansas

Seymour Rosenberg
Department of Psychology
Rutgers University
New Brunswick, New Jersey

Neal S. Rubin
Department of Psychiatry
University of Illinois College of Medicine
Michael Reese Medical Center
Chicago, Illinois

Nina R. Schooler
Western Psychiatric Institute and Clinic
University of Pittsburgh
Pittsburgh, Pennsylvania

C. R. Snyder
Department of Psychology
University of Kansas
Lawrence, Kansas

Will D. Spaulding
Department of Psychology
University of Nebraska, Lincoln
Lincoln, Nebraska

Herbert E. Spohn
Director of Research
Menninger Foundation
Topeka, Kansas

Richard A. Steffy
Department of Psychology
University of Waterloo
Waterloo, Ontario, Canada

Eckart R. Straube
Department of Psychiatry
University of Tübingen
Tübingen, Germany

David Vollick
Department of Psychology
University of Western Ontario
London, Ontario, Canada

Irwin Waldman
Department of Psychology
University of Minnesota
Minneapolis, Minnesota

Merilyne Waldo
Department of Psychiatry
University of Colorado Health Sciences
    Center
Denver, Colorado

SCHIZOPHRENIA

Heritage of the Schizophrenia Concept

RUE L. CROMWELL

The term "schizophrenic psychoses" was coined in the writings of Eugen Bleuler (1911/trans., 1950). Like all elements of our language, it came to us with the cultural influences that reflect the times. Before the present book examines some of the ideas and understandings at the forefront of schizophrenia research and treatment, a brief look at aspects of this heritage is appropriate.

Eugen Bleuler's father was a farmer in Zøllikon, near Zürich, Switzerland. During his time only the sons of nobility and aristocracy were considered appropriate for colleges and universities—and a farmer was hardly viewed with such status. However, there arose an interest among the common people with respect to education and opportunities for their children. Eugen's father, together with neighboring farmers, began to collect books, build libraries in their homes, and conduct informal seminars in order to prepare their children for higher education. So it was that Eugen Bleuler (1857–1939), in this climate of constructive interest, broke traditional barriers and entered medical school.

A major mental hospital, the Burghølzli, had been established in 1870 in the Zürich area. No psychiatry training had been established, so psychiatrists were "imported" from Germany. These psychiatrists did not know the local dialect, and communication with patients was poor. (Apparently, the finer aspects of meaning were not considered essential then for effective diagnosis and patient care. It seemed to be enough to understand the gross features of the disorder.) As a consequence, personal needs of the patients, independent of the mental illness, were not met—and not even understood.

Relatives of the patients became concerned about this failure in personal understanding and care. They exerted pressure to acquire someone who could understand the patients. A young local medical student was summoned for this role. This young student was Eugen Bleuler. Thereby, Bleuler was introduced to the mentally ill—prior to didactic training about mental illness.

Given this assignment, Bleuler spent innumerable hours sitting with, walking with, and listening to patients. In fact, he worked with them all day long. Unquestionably, it was from this rich background that his new concept, schizophrenic psychoses, evolved.

Bleuler thought of schizophrenia from the perspective of the patient's subjective state. He did not hesitate to infer that each patient, even the most humble or unexpressive, had thoughts and feelings. Bleuler observed how these thoughts and feelings could "break apart" (i.e., fail to relate to each other or to reality). Loose associations of one thought to another, the lack of accompaniment of the expected feeling (affect) with a thought, the loss of confidence to assert an abstract thought (i.e., the ambivalence), the unique personal meaning attributed to some thoughts (i.e., the autism)—all these were the stuff of what Bleuler, from his long hours of listening and conversing, came to view as the essence of schizophrenia. Indeed, for him it was a phrenic, not a cephalic, disorder.

Although Bleuler came to his understandings from firsthand clinical observation, his ultimate views did not reject those of Emil Kraepelin in Germany. Kraepelin had introduced dementia praecox in his 1896 textbook (see Diefendorf, 1923), with emphasis on the course of the disorder rather than on common symptom features. Bleuler fully acknowledged this development (E. Bleuler, 1911):

By the presence of the symptom complex so selected and defined (by Kraepelin) the great group of dementia praecox is characterized as a unit. . . . A closer examination shows that, in fact, all these cases have much in common, that they are clearly marked off from other types of mental disease. (p. 3)

Thus, we are left with no alternative but to give the disease a new name . . . schizophrenia. . . . For the sake of convenience I use the word in the singular although it is apparent that the group includes several diseases. (p. 8)

Apparently the acknowledgment and respect between Kraepelin and Bleuler was mutual. Kraepelin, a man of "higher origins" who was comfortable in the presence of nobility, often took his summer vacations in Italy. On the way he was known to stop off as a guest with the Bleuler family. He brought with him each time a suitcase of clinical case folders. Eugen's son, Professor dr. Med. Manfred Bleuler,[1] who succeeded his father as head of the Burghølzli, recalls that his father and Kraepelin would sit examining and discussing these clinical cases. Then, as Kraepelin returned from Italy, the event was repeated.

Thus, Kraepelin and Bleuler were on the same quest. Each knew that the understand-

ing of the disorder had to go beyond such things as hallucinatory or delusional report, disordered expression of thought, or catatonic motor features. Both believed that an organic basis would probably be shown to exist. Both accepted the possibility of a familial contribution in at least some cases. Both struggled with the unitary versus multiple nature of the disorder. As for subtle biobehavioral features, Kraepelin noted: "Ordinary external impressions are correctly apprehended, the patients being able to recognize their environments and to comprehend most of what takes place about them. Yet accurate tests show that very brief stimuli are not well apprehended" (Diefendorf, 1923, p. 222). Eugen Bleuler undoubtedly agreed.

Being privy only to the chronic patients who remained in contact with the clinic, both Kraepelin and Bleuler viewed the disorder as poor in prognosis, if not incurable. It was left to Bleuler's son (M. Bleuler, 1978) to shed a more optimistic light on this issue through long-term follow-up of patients, many of whom were long separated from the hospital. What, then, characterizes the difference between these two brilliant clinicians? In response to this question, Manfred[1] recounts the following incident.

One evening, when Manfred was a child, his father came home from the clinic at the end of the day. At the dinner table his father reflected on a catatonic woman he had seen that day. She was severely impaired and had not spoken for many months. Nevertheless, the elder Bleuler sat with her in her mute state. As he did so, she fixed her eyes on Bleuler's wedding ring. She reached out and gently touched it with one finger. She withdrew her hand and fleetingly looked at her doctor before gazing away.

As the elder Bleuler sat at the dinner table, he inferred what may have been happening in her thoughts. It was as if she were saying, "I know what that is. I was once married. I once had a wedding ring also. I was once a person of dignity. I was once loved. I have known that. But here I am now, a person of stone." And such a conclusion, according to Manfred Bleuler, was

1. Based on personal communication with Manfred Bleuler at his home in Zøllikon, Switzerland, on June 26, 1986. Acknowledgment is offered to Professor Bleuler for editing this manuscript and for reminding me to express his father's concept in the plural (i.e., schizophrenic psychoses).

a difference between his father and Emil Kraepelin. In the following paragraphs that difference is pondered.

THE CULTURAL HERITAGE

Terms in our language are severally influenced by the ideas and values of the civilization that led to them. The term "schizophrenia" is no exception. Just as the flow and evolution of civilized thought and value helped shape the term, so will succeeding events doubtlessly change its meaning and use. Thus, how we view schizophrenia now marks a point in time. Perhaps only a few of these antecedent influences are detectable, but some are worthy of comment.

Observation

The first major trend, which laid the groundwork not only for our concept of schizophrenia but for all other scientific and secular bodies of knowledge, came almost 800 years before the time of Bleuler. It was an assertion that independent inquiry is necessary to arrive at the truth. In medieval times, the church was the repository of most formal knowledge. More importantly, the understanding of the world was assumed to follow only from religious faith. For example, Anselm expressed the long-standing view, "I must believe in order that I may understand." A pivotal change occurred in 1122 when Peter Abelard made the shocking counter-assertion, "I must understand in order that I may believe." He further stated, "By doubting we come to questioning, and by questioning we perceive the truth" (see Clark, 1969, p. 44). Although Abelard's major life work focused on examining alternative premises in rational (deductive) logic, his challenges paved the way for formal inquiry of all kinds—for empirical methods such as clinical observation and for other scientific methodology, including research design and data analysis. Like Galileo 500 years later, who advanced the scientific (inductive) method, Abelard was repeatedly in trouble with the church for his views.

By the time of Bleuler, however, the importance of observing was taken for granted, and the keenness of clinical observation is well portrayed by both Kraepelin and Bleuler. Yet this historical shift in how we approach knowledge required centuries. Perhaps it was best and most simply summarized by I. P. Pavlov (1849–1936), a Russian contemporary of Bleuler: "Observation—and, again, observation" (W. N. Kellogg, personal communication, 1947).

Humanism

Along with the increased emphasis on reason, and later on sensory experience, as the basis for acquiring knowledge, the importance of the human being as such came to be recognized. The human being became recognized as both the instrument and object of the knowledge search. This trend, in fact, was not independent of the one toward observation. Instead, the shift toward inquiry placed greater emphasis on the individual—his or her doubting and subsequent investigation. This humanistic trend was first demonstrated by a revival of earlier Greek and Roman writings during the 1400s; it later became coordinated with the scientific and political revolutions of the 1600s. Scientific and technological discoveries led to greater industry and commerce, which required a middle class to manufacture and to buy. The emerging middle class came to question whether God gave kings and nobility the divine right to govern. They tended instead to conclude that God gave "natural rights" to the people, who then by social contract assigned powers of sovereignty to the kings and political leaders (e.g., Jefferson, 1776; Paine, 1791). Such issues were soon taken to the battlefield in England, France, and America.

Within this context of the events of the prior 300 or 400 years, it is not surprising that the right of a Swiss farm boy to receive an education was a point of concern. Likewise, it is not surprising that the rights and welfare of the mentally ill became a focus of attention. At the beginning of the humanistic movement only the aristocratic, the highly educated, and clergy merited such concern. By stages, however, the concern for welfare has penetrated to the middle class, the urban poor (Dickens' time), slaves, and women. The trend continues.

The same trend, away from figures of deity and sainthood toward common humanity, is well reflected in art. In the early 1500s the Venetian painter Giorgione (1477–1510) perhaps disturbed the course of history by painting *Ritratto di Vecchia* (*col tempo*) (Academy of Fine Arts, Venice, Italy). It depicts a poor and old, powerless, fear-laden woman, apparently battered and abused "with time" and circumstance, who appears to have been a beauty in her earlier years. For such a work of art to appear amidst representations of the deity, biblical icons, and royal portraits (not to mention portraits of rich merchants a century later) spoke to the changing conceptualization of dignity and worth.

Meanwhile, the role of the church as the guide and repository for the pursuit of knowledge was waning. New scientific findings were increasingly difficult to reconcile with old theology. So too were the new rational ideas. For example, the writings of Descartes (1596–1650), a devout Catholic, were banned by the church because they relied too heavily on reason.

Subjective Feeling and Thought

Another trend reflected in Eugen Bleuler's concept of schizophrenia is the recognition of internal feeling, thought, tension, and conflict. To pinpoint the various possible influences leading to this trend perhaps defies accuracy. After reason, and then observation, began to replace church authority as the basis for understanding humankind, a period of time came in which it was thought sufficient to understand people simply as reasoning and logical entities. Then, during the century preceding Eugen Bleuler's, more writers began to reject this simplistic view of people. About 50 years before Bleuler's time, Dostoyevski began asserting that the rational nature of people was only a veneer, that they were more completely

characterized by inner emotional turmoil and impulses. Only about 20 years before Bleuler's major work, Nietzsche was taking great delight in attacking as absurd every conceivable value and premise that characterized the rational person or to which the rational person dearly held. To Nietzsche, people were best explained by an underlying motive, devoid of rational decision. This motive was for power (or, if you will, internal locus of control) in anticipating event outcomes. "Rational truths" were flimsy artifacts. Finally, concurrent with Bleuler came Freud, who changed and extended beyond Nietzsche the idea of underlying motives about which the person does not rationally decide.

Because these events emphasized the existence of an "inside world" as well as an external environment, the stage was set to ask which was given the most attention by the individual. It is here that a contemporary of Eugen Bleuler, Carl G. Jung, made a contribution by introducing the concept of introversion–extraversion. Then, a young physician who studied with Bleuler himself, Hermann Rorschach, utilized an ink blot test to measure, among other things, the *Erlebnistypus,* this dimension of responsiveness to internal versus external stimuli.[2]

However, these existential thinkers immediately preceding Bleuler cannot be counted as the first to introduce the importance of subjective feeling and thought. For centuries poetry and song have been accepted as exceeding prose, and art as exceeding words, in expressing these inner experiences. In addition to Giorgione, Van Eyck, 400 years before Bleuler, was recognized for his sensitive portrayal of the human face as reflecting the inner personality. The poetry of Shakespeare followed 100 years later. Then some 50 years after that,

2. It is appropriate to note that when Hermann Rorschach was developing the ink blot test while working with Eugen Bleuler, he asked Manfred (b. 1903), Eugen's son and then a grammar school pupil, if he would show the ink blot cards to his schoolmates and report their responses. Manfred complied. Thus, Manfred Bleuler may be recorded as the first person to administer Rorschach's test systematically to hundreds of children.

Rembrandt (1607–1669) excelled all others in his ability to reveal sympathetically on canvas the diversity of internal states in the faces of his subjects.

Having recounted these possible historic influences, one must not ignore the final major force. Eugen Bleuler began his study of schizophrenia with observation and interaction, not with text and tutorial. If approached in this way, does not schizophrenia demand to be understood in terms of subjective thoughts and feelings? With the elusive falling away of rational structures, what is left to observe and describe?

Dualistic Explanation

The recourse to the subjective took Bleuler's concept of schizophrenia inevitably into the problems of dualistic explanation. Because this age-old issue continues as a theoretical and linguistic troublemaker in concepts such as schizophrenia, it especially merits attention here.

The origin of considering mind and body as separate entities can easily be conjectured. Primeval individuals needed explanations for why people quit behaving at death as well as why they might show unexpected or aberrant behavior. From the primeval to the present, religion has needed a language to help account for transition to the hereafter. From such bodies of thought, the concept of mind has served a sound functional purpose and has become embedded in the common language. The trouble began only after a specialized language was needed for scientific purposes.

If science, as by definition, is a body of knowledge based on the observable, the terms used in science should meet one of two requirements. They should either (a) refer (by denotation, counting, or measuring) to something that is observable, or, if referring to phenomena outside the realm of direct observation, they should (b) be anchored to some observable event that provides an indirect measure. For science to be a repository of public knowledge (a repository not only of terms and their definitions but also of antecedent–consequent

and coordinate relationships among them), a third requirement (c) occurs: the terms and their referents must be not only observable but also "publicly shared observable." This third requirement in particular has created confusion because of privately held observations. It is freely assumed that both the scientific observer and the subject have these unshared private experiences. Bleuler freely assumed this in schizophrenia. Yet, for sound rules of repository, our observations must be reduced to propositions shareable with and subject to the critical scrutiny of others. How fortunate are the physicists, who deal with a subject matter that does not talk and thereby reveal subjective thoughts and feelings!

As viewed through history, dualistic explanation has taken many forms. Mind, for example, has usually been defined as outside the realm of physical time and space measurements. It has been (and sometimes still is) considered the determinant of bodily action (or else an inevitable or necessary correlate thereof). Such a proposition is a dualistic explanation and thus unacceptable in scientific language. The common thread of all dualistic explanations is a nonobservable posited as determining an observable.

In attempting to understand the problem of dualistic construction in the enterprise of behavioral science and mental health, a review of the classical concepts of dualism is fairly uninformative. Thinkers such as Democritus, Plato, Aristotle, and later, Descartes, Leibniz, Hobbes, and still later Freud, used creative brushstrokes in their dualistic explanations and, except for Hobbes, were in no way attentive to the guidelines necessary to an efficient scientific language. Spinoza proposed a monistic universe that had two levels of descriptive language, the physical language and the mental language. This was a significant step, but the vestiges of the traditional dichotomy would still encumber the hypothetico-deductive, cross-disciplinary, and repository requirements of modern science.

Psychology, as a laboratory science beginning in the 1800s, was defined as the study of consciousness. So, at the outset, its conception was manifestly dualistic. By the turn of the century, however, scientific psychology was becoming sensitive to its dualistic problems. In 1904, William James wrote:

For twenty years past I have mistrusted "consciousness" as an entity; for seven or eight years past I have suggested its non-existence to my students, and tried to give them its pragmatic equivalent in realities of experience. It seems to me that the hour is ripe for it to be openly and universally discarded. (James, 1904, pp. 477–478)

Indeed it was discarded, because, 1 year after James' death and in the same year of Bleuler's text, John B. Watson in 1911 proposed behavior as the subject matter of psychology. With the change to an objective subject matter like other sciences, however, Watson did not solve the problem of dualistic explanation:

Human psychology has failed to make good its claim as a natural science. Due to a mistaken notion that its fields of facts are conscious phenomena and that introspection is the only direct method of ascertaining these facts, it has enmeshed itself in a series of speculative questions which, while fundamental to its present tenets, are not open to experimental treatment. . . . Psychology, as the behaviorist views it, is a purely objective, experimental branch of natural science which needs introspection as little as do the sciences of chemistry and physics. . . . It can dispense with consciousness in a psychological sense. . . . This suggested elimination of states of consciousness as proper objects of investigation in themselves will remove the barrier from psychology which exists between it and the other sciences. The findings of psychology become the functional correlates of structure and lend themselves to explanation in physio-chemical terms. (Watson, 1913, pp. 176–177)

Instead of positing mind or consciousness as the basis of behavior, Watson posited physicochemical events. At that time, as in many respects today, such events lacked the operational referents, direct or indirect, necessary to meet the aforementioned requirements. Thus, to posit physicochemical events, rather than mind or consciousness, as the determining basis of behavior was, in effect, substituting a manifest with a latent dualism. That is, unobservables are used to explain observables. Furthermore, because introspection was rejected as a scientific method, it would have been impossible for Watsonian behaviorism to have accommodated Bleuler's keen insights about schizophrenia. This is only one instance of a legitimate problem being avoided because things subjective were declared of no scientific interest. Nevertheless, the original stance in behaviorism remained. Pratt, espousing the Watson view, stated it even more strongly: "What psychology strives to do, all that it could ever want to do, is to explain the self in terms of physiological conditions, among which those responsible for perception and memory would play a significant role" (Pratt, 1939, p. 39).

Needless to say, others detected this dualistic fallacy. Skinner (Ferster & Skinner, 1957) attempted to resolve it by designing a theory of environmental (rather than organismic) control and by adopting two fundamental assumptions from Charles Darwin: (a) multiple and random generation, and (b) selective survival. Instead of referring to a species change over time, Skinner applied these assumptions to the behavioral repertoire of single individuals. Individuals, as a basic given, were assumed capable of random and variable behavior. Through life circumstances some of these behaviors are reinforced by the environment and some are not. If reinforced, the behavior has an increased probability of being repeated (surviving). If not reinforced, the behavior will move toward extinction. Thus, Skinner explained the determinants of behavior not on the basis of mind or consciousness, not on the basis of Watson's remote physicochemical events, but instead on the basis of environmental reinforcers.

With both the behaviors and the reinforcers in a denotable universe of time and space, Skinner's theory was free of dualism. Much efficient headway was thereby gained in studying how certain behaviors become modified. However, the theory did not provide for individual difference constructs. The same parametric rules applied to all. No provision existed for cognitive, biological, genetic, or other organismic factors that could predict that different individuals might respond differently to the behavior-reinforcer conditions. Bleuler posited schizophrenia as an individual difference construct—one in which internal and external events did not follow the same nomothetic rules as with normal individuals. Consequently, Skinner's theory has not provided fertile ground to advance knowledge about schizophrenia.

Kantor (1947, 1959) also sensed the problems of early scientific psychology and of Watson's theory. Moreover, he did not accept Skinner's resolution. In his metascientific formulation he was concerned that dualism be avoided but that legitimate areas of inquiry for psychology not be ruled out. Kantor's formulation depicted four steps in the scientist's enterprise, from observation to conclusion. The first step assumed the subject matter of all sciences to be denotable and shareable events within a time–space field. In other words, inferences, such as disordered thought, are constructions of events, not the events themselves. Kantor saw psychology as an arbitrary division of labor that attends primarily to events of interaction between organisms and stimulus objects in this time–space field. (Indeed, he called his theory interbehaviorism.) Unlike Skinner, both organismic and environmental variables, if operationally defined, were acceptable. Moreover, the antecedent–consequence relation could be hypothesized in either direction, not just from environment to organism.

Kantor assumed, second, that the scientist creates a record of these observations (after appropriate denoting, counting, or measuring), and, third, that this record is submitted to analysis and further reduction through mathematics and logic. Finally, the scientific observer construes the event. This construction is a verbal proposition or mathematical formula that relates two or more observed variables in antecedent–consequent or correlative relationship. The construction also notes the field and biographic setting where the observation occurred. Thereby, the construction is suitable for the scientific repository; it can be scrutinized and potentially replicated by others.

Much is accomplished in this simple formulation. Dualism is discarded, because only observables may be related to observables. Skinnerian behavior analysis is fully acceptable but only as one class of organism–environment interaction and construction. Subjective inferences, such as the subjectively held thoughts and feelings Bleuler described, are fully accepted. They are accepted not as events (i.e., what the patient said and did) but as constructions of events. They are scientifically acceptable so long as they, as variables, enter into reliable relationships with other variables derived from the event field. Introspection, like other observational techniques, is thereby fully accepted if it can be reliably reported, recorded, related to other variables, and replicated.

Of importance, Kantor would emphasize the denotation of what was actually observed, which gave rise to these constructions couched in subjective language. He would contend that such constructions survive, as do all others in science, until some alternative construction accounts for more events or accounts for given events with higher levels of predictability.

After recounting how introspective reporting of thoughts and feelings is acceptable in Kantor's (1947, 1959) formulation, it is also important to describe the aspects that are unacceptable. One popular example is to assume that the subjectively held experiences of an observed individual predetermine how he or she is going to behave. In spite of the value of subjective thoughts and feelings as useful constructs to relate to other variables, this particular construction is dualistic. The unobservable predetermines the observable. As dualistic, it is a nonheuristic cul-de-sac that retards the advancement of knowledge.

Some of the features of Kantor's (1947, 1959) formulation can be illustrated by the "rain god paradox." Let us assume a primitive tribe interprets dark, low-lying clouds to indicate that the rain gods are angry. When angry, the rain gods will create thunder, lightning, and rain. As applied to the Kantorian formulation, a construction that links "dark, low-lying clouds" to increased probability of "thunder, lightning, and rain", is not dualistic. Observables are linked to observables. The hypothesized relationship is analyzable, construable, and replicable. (Looking back a century from now, it is possible that many of the current formulations will be viewed as being of this caliber!) Certainly, contemporary thinking would view the theory as primitive and would believe that newer meteorological formulations would improve and broaden predictions. All constructions, both primitive and contemporary, are arbitrary, and the testable formulation arising from rain gods, although not expected to survive, is nevertheless legitimate.

However, other aspects of the rain god formulation illustrate unacceptable scientific language. The premise that rain gods cause the dark clouds (or cause the rainy aftermath) is indeed dualistic. Such propositions have unobservables that determine observables. The field of mental health is plagued with such formulations, albeit they are more subtle.

Another fallacy often concurrent with dualism is the assumption that the construction causes the event: "Why does this person have hallucinations and thought disorder?" "Because he is schizophrenic." If schizophrenia is defined in terms of these same symptoms, it cannot also cause them. A map that defines a territory does not cause the territory to occur. The word "chair" does not cause the object chair to occur.

Neurochemical, psycholinguistic, sociological, and other organismic variables are not only acceptable in Kantor's (1947, 1959) formulation but are needed in cross-disciplinary research. As long as the variables therefrom yield testable hypotheses, they are acceptable to the language of science. These systems of constructs, associated with different disciplines, are often referred to as levels of description, as determined by the relative molarity versus molecularity of their constructs. Molarity versus molecularity is defined by the relative amount of time and space required to denote the construct.

Range of Convenience

Kelly (1955), who argued that individual personalities as well as scientists are in the business of building construct systems, stated clearly the notion that different constructs (and systems of constructs) have different ranges of convenience. That is, concepts, like other tools, are suited for certain purposes. A particular problem, such as understanding schizophrenia, may be outside the range of convenience of certain constructs. Thus, these constructs are of no value in understanding that problem. In contrast, through creativity or serendipity, some constructs are discovered to have a range of convenience that was not originally suspected. The investigation of schizophrenia has been approached on a number of different levels of construction, and which levels ultimately have the greatest value is yet to be determined.

Reductionism

The concept of range of convenience challenges the assumption of reductionism. Reductionism, a logical fallacy different from but sometimes co-existent with dualism, assumes that the explanation most preferable is always the one based on the most molecular level of description. An extreme form of reductionism would maintain that more molecular levels of description actually cause the more molar levels of description. From this view, all we need to study is the biological, genetic, biochemical, and finally the physicochemical correlates of schizophrenia. By such progression we would thereby understand it. Notions of range of convenience and level of predictability are set aside. This logical fallacy is still inherent in the thinking of many investigators of schizophrenia and of other psychiatric disorders.

Indeed, some problems require that the scientist move to a more molecular level for adequate solution. In such cases the move toward molecularity does not involve the fallacy of reductionism. Only when molecular constructions are made at the expense of predictive adequacy and range of convenience is the reductionistic fallacy committed.

Historically, methods and technology for the more molecular constructs have usually advanced first. Perhaps they were relatively less threatening to medieval religious convictions. If methods and knowledge for molar constructs had developed first, molarity would have been deemed most basic. That is, the logical fallacy could have gone in the reverse direction. For the time being, in schizophrenia research, it would appear fruitful to adhere to the notion that different constructs have different ranges of convenience and that level of predictability, not molecularity (i.e., the more biological), is the ultimate criterion to advance understanding.

Often overlooked is the alternate fallacy of expansionism. One can assume that the more molar construction is always preferable. Molecular constructions are thereby excluded. Again, it may be that some problems of schizophrenia can achieve optimal predictability when molar constructs are employed. However, to say, for example, that the family system or the rejection of unwanted behavior by society is the only basis by which to understand schizophrenia would indeed be expansionistic.

Mind

Quite separate from the issue of dualistic fallacy, a comment on the use of the term "mind" is appropriate. The dualistic usage of mind, that mental state predetermines overt behavior, is only one way in which mind is currently used. Many choose to use the term outside scientific construct systems. There is no sound tenet that holds that other construct systems, such as religion

and law, should be subordinate to the scientific. So, the guidelines here do not apply to such usages. In contrast, many use the term within scientific parlance. Some fear that giving up the concept means giving up data from subjective impressions. Some fear that giving up the concept represents a step backward from the humanistic, compassionate view of the dignity and worth of people. Some are simply inattentive to or careless about rigorous rules of language within science. Needless to say, all these reasons would be rejected by Kantor's (1947, 1959) formulation.

Others have attempted to redefine "mind" monistically as a generic term referring to behavior—or else, anything that is not brain and brain function. Still others use it as a rough equivalent for anything cognitive or affective or motivational. Some positively assert the use of "mind" because of the need, well documented by Joseph Campbell (1988), for something mystical and mythic outside the rigors of modern science. The uses of the term "mind" are so varied that scientific objection to it must range from its being obstructive to being merely useless excess baggage in scientific language.

Clearly, the use of "mind" is well fixed in our common language. Moreover, most people fear giving up the conceptual ground on which they stand. As George Bernard Shaw has suggested, people are immediately willing to give up an obsolete instrument, such as a wooden plow or hand-cranked car, but they are most unwilling to give up an obsolete idea or concept (Shaw, 1907, pp. 140–141). Only occasionally do we try. As one of my students once said, "If you think I believe in mind–body dualism, you are out of your behavior."

Schizophrenia, as we view it today, is a complex of problems requiring many levels of description and investigation. To identify logical fallacies, such as have been described above, among the investigations of schizophrenia requires very little effort. This is all the more reason we should be mindful of the roots and heritage of the concept with which we deal.

ABOUT THIS BOOK

In the foregoing sections an attempt has been made to show that the term "schizophrenia" is a product of its time, that it benefited from the advances in our cultural heritage, and that it shares some of the problems yet to be resolved in our cultural heritage. It is not an age-old concept. It emerged in the same year as the Chevrolet car, the Indianapolis Speedway Races, the abandonment of horse-drawn double-decker buses in London, the invention of the "self-starter" for motor cars, Irving Berlin's song "Alexander's Ragtime Band," Rorschach's ink blot test, and behaviorism, all products of their time as well. Clearly, the worldwide adoption of the term "schizophrenia" attests to the need to demark this particular area of human suffering.

The purpose of this book is to present what is in the forefront of our understanding of schizophrenia eight decades later. In doing so, six strategies are especially notable. Sober judgment would suggest that a combination and integration of these strategies, rather than one bandwagon approach, will move knowledge of schizophrenia ahead.

The first strategy, apparent across the various contributors, is that the classifying and tracking of symptoms over time are as important now as Kraepelin and Bleuler initially assumed. Stated negatively, much is likely lost by considering together all types of symptoms and all courses of the disorder. Negative versus positive symptoms and the differential course of reactive and process subclasses of the disorder are especially of current concern.

A second strategy assumes that the genetics of schizophrenia is especially important. Of course, as a counterpoint, if monozygotic twins discordant for schizophrenia are considered, all the variance accounting for their individual differences is environmental. Nevertheless, it is widely accepted that an important genetic contribution does exist. At the forefront are concerns about whether a poly-, oligo-, or monogenic model for schizophrenia is most appropriate. An-

other concern regards what is actually transmitted genetically. Is it a factor directly responsible for the syndrome itself? Or, does it consist of one or more pathogenic traits, each of which has its separate genetic distribution and each of which plays a role in the stress–vulnerability interaction that determines who precipitates with the disorder?

A third strategy assumes that the earliest and most simple level of functioning in the boundary area between behavior and neuroscience will reveal insight into events from which the later and full clinical manifestations of schizophrenia follow. Included within this strategy are questions about the psychophysiology of orienting, the neural gating of simple sensory stimuli, the neurochemistry related to neuroleptically relevant transmitters, and the imaging to reflect brain metabolism and structure peculiar to schizophrenia.

A fourth strategy, separate from the biological, is that of examining conceptual structure. Conceptual structure is the formal way in which the individual organizes information arising from the vicissitudes of life experience. New mathematical methods for analysis of conceptual matrices (grids) may allow insight into why some individuals develop schizophrenia and others, equally vulnerable, do not.

A fifth strategy assumes that immediate processing of sensory data provides the fundamental basis from which the more complex clinical manifestations of schizophrenia later follow. Concerns here have focused on reaction time crossover, eye tracking, visual memory, and the capacity versus deficit model of impaired processing.

The sixth strategy assumes that insights will emerge simply from the careful examination of current treatment modalities. How do neuroleptic drugs have their effect? Why does family (more than individual) therapy appear to be a significant coordinate treatment with pharmacotherapy? What works in the rehabilitation of chronically ill patients? These questions are important not only to seek relief for patients but also to pinpoint what antecedent (etiological) factors exist. Accordingly, still newer treatments and preventions may follow.

The chapters that follow come from a community of investigators who accept and respect all of these strategies and who have chosen to advance particular ones.

REFERENCES

Bleuler, E. (1911). *Dementia Praecox oder die Gruppe der Schizophrenien*. Leipzig: Deuticke. (Bleuler, E. [1950]. *Dementia praecox or the group of schizophrenias* [J. Zinkin, Trans.]. New York: International Universities Press.)

Bleuler, M. (1978). *The schizophrenic disorders: Long-term patient and family studies*. (S. M. Clemens, Trans.). New Haven, CT: Yale University Press.

Campbell, J. (1988). *The power of myth*. New York: Doubleday.

Clark, K. (1969). *Civilisation*. New York: Harper & Row.

Diefendorf, A. R. (1923). *Clinical psychiatry: A textbook for students and physicians*. New York: Macmillan. (Abstracted and adapted from Kraepelin, E. [1896]. the Fifth *Lehrbuch der Psychiatrie* [5th German ed.]. Leipzig: Verlag von Johann Ambrosius Barth.)

Ferster, C. B., & Skinner, B. F. (1957). *Schedules of reinforcement*. New York: Appleton-Century-Crofts, Inc.

James, W. (1904). Does "consciousness" exist? *Journal of Philosophy, Psychology, and Scientific Methods, 1*, 477–491.

Jefferson, T. (1776). *The declaration of independence*. Washington, DC: National Archives.

Kantor, J. R. (1947). *Problems of physiological psychology*. Bloomington, IN: Principia Press.

Kantor, J. R. (1959). *Interbehavioral psychology* (2nd ed.). Bloomington, IN: Principia Press.

Kelly, G. A. (1955). *The psychology of personal constructs*. New York: Norton.

Paine, T. (1791). *Rights of man: Being an answer to Mr. Burke's attack on the French Revolution*. Baltimore: David Graham.

Pratt, C. C. (1939). *The logic of modern psychology*. New York: Macmillan.

Shaw, G. B. (1907). *Major Barbara*. New York: Penguin Books.

Watson, J. B. (1913). Psychology as a behaviorist views it. *Psychological Review, 20*, 158–177.

Part I

NEUROANATOMICAL CONCEPTIONS
AND RESEARCH

2

Left Globus Pallidus Hyperactivity and Right-Sided Hemineglect in Schizophrenia

TERRENCE S. EARLY

Evidence for anatomical and cognitive dysfunction of the left hemisphere in schizophrenia has been found in two separate studies. In the first study (Early, Reiman, Raichle, & Spitznagel, 1987), positron emission tomography (PET) was used to demonstrate an abnormally high ratio of regional to whole brain cerebral blood flow (CBF) in the left globus pallidus of neuroleptic-naive patients. In the second study, schizophrenic patients demonstrated abnormal orienting to right visual hemispace, again consistent with an abnormality of the left hemisphere (Posner, Early, Reiman, Pardo, & Dhawan, 1988). These findings may be related by a theory of the pathophysiology of psychosis based on an association between striatopallidal hyperactivity and hemineglect.

In contrast to prevailing theories of dopaminergic excess, these results suggest that schizophrenic patients have a dysregulation that is functionally equivalent to *decreased* dopaminergic input to nonmotor parts of the left basal ganglia. Thus, schizophrenic patients are similar to patients with hemiparkinsonism involving the left striatum, with the difference that only nonmotor parts of the striatum (relatively spared in Parkinson's disease [Agid, Javoy-Agid, & Ruberg, 1987]) are involved. Literature is reviewed that suggests that neuroleptic medications might work by restoring symmetry to striatal function (Bracha, Schultz, Glick, & Kleinman, 1987; Gruzelier & Hammond,

1979; Jerussi & Taylor, 1982; Tan & Gurgen, 1986; Tomer, 1989; Tomer & Flor-Henry, 1989).

PET Studies of Neuroleptic-Naive Schizophrenic Patients

The role of left basal ganglia dysfunction in the pathophysiology of schizophrenia was suggested following a PET study of newly diagnosed schizophrenic patients. Unlike most PET studies, never-medicated patients were studied to eliminate the possibility of long-lasting effects of antipsychotic medication. In addition, a method of anatomical localization was used that permitted objective, accurate, and reliable localization of small regions of interest such as the globus pallidus (Fox, Fox, Raichle, & Burde, 1985). Most studies have not reported values for globus pallidus metabolism because of the difficulty in localizing this structure. Finally, the problem of false-positive error resulting from multiple comparisons was avoided by replicating results of the exploratory study in a separate population. In the first phase of this study, regional cerebral blood flow (rCBF) was measured in 5 patients with schizophrenia and 10 normal control subjects. An analysis of 17 bilateral regions indicated an abnormally high ratio of left globus pallidus to whole brain blood flow in the patient population. In the replication phase, rCBF was measured in 5 additional never-medicated patients and 10 additional control subjects for the globus pallidus and frontal regions alone. Analysis of the globus pallidus region confirmed the finding of an abnormally high ratio of left globus pallidus to whole brain blood flow. Results from this study are presented in Figure 2.1.

The finding probably reflects increased neuronal activity of projections to the left globus pallidus. Major projections include the caudate, putamen, nucleus accumbens, and subthalamic nucleus. These results are compatible with an abnormality of the left mesolimbic dopaminergic system. However, these results are not compatible with prevailing notions of excessive dopaminergic activity in schizophrenia, because a lesion of dopaminergic neurons will produce hyperactivity of the left globus pallidus.

Hemineglect

In a separate project, patients were studied with a task that measures the ability to direct the "attentional spotlight" within the visual field (see Figure 2.2). Patients were slow to respond to targets in the right visual field following an invalid cue in the left visual field. Valid cues preceding targets in the left or right field resulted in no asymmetry. If uncued, patients were much slower to respond on the right. In fact, *all* patients were slower to respond to a right visual field target following a left visual field cue than in the opposite situation. This impaired ability to orient to right hemispace is similar to that seen in patients with hemineglect resulting from a stroke. Because each subject served as his or her own control in the comparison of right-sided to left-sided performance, the finding could not be accounted for by any general deficiency in understanding instructions or lack of motivation.

The globus pallidus abnormality and right

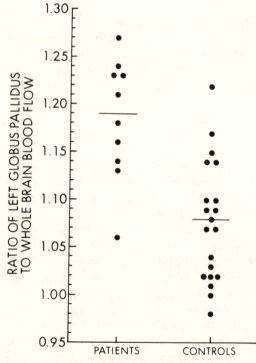

Figure 2.1. The ratio of left globus pallidus to whole brain blood flow in 10 never-medicated patients with schizophrenia and 20 normal control subjects. The mean for each group is indicated by a horizontal line.

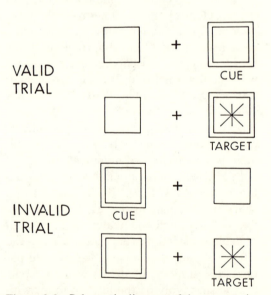

Figure 2.2. Schematic diagram of the covert visual orienting task. The cue is brightening of one of the boxes, which directs attention to that side. The cue-to-target interval is too short for eye movements to occur. Subjects respond by pressing a button as rapidly as possible following the occurrence of the target (a star). The task measures the ability to direct attention within each visual hemifield.

hemispatial orienting impairment both suggest left hemispheric dysfunction. A form of left hemispheric dysfunction that could account for the behavioral results is suggested by animal studies concerning the anatomy of attentional systems.

REVIEW OF BASAL GANGLIA STRUCTURE AND FUNCTION

The basal ganglia are a mass of gray matter structures at the base of the brain, including the striatum, globus pallidus, subthalamic nucleus, and substantia nigra (see Nauta, 1989, Nauta & Domesick, 1984, for reviews). The striatum can be subdivided into dorsal striatum (caudate and putamen) and ventral striatum (nucleus accumbens and olfactory tubercle). All regions of the cortex project to striatum (Pycock & Phillipson, 1984). Cortical and subcortical regions are connected as a series of multiple topographically organized loops involving connections between the cortex, striatum, globus pallidus, thalamus, and then back to the cortex (Alexander, DeLong, & Strick, 1986). Projections from separate cortical regions remain separated throughout the loop (Alexander et al., 1986). Dopaminergic input originates in the substantia nigra–ventral tegmental area complex and projects to all regions of the striatum (Pycock & Phillipson, 1984). It is thought that the dopaminergic input has a modulatory rather than information-carrying role (Iversen, 1984). Dopamine facilitates processing but does not engage in fast point-to-point information transfer.

The caudate nucleus receives input from the associative cortex, and the putamen receives input from sensory, motor, and premotor areas. The caudate and putamen both project to the dorsal globus pallidus (or dorsal pallidum) and from there to separate thalamic nuclei, then back to the cortex. Individual corticostriatopallidothalamic loops have separate functions. Thus, the caudate nucleus is more involved in complex cognitive activities and the putamen has a greater

role in motor programming (Alexander et al., 1986).

The ventral striatum receives input from limbic cortical regions, including the anterior cingulate gyrus, insula, entorhinal cortex, hippocampus, and amygdala (Heimer, Alheid, & Zabortsky, 1985; Nauta, 1989). Projections from the ventral striatum are directed to the ventral pallidum. The ventral pallidum in turn projects to the mediodorsal nucleus of the thalamus, substantia nigra–pars compacta, ventral tegmental area (VTA), lateral habenular nucleus, and amygdala (Nauta, 1989; Nauta & Domesick, 1984). Projections from the mediodorsal nucleus of the thalamus return to the anterior cingulate cortex (Alexander et al., 1986). Overall this system is connected with sites in the limbic system that are involved in drive regulation, emotional behavior, and homeostatic control of the internal environment.

Dopaminergic input to the basal ganglia consists of two pathways, the mesolimbic projection and the nigrostriatal projection. The mesolimbic pathway originates in the VTA and projects to the nucleus accumbens and olfactory tubercle and to other sites in the limbic system and cortex. The nigrostriatal pathway originates in an area adjacent to the VTA known as the substantia nigra and terminates in the caudate and putamen. These projections inhibit the excitatory influence of glutamatergic cortical neurons that terminate on γ-aminobutyric acidergio (GABAergic) projections to the globus pallidus (Graybiel, 1984).

The overall organization of three major loops in the basal ganglia is pictured schematically in Figure 2.3, which includes information on neurotransmitters and the inhibitory or excitatory nature of the projection. The model postulates that unmedicated schizophrenic patients have left striatopallidal hyperactivity and right-sided hemineglect. These core features are the major constraint on the possible number of lesions that could result in psychosis. My colleagues and I speculate that these findings are due to impaired function of a cortic-

BASIC PLAN

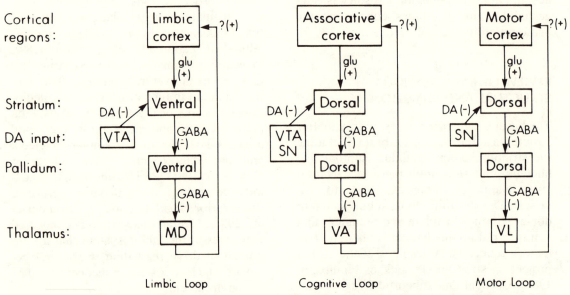

Figure 2.3. The three major loops in the basal ganglia. (Key to abbreviations: DA, dopamine; glu, glutamate; VTA, ventral tegmental area; GABA, γ-aminobutyric acid; MD, mediodorsal nucleus of the thalamus; VTA-SN, ventral tegmental area–substantia nigra; VA, ventral anterior nucleus; SN, substantia nigra; VL, ventrolateral nucleus.)

ostriatopallidothalamic circuit. This type of impairment can be seen following a lesion of dopaminergic innervation to nonmotor striatum, which is associated with increased firing of striatopallidal neurons and increased flow and metabolism in the globus pallidus. Other lesions could possibly give the same results, and indeed all might conceivably be causes for schizophrenia. Finally, medications may alter or reverse this abnormality.

The fact that hemiparkinsonian patients are not schizophrenic is compatible with the documented relative sparing of dopaminergic input to the caudate and nucleus accumbens in Parkinson's disease. Neuropathological studies of patients with Parkinson's disease indicate that symptoms are seen when about 70% to 80% of dopaminergic innervation is lost (Agid et al., 1987). Feedback mechanisms such as dopamine receptor supersensitivity may be able to compensate for the deficit prior to the loss of this critical amount. In cases of hemipar-

kinsonism, the affected side shows greater than 80% loss of dopaminergic innervation. In contrast, the side of the brain ipsilateral to the affected side always has less than 75%. Thus, function is likely to be preserved in the ventral striatal system until much later in the disease.

Thus, it is entirely plausible that a disease could involve only nonmotor corticostriatopallidothalamic loops. One way in which impaired function of this type is known to occur is through a striatal dopaminergic deficiency. This deficiency could be caused by the death or sustained functional inhibition of dopaminergic neurons projecting to the striatum as a result of some other lesion. One example of the latter would be increased dopaminergic input to the left amygdala, as has been reported in a replicated neuropathological study of schizophrenic patients (Reynolds, 1983, 1987). Dopaminergic stimulation of the amygdala inhibits dopamine turnover in the nucleus accumbens (Louilot, Simon, Taghzouti, &

LeMoal, 1985), which could result in a functional lesion of this projection.

Another possible cause for striatopallidal hyperactivity and hemineglect could be a frontal cortex lesion. Hosokawa, Motohiro, Aiko, and Shima (1985) have reported that unilateral frontal cortical ablations result in an ipsilateral increase in deoxyglucose metabolism in the globus pallidus and ipsilateral circling. Thus, a left frontal cortex lesion might give the core features presented here. The exact anatomical cause and the role of dopaminergic innervation in these results is not known, but other studies have clearly implicated striatal dopaminergic systems in neglect resulting from a frontal cortex lesion (Corwin et al., 1986).

The Rotating Rodent Model

"The pallidum [is] an activating center for locomotion and turning attention, as though fascinated, towards an object or event appearing from the contralateral side" (Hassler, 1978). Recent research has stressed the involvement of the basal ganglia in nonmotor functions such as attention (Schallert & Hall, 1988), sensory functions (Lidsky, Manetto, & Schneider, 1985), and cognition (Jayaraman, 1987). The rotating rodent model provides evidence for this evolving concept of basal ganglia function. In this experimental model, lesions are made in the ascending dopaminergic projections on one side, involving the substantia nigra, pars compacta, VTA, or median forebrain bundle. The lesions result in combinations of motor, attentional, and postural asymmetries.

Motor responses to destruction or stimulation of the ascending dopaminergic projections involve intentional neglect (decreased initiation of contralateral movements), contralateral slowing, and abnormalities in the patterning of motor behavior. Animals circle ipsilaterally with respect to the lesion (Pycock, 1980) because they do not initiate motor activity toward the "bad" side of space contralateral to the lesion (Carli, Evendon, & Robbins, 1985).

These animals also demonstrate sensory hemineglect (Marshall, 1979; Marshall & Gotthelf, 1979; Marshall, Berrios, & Sawyer, 1980; Schallert, Upchurch, Wilcox, & Vaughn, 1983) contralateral to the side of the lesion. Thus, the animals orient to the side of space that inputs to the nonlesioned striatum. Sensory hemineglect seen immediately following a unilateral 6-hydroxydopamine (6-OHDA) lesion is replaced by extinction only with double simultaneous stimulation (Schallert et al., 1983), which may be followed by recovery if the lesion is not too extensive. Like turning, this contralateral neglect can be changed to ipsilateral neglect with apomorphine (Marshall & Gotthelf, 1979), suggesting that receptor up-regulation may be involved. Bilateral lesions lead to a severe avolitional state characterized by akinesia, aphagia, and adipsia (Ross & Stewart, 1981; White, 1986).

A permanent attentional deficit can also be demonstrated in unilaterally lesioned rodents (Schallert & Hall, 1988). Rats do not disengage attention from an ongoing oral behavior (such as eating) to respond to vigorous stimulation contralateral to the lesion. At the end of the eating bout, they display normal responsiveness to stimulation of the bad side. The disengage deficit has not been localized but is also produced by selective dopaminergic lesions of the median forebrain bundle. It can be dissociated from the motor hemineglect component because it is present in some rats who have completely recovered from the hemineglect and it is apparently not due to extinction.

Unilateral dopaminergic lesions are followed by metabolic alterations (Brown & Wolfson, 1983; Kelly, Graham, & McCulloch, 1982; Kozlowski & Marshall, 1980; Trugman & Wooten, 1986; Wooten & Collins, 1981, 1983) that include increased metabolism over the globus pallidus and the development of dopamine receptor supersensitivity on the side of the lesion (Heikkila, Shapiro, & Duvoisin, 1981).

The CBF and cerebral glucose metabolism in a given region of brain tissue are thought to reflect metabolism in the terminal fields, rather than in the cell bodies of neurons within the region (Raichle, 1987;

Schwartz et al., 1979). Thus regional metabolism reflects the firing rate of (inhibitory or excitatory) neurons projecting to that region. A lesion of the substantia nigra, VTA, or striatum results in increased metabolism in the globus pallidus on the lesioned side (Wooten & Collins, 1981, 1983). The increase in metabolic activity persists at least 104 days in rodents following 6-OHDA and at least 150 days in primates following methylphenyltetrahydropyridine (Porrino et al., 1987). These alterations in local metabolism can be understood on the basis of anatomical connectivity. A selective lesion of the dopaminergic projections to the basal ganglia disinhibits the GABAergic projection to the globus pallidus. The increased firing of this projection is reflected in increased metabolic activity in the terminal fields in the pallidum.

A final component of the rotating rodent model is the development of dopamine receptor supersensitivity. Severing dopaminergic input increases the number of postsynaptic receptors in the striatum of the lesioned side. This may account for the recovery experienced by some animals following the lesion and can be seen as an adaptive response that compensates for the reduction in dopaminergic input. Supersensitivity results in different rotational responses to direct and indirect dopaminergic agonists (Pycock, 1980; Wooten & Collins, 1981, 1983). The direct dopaminergic agonist apomorphine causes circling contraversive to the lesion; the rats have greater dopaminergic stimulation on the lesioned side as a result of the receptor supersensitivity and consequently orient toward the contralateral space. The indirect agonist amphetamine, which depends on endogenous stores of dopamine, causes the opposite imbalance and ipsiversive circling.

Summary of animal studies. Rats with unilateral lesions of the ascending striatal dopaminergic projections have the following abnormalities:

1. Increased metabolism in the ipsilateral globus pallidus.

2. A multifaceted hemineglect syndrome that includes:
   a. Contralateral motor neglect, indicated by a tendency to turn ipsilaterally and by a reduction in all contralaterally directed behaviors.
   b. Contralateral sensory neglect and extinction.
   c. A permanent difficulty disengaging attention from ongoing oral behavior to shift attention to the side contralateral to the lesion that is distinct from the sensory neglect.
3. Dopamine receptor supersensitivity on the side of the lesion, leading to opposite turning with indirect and direct dopaminergic agonists.

HUMAN STUDIES

Evidence for subtle right-sided hemineglect in schizophrenic patients is available from a number of other studies. Results of the visual orienting study have been replicated by Potkin, Swanson, Urbanchek, Carreon, and Bravo (1989). They also found that patients had fewer eye fixations in right hemispace when scanning a visual form. The number of fixations in left visual hemispace was normal.

Torrey (1980) found evidence for right-sided neglect in schizophrenic patients using the face–hand test and a test for graphesthesia. Manshreck and Ames (1984) replicated the observation of poorer right-handed performance on graphesthesia and also demonstrated on tests of stereognosis right-handed impairments that correlated with measures of thought disorder. Mild right-sided neglect may potentially explain a great deal of the literature on left hemispheric cognitive dysfunction in schizophrenia.

Schizophrenic patients also demonstrate a form of motor behavior similar to the turning behavior seen in animals with motor hemineglect. A rotometer was used to measure turning preferences in human subjects. Hemiparkinsonian patients were found to turn in the expected direction—toward the side of the damaged striatum (Bracha et al., 1987). When this test was applied to drug-free schizophrenic patients, all patients showed a turning preference to the left (Bracha, 1987). This was in contrast to the normal subjects, who on the whole turned as frequently to either side. Although the authors suggested that their finding was likely to reflect *overactivity* of dopaminergic projections to the right striatum, I suggest that it could reflect *underactivity* of dopaminergic projections to the left. Medication apparently normalizes the turning preference in the patients.

Two groups have published conflicting results of PET studies using different dopamine receptor ligands and tracer-kinetic models to measure dopamine receptor binding in drug-naive schizophrenic patients. Wong et al. (1986) reported an increase in maximum binding and the dissociation constant in schizophrenic patients but did not report measures of asymmetry. Farde et al. (1987) did not find increased maximum binding or dissociation constant but did find a reversal in the normal right-greater-than-left binding in 4 of 16 schizophrenic patients. Increased receptor number over the left striatum could be a consequence of decreased dopaminergic input.

Phenomenology and Thought Disorder in Schizophrenia

A type of thought disorder commonly seen in schizophrenia is derailment, defined by Andreason (1979) as "a pattern of spontaneous speech in which the ideas slip from one track onto another that is clearly but obliquely related, or onto one that is completely unrelated." With derailment, the *linear,* goal-directed nature of speech is disrupted by frequent divergence from the semantically meaningful (if idiosyncratic) goal. In the process of starting the thought, there is a slippage off topic that may be only partial, in which case the next thought fragment seems somewhat related, or may be complete. Meaning is lost from speech because the main topic cannot be referred to constantly.

These deficits of language and thought suggest a failure to exercise a selective control over the semantic relations of words. This possibility was explored in a neuropsychological test that required subjects to select and act on either a word or a nonlinguistic symbol. The person is required to press one of two keys as quickly as possible according to directions indicated by either an arrow pointing left or right or the word "left" or "right" presented visually on the center of a cathode ray tube. On pure trials only an arrow or a word is presented; on mixed trials both are presented and the irrelevant one may either agree or disagree with the instructed direction.

Normal subjects are about equally fast with either arrow or word and show mutual interference between the two. Patients with lesions of the left cerebral hemisphere are faster with the arrow stimulus than the word and get much more interference of the arrow on the word than the reverse (Posner et al., 1988). Patients with lesions of the right cerebral hemisphere are faster with the word stimulus and get more interference of a conflicting word on the arrow than the reverse. Schizophrenic patients show the pattern of deficits found in patients with left hemisphere lesions. They are very slow and make many errors with the word stimulus, particularly when it competes with an arrow in the opposite direction. Following therapy, the patients tend to show more normal performance with the word stimulus.

These results suggest that the abnormality seen in schizophrenic patients either may be due to reduced access of the word to left hemisphere mechanisms that code its meaning or may be an impairment in the ability of the person to attend selectively to the word meaning. Although these are both complex functions, the tests involve only a single word on each trial and thus indicate that the deficit does not depend on higher level emotional, syntactic mechanisms or on sustained attention. The deficit can be demonstrated within a single verbal instruction. Moreover, the clear effect of neuroleptics in improving word processing as well as the high educational attainments of the patients indicate that the word deficit is not due to impaired reading ability.

Recently, the neural systems involved when normal subjects process words to derive their semantics have been studied in detail with PET imaging of CBF (Petersen, Fox, Posner, Mintun, & Raichle, 1988). The results of these studies have been in general accord with results obtained from cognitive experiments with normal and brain-injured subjects. They suggest that the semantic processing of individual visual and auditory words activates an area of the left dorsolateral prefrontal cortex (DLPFC). Weinberger (1986) has shown bilaterally increased CBF in this region in normal subjects during the Wisconsin card sorting task, a neuropsychological task performed poorly by patients with DLPFC lesions. Schizophrenic patients are impaired on this task and do not show increased CBF to the DLPFC during this task, a finding that is shared by patients with Parkinson's disease (Weinberger, 1986).

Single-cell recording in nonhuman primates has identified this area with representation of information when the information is not physically present (Wurtz, Goldberg, & Robinson, 1980). Tests of delayed alternation depend on this ability and are impaired by selective dopaminergic lesions of the prefrontal cortex (Brozowski, Brown, Rosvold, & Goldman, 1979) or VTA (Simon, Scatton, & LeMoal, 1980). The ability to direct behavior on the basis of self-generated (as opposed to perceived) representations demonstrated in these studies in primates is compatible with a role in semantic processing in humans.

A second area active during processing of word stimuli, but also in nonlinguistic active processing tasks, lies on the midline of the cerebral hemispheres and includes the anterior cingulate gyrus (area 24) and the supplementary motor cortex (medial area 6). The anterior cingulate has long been implicated in attention, and lesions in this area can result in hemineglect or an avolitional state known as akinetic mutism (Damasio & Van

Hoesen, 1983). The midline system is closely connected to the basal ganglia and receives input from the nucleus accumbens (via the mediodorsal nucleus of the thalamus) and from the DLPFC.

The DLPFC and the midline areas are closely interconnected anatomically. The PET data indicate that these regions function together in processing the semantics of visual words. Thus, I suggest that lesions of the striatum may act on the midline system to reduce the ability of the schizophrenic subject to select semantic information. Studies of schizophrenic patients in semantic tasks (Done & Frith, 1984) have frequently been used to argue that schizophrenics show normal activation of semantics but cannot select the appropriate information or inhibit inappropriate activations. The functions of semantic selection and inhibition have long been assigned to attention based on studies of normal persons processing word stimuli (Neely, 1977; Posner et al., 1988). An anatomical model of a deficit in midline systems resulting from inappropriate activation from the basal ganglia provides a basis for observations on language abnormalities in schizophrenic patients that have been prominent in the literature for more than 20 years.

Apart from the formal thought disorder, typical symptoms of schizophrenia include auditory hallucinations, ideas of control, thought insertion, and thought withdrawal. These symptoms may be considered internal generation and perception of speech and cognitive action programs, resulting in a form of control of cognitive processing that is perceived as being alien or not self-directed. One way to attempt to understand these symptoms is by analogy to intentional motor behavior.

Intentions are mental activities that are goal directed, volitional, and associated with a sense of mental effort. In studies of motor function, the neuronal basis for intentional behavior is investigated by carefully scrutinizing brain activity that occurs prior to voluntary movement in areas of the brain that have important connections to parts of the brain implicated in movement, such as the putamen and primary motor cortex. Intentional activity is seen when one *prepares* to move, even if the movement is not completed. One particular region, the supplementary motor area (SMA), has emerged as a particularly likely site for the major generator of intentional motor behavior (Goldberg, 1985).

The model is supported by research involving lesioning, electrical stimulation, electrophysiological techniques that include surface electroencephalography (EEG) and implanted electrodes, and studies of CBF and cerebral glucose metabolism during motor activity. Lesions in the area produce a hypointentional state characterized by akinesia and mutism (Jonas, 1981), and stimulation produces complex motor behavior and occasionally vocalization (Weisendenger, 1984). Surface EEG reveals a slow downward potential over this region, known as the readiness potential, that precedes spontaneous voluntary behavior (Deecke, Kornhuber, Lang, Lang, & Schreiber, 1985). Similar evidence for activation of this region prior to the initiation of motor activity is provided by studies of CBF and metabolism (Fox et al., 1985) and implanted electrodes (Okano & Tanji, 1987). Involvement in cognitive intentional activity has also been suggested as well and supported by evidence of activation in this area during imagined motor activity (Roland, Meyer, Lassen, & Skinhoj, 1980).

A particularly striking aspect of the involvement of the SMA in intentional activity is provided by case reports of the "alien hand phenomenon" observed in the right hand following infarctions of the left SMA (Goldberg, Meyer, & Toglia, 1981). The patients found their right hands engaging in autonomous motor activity that was not consciously intended. This phenomenon has also been reported in split-brain patients, in whom far more than the alien hand phenomenon has been demonstrated. Following commissurotomy, the left and right hemispheres of split-brain patient express different beliefs, emotional reactions, and preferences (Gazzaniga, 1985). These patients demonstrate that it is possible for a brain to have two separate generators of intentional cognitive activity. In these patients the left hemisphere controls language and motor activity. The differing intentions of the right hemisphere are usually uncovered only with careful testing. The corpus callosum is suggested to have an inhibitory role on homologous cortical regions of the right hemisphere that may be important for the experience of mental and behavioral unity.

The functions of the midline frontal regions (SMA and possibly anterior cingulate cortex) are expressed through projections to the striatum (Goldberg, 1985) and are dependent on striatal dopaminergic input (Jurgens, 1984; Ross & Stewart, 1981). Deficient dopaminergic input to nonmotor parts of the left striatum would be expected to impair these functions, perhaps interfering with a normal pattern of left hemispheric dominance for these command functions. This impairment of dominance could result in a release of function by homologous regions of the right hemisphere, leading to partial control of processing by the right hemisphere and the generation of autonomous cognitive programs that interfere with those generated by the left.

A very similar model has been articulated by Frith and Done (1988). They distinguished between "stimulus intentions" (thoughts generated by external stimuli) and "willed intentions" (internally generated thoughts) associated in the motor domain with the arcuate premotor area and SMA, respectively. They postulated that schizophrenic patients have an impairment in the corollary discharge that normally would inform an organism that a given stimulus intention was self-generated. The model my colleagues and I developed differs in that we conceive of a separate center for the generation of intentional cognitive action programs. A central feature of both models is the need to account for information that is perceived as alien.

The akinesia of the negative-symptom schizophrenic patient is also similar to akinesia seen with SMA or anterior cingulate cortex lesions, and suggests that decreased as well as conflicting volitional cognitive activity might be accounted for by the model. Thus, the negative symptoms would in fact be due to a dopamine deficiency, as has been suggested. This account, although admittedly speculative, proposes a different way of thinking about psychopathology that has the advantage of being anatomically specified.

Summary of Human Studies

Patients with schizophrenia have a number of features in common with animals that have had selective unilateral lesions of the ascending dopaminergic projections to striatum. These include:

1. Increased blood flow in the left globus pallidus.
2. Evidence for right-sided sensory neglect provided by multiple studies in the laterality literature.
3. An impairment in the ability to disengage attention in order to attend to the right visual field.
4. Contralateral motor neglect, indicated by a tendency to turn to the left (e.g., counterclockwise).
5. Possible evidence for dopamine receptor supersensitivity in the left striatum of never-medicated patients.
6. Language deficits that represent a higher level abnormality of lateralized attention.

LEFT-SIDED TEMPORAL LOBE EPILEPSY AND PSYCHOSIS

A good theory has the power to explain a great deal of existing data and generate other falsifiable predictions. The model suggests a possible explanation for the association of psychosis with left-sided temporal lobe epilepsy. Although there is still some controversy regarding this issue, there is considerable evidence that patients with epilepsy due to a seizure focus in the left temporal lobe are particularly prone to develop psychotic illness. According to the model outlined here, this would be expected

to result from destruction of the ascending dopaminergic projections of the left hemisphere.

There are direct projections from the amygdala and hippocampus to the ipsilateral nucleus accumbens. The neurotransmitter in this pathway is probably glutamate, which is an excitatory transmitter known to cause cell death with repeated application in certain experimental paradigms. In the kindling model of partial complex seizures, repeated subconvulsive chemical or electrical stimulation of various sites in the temporal lobes eventually gives rise to partial seizures. Kindling the amygdala with ferric chloride injection (Csernansky, Csernansky, Bonnett, & Hollister, 1985) results in ipsilateral striatal dopaminergic receptor supersensitivity and a contralateral turning bias following the administration of apomorphine (also seen following 6-OHDA lesions). Electrical kindling produces effects on turning behavior consistent with damage to the ipsilateral dopaminergic striatal input (Mintz, Tomer, Houpt, & Herberg, 1987).

DISEASE HOMOGENEITY

One of the more striking aspects of the data reviewed here is the uniformity of evidence for left hemispheric abnormalities in schizophrenic patients. All of the patients tested demonstrated right hemispatial abnormalities in visual orienting, turning, and visual fixations. It is possible that a variety of neuronal lesions could result in the asymmetrical dopaminergic hypofunction suggested here as the final common pathway for psychosis. The pathway involved should give the metabolic and behavioral abnormalities described above in selectively lesioned animals.

THERAPEUTIC IMPLICATIONS

Dopamine turnover in the two nigrostriatal pathways is reciprocally regulated such that electrical or pharmacological stimulation of one side causes inhibition of the other (Glowinski, Besson, & Cheramy, 1984). This reciprocal regulation of dopamine turnover may be important for interhemispheric interaction and also suggests a potential mechanism of action for antipsychotic medications compatible with the model outlined here. Antipsychotics may work by reducing the postulated abnormal asymmetry in striatal dopaminergic input.

There are data that suggest that antipsychotic medications do have a lateralized effect. Neuroleptic treatment is associated with a shift in EEG voltage to the left (Serafetinedes, 1973), lateralized alterations in visual evoked potentials (Myslobodsky, Mintz, & Tomer, 1983), and a reversal in the asymmetry of the Hoffman reflex (an electromyographic measure) (Tan & Gurgen, 1986). Patients have poorer performance in the right hemispace on a letter cancellation test and on a form sorting task when unmedicated, and treatment reverses the side of deficit (Tomer, 1989; Tomer & Flor-Henry, 1989). All of these findings are consistent with neuroleptic-induced inhibition of the right hemisphere.

Other suggestive results are available in one study concerning the effects of acute treatment with haloperidol on lateralized dopamine turnover (Jerussi & Taylor 1982). Normal rats were tested for circling behavior and found to have higher levels of DOPAC (a dopamine metabolite) in the striatum ipsilateral to the direction of rotation. Rats acutely treated with haloperidol demonstrated the reverse asymmetry in striatal DOPAC levels.

One interesting therapeutic implication is suggested by the rodent literature. Unilaterally lesioned rodents develop receptor supersensitivity on the side of the lesion, resulting in enhancement of the neglect with indirect dopaminergic agonists such as apomorphine (Pycock, 1980). The beneficial response to direct agonists is highly dose dependent, with initial correction of the neglect at low doses followed by stereotypy at higher doses. If the proposed anatomical lesion that is associated with the cognitive deficits in schizophrenia is also associated with receptor supersensitivity, direct dopaminergic agonists would have antipsychotic effects that should be much better than those of indirect agonists. Apomorphine has

been demonstrated to have beneficial effects on the positive symptoms of schizophrenia (Costall & Naylor, 1986). The antipsychotic effects of apomorphine have been attributed to preferential effects on release-inhibiting presynaptic dopamine autoreceptors at low doses. The model of striatal dopamine hemideficiency provides another explanation for this effect. Low doses of direct agonists should be a fairly beneficial treatment, at least in schizophrenic patients who have receptor up-regulation. Dosage might be a very important factor because, in the motor system, reversal of turning preference is replaced by stereotypy at slightly higher doses.

SUMMARY

Schizophrenic patients have a variety of metabolic and behavioral features suggestive of impairment of nonmotor corticostriatopallidothalamic projections of the left hemisphere. The most well-studied analogue of this model is provided by animals that have had selective unilateral lesions of dopaminergic projections to the striatum. A dopamine hemideficiency model explains a great deal of available data concerning cognitive abnormalities in schizophrenia and suggests a large number of additional testable hypotheses. The uniformity of evidence for lateralized cognitive dysfunction reviewed in this chapter suggests that schizophrenia might be a much more homogeneous disorder than has been previously supposed, and emphasizes the importance of right–left comparisons in brain research.

ACKNOWLEDGMENTS

This research was supported by the McDonnell Center for Studies in Higher Brain Function via the National Institutes of Health Grant HL13851 from the National Heart, Lung, and Blood Institute; and by the National Alliance for Research on Schizophrenia and Depression Grant "1989 NARSAD Young Investigator Award Recipient."

REFERENCES

Agid, Y., Javoy-Agid, F. J., & Ruberg, M. (1987). Biochemistry of neurotransmitters in Parkinson's disease. In C. V. Marsden & S. Fahn (Eds.), *Movement disorders 2* (Vol. 2, pp. 166–230). London: Butterworth & Co Publishers.

Alexander, G. E., DeLong, M. R., & Strick, P. L. (1986). Parallel organization of functionally segregated circuits linking basal ganglia and cortex. *Annual Review of Neuroscience, 9,* 357–381.

Andreason, N. C. (1979). Thought, language, and communication disorders. *Archives of General Psychiatry, 36,* 1315–1321.

Bracha, H. S. (1987). Asymmetric rotational (circling) behavior, a dopamine asymmetry: Preliminary findings in unmedicated and never-medicated schizophrenic patients. *Biological Psychiatry, 22,* 995–1003.

Bracha, H. S., Schultz, C., Glick, S. D., & Kleinman, J. E. (1987). Spontaneous asymmetric circling behavior in hemi-Parkinsonism: A human equivalent of the lesioned-circling rodent behavior. *Life Sciences, 40,* 1127–1130.

Brown, L. L., & Wolfson, L. I. (1983). A dopamine-sensitive striatal efferent system mapped with (^{14}C)-deoxyglucose in the rat. *Brain Research, 261,* 213–229.

Brozowski, T. J., Brown, R. M., Rosvold, H. E., & Goldman, P. S. (1979). Cognitive deficit caused by regional depletion of dopamine in prefrontal cortex of rhesus monkey. *Science, 205,* 929–932.

Carli, M., Evendon, J. L., & Robbins, T. W. (1985). Depletion of unilateral dopamine impairs initiation of contralateral actions and not sensory attention. *Nature, 313,* 679–682.

Corwin, J. V., Kanter, S., Watson, R. T., Heilman, K. M., Valenstein, E., & Hashimoto, A. (1986). Apomorphine has a therapeutic effect on neglect produced by unilateral dorsomedial prefrontal cortex lesions in rats. *Experimental Neurology, 94,* 683–698.

Costall, B., & Naylor, R. J. (1986). Neurotransmitter hypothesis of schizophrenia. In P. B. Bradley & S. R. Hirsch (Eds.), *The psychopharmacology and treatment of schizophrenia* (p. 135). Oxford, England: Oxford Medical Publications.

Csernansky, J. G., Csernansky, C. A., Bonnett, K. A., & Hollister, L. E. (1985). Dopaminergic supersensitivity follows ferric chloride-induced limbic seizures. *Biological Psychiatry, 20,* 723–733.

Damasio, A. R., & Van Hoesen, G. W. (1983). Emotional disturbance associated with focal lesions of the limbic frontal lobe. In K. Heilman & P. Satz (Eds.), *Neuropsychology of human emotion* (pp. 85–110). New York: Guilford Press.

Deecke, L., Kornhuber, H. H., Lang, W., Lang, M., & Schreiber, H. (1985). Timing function of the frontal cortex in sequential motor and learning tasks. *Human Neurobiology, 4,* 143–154.

Done, J. D., & Frith, C. D. (1984). The effect of context during word perception in schizophrenic patients. *Brain and Language, 23,* 318–336.

Early, T. S., Reiman, E. M., Raichle, M. E., & Spitznagel, E. L. (1987). Left globus pallidus abnormality in never-medicated patients with schizophrenia. *Proceedings of the National Academy of Sciences (U.S.A.), 84,* 561–563.

Farde, L., Weisel, F. A., Hall, H., Halldin, C., Stone-Elander, S., & Sedvall, G. (1987). No D2 receptor increase in PET study of schizophrenia (Letter). *Archives of General Psychiatry, 44,* 671.

Fox, P. T., Fox, J. M., Raichle, M. E., & Burde, R. M. (1985). The role of the cerebral cortex in the generation of voluntary saccades: A positron emission tomography study. *Journal of Neurophysiology, 54,* 348–369.

Frith, C. D., & Done, D. J. (1988). Towards a neuropsychology of schizophrenia. *British Journal of Psychiatry, 153,* 437–443.

Gazzaniga, M. S. (1985). *The social brain.* New York: Basic Books, Inc.

Glowinowski, J., Besson, M. J., & Cheramy, A. (1984). Role of the thalamus in the bilateral regulation of dopaminergic and GABAergic neurons in the basal ganglia. *CIBA Foundation Symposium, 107,* 150–163.

Goldberg, G. (1985). Supplementary motor area structure and function: Review and hypothesis. *Behavioral Brain Science, 8,* 567–616.

Goldberg, G., Meyer, N. H., & Toglia, J. Y. (1981). Medial frontal cortex infarction and the alien hand sign. *Archives of Neurology, 38,* 683–686.

Graybiel, A. (1984). Neurochemically specified subsystems in the basal ganglia. *CIBA Foundation Symposium, 107,* 114–149.

Gruzelier, J., & Hammond, N. V. (1979). The effect of CPZ upon psychophysiological, endocrine, and information processing measure in schizophrenia. *Journal of Psychiatric Research, 14,* 167–182.

Hassler, R. (1978). Striatal control of locomotion, intentional actions and of integrating and perceptive activity. *Journal of the Neurological Sciences, 36,* 187–224.

Heikkila, R. E., Shapiro, B. S., & Duvoisin, R. C. (1981). The relationship between loss of dopamine nerve terminals, striatal (^{3}H)spiroperidol binding and rotational behavior in unilaterally 6-hydroxydopamine-lesioned rats. *Brain Research, 211,* 285–292.

Heimer, L., Alheid, G. F., & Zabortsky, L. (1985). Basal ganglia. In *The rat nervous system* (pp. 37–86). Sydney, Australia: Academic Press.

Hosokawa, S., Motohiro, K., Aiko, Y., & Shima, F. (1985). Altered local cerebral glucose utilization by unilateral frontal cortical ablations in rats. *Brain Research, 343,* 8–15.

Iversen, W. S. D. (1984). Behavioral aspects of the corticosubcortical interaction with special reference to frontostriatal relations. In F. Reinoso-Suarez & C. Ajmone-Maisan (Eds.), *Cortical integration* (pp. 237–254). New York: Raven Press.

Jayaraman, A. (1987). The basal ganglia and cognition: An interpretation of anatomical connectivity patterns. In *The basal ganglia and behavior: Sensory aspects of motor function* (pp. 149–160). Toronto: Hans Huber Publishers.

Jerussi, T. P., & Taylor, C. A. (1982). Bilateral asymmetry in striatal dopamine metabolism: Implications for pharmacotherapy of schizophrenia. *Brain Research, 246,* 71–75.

Jonas, S. (1981). The supplementary motor region and speech emission. *Journal of Communication Disorders, 14,* 349–373.

Jurgens, U. (1984). The efferent and afferent connections of the supplementary motor area. *Brain Research, 300,* 63–81.

Kelly, P., Graham, D. I., & McCulloch, J. (1982). Specific alterations in local cerebral glucose utilization following striatal lesions. *Brain Research, 233,* 157–172.

Kozlowski, M. R., & Marshall, J. F. (1980). Plasticity of (^{14}C)2-deoxy-D-glucose incorporation into neostriatum and related structures in response to dopamine neuron damage and apomorphine replacement. *Brain Research, 7,* 167–183.

Lidsky, T. I., Manetto, C., & Schneider, J. S. (1985). A consideration of sensory factors involved in motor functions of the basal ganglia. *Brain Research Reviews 9,* 133–146.

Louilot, A., Simon, H., Taghzouti, K., & LeMoal, M. (1985). Modulation of dopaminergic activity in the nucleus accumbens following facilitation or blockade of the dopaminergic transmission in the amygdala: A study by *in vivo* differential pulse voltammetry. *Brain Research, 346,* 141–145.

Manshreck, T. C., & Ames, D. (1984). Neurologic features and psychopathology in schizophrenic disorders. *Biological Psychiatry, 19,* 703–719.

Marshall, J. F. (1979). Somatosensory inattention after dopamine-depleting intracerebral 6-OHDA injections: Spontaneous recovery and pharmacological control. *Brain Research, 177,* 311–324.

Marshall, J. F., Berrios, N., & Sawyer, S. (1980). Neostriatal dopamine and sensory inattention. *Journal of Comparative and Physiological Psychiatry, 94,* 833–846.

Marshall, J. F., & Gotthelf, T. (1979). Sensory inattention in rats with 6-hydroxydopamine-induced degeneration of ascending dopaminergic neurons: Apomorphine-induced reversal of deficits. *Experimental Neurology, 65,* 398–411.

Mintz, M., Tomer, R., Houpt, S., & Herberg, L. J. (1987). Amygdala kindling modifies interhemispheric dopaminergic asymmetry. *Experimental Neurology, 96,* 137–144.

Myslobodsky, M. S., Mintz, M., & Tomer, R. (1983). Neuroleptic effects and the site of abnormality in schizophrenia. In *Hemisyndromes: Psychology, neurology, psychiatry* (pp. 347–388). New York: Academic Press, Inc.

Nauta, W. J. H. (1989). Reciprocal links of the corpus striatum with the cerebral cortex and limbic system: A common substrate for movement and thought? In J. Mueller (Ed.), *Neurology and psychiatry: A meeting of minds* (pp. 43–63). Basel: Karger.

Nauta, W. J. H., & Domesick, V. (1984). Afferent and efferent relationships of the basal ganglia. *CIBA Foundation Symposium, 107,* 3–29.

Neely, J. H. (1977). Semantic priming and retrieval from lexical memory: Roles of inhibitionless spreading activation and limited-capacity attention. *Journal of Experimental Psychology: General, 106,* 226–254.

Okano, K., & Tanji, J. (1987). Neuronal activities in the primate motor fields of the agranular frontal cortex preceding visually triggered and self-paced movement. *Experimental Brain Research, 66,* 155–166.

Petersen, S. E., Fox, P. T., Posner, M. I., Mintun, M., & Raichle, M. E. (1988). Positron emission tomographic studies of the cortical anatomy of single word processing. *Nature, 331,* 585–589.

Porrino, L. J., Burns, R. S., Crane, A. M., Palombo, E., Koplin, I. J., & Sokoloff, L. (1987). Changes in local cerebral glucose utilization associated with Parkinson's syndrome induced by 1-methyl-4-phenyl-1,2,3,6-tetrahydropyridine (MPTP) in the primate. *Life Sciences, 40,* 1657–1664.

Posner, M. I., Early, T. S., Reiman, E. R., Pardo, P. J., & Dhawan, M. (1988). Asymmetries in hemispheric control of attention in schizophrenia. *Archives of General Psychiatry, 45,* 814–821.

Potkin, S. G., Swanson, J. M., Urbanchek, M., Carreon, D., & Bravo, G. (1989). Right visual field deficits in reaction time after invalid cues in chronic and never-medicated schizophrenics compared to normal controls. *Biological Psychiatry, 25,* 74A–79A.

Pycock, C. J. (1980). Turning behavior in animals. *Neuroscience, 5,* 461–514.

Pycock, C. J., & Phillipson, O. T. (1984). A neuroanatomical and neuropharmacological analysis of basal ganglia output. In L. I. Iverson, S. D. Iversen, & S. H. Snyder (Eds.), *Handbook of psychopharmacology* (Vol. 18, pp. 191–228). New York: Plenum Press.

Raichle, M. (1987). Circulatory and metabolic correlates of brain function in normal humans. In F. Plum (Ed.), *Handbook of physiology—revised, Section 1. The nervous system,* Vol. 5: Higher functions of the brain (pp. 643–674). Washington, DC: American Physiological Association.

Reynolds, G. P. (1983). Increased concentrations and lateral asymmetry of amygdala dopamine in schizophrenia. *Nature, 305,* 527–529.

Reynolds, G. P. (1987). Post-mortem neurochemical studies in human postmortem brain tissue. In H. Hafner, W. F. Gattaz, & W. Janzarik (Eds.), *Search for the causes of schizophrenia* (pp. 236–240). Heidelberg: Springer.

Roland, P. E., Meyer, E., Lassen, N. A., & Skinhoj, E. (1980). Supplementary motor area and other cortical areas in organization of voluntary movements in man. *Journal of Neurophysiology, 43,* 118–136.

Ross, E. D., & Stewart, R. M. (1981). Akinetic mutism from hypothalamic damage: Successful treatment with dopamine agonists. *Neurology, 31,* 1435–1439.

Schallert, T., & Hall, S. (1988). ''Disengage'' sensorimotor deficit following apparent recovery from unilateral dopamine depletion. *Behavioural Brain Research, 30,* 15–24.

Schallert, T., Upchurch, M., Wilcox, R. E., & Vaughn, D. M. (1983). Posture-independent sensorimotor analysis of inter-hemispheric receptor asymmetries in neostriatum. *Pharmacology, Biochemistry and Behavior, 18,* 753–759.

Schwartz, W. J., Smith, C. B., Davidsen, L., Savaki, H., Sojoloff, L., Mata, M., Fink, D., & Gainer, H. (1979). Metabolic mapping of functional activity in the hypothalamoneurohypophysial system of the rat. *Science, 205,* 723–725.

Serafetinedes, E. A. (1973). Voltage laterality in the EEG of psychiatric patients. *Diseases of the Nervous System, 34,* 190–191.

Simon, H., Scatton, B., & LeMoal, M. (1980). Dopaminergic A10 neurones are involved in cognitive functions. *Nature, 286,* 150–151.

Tan, U., & Gurgen, F. (1986). Modulation of spinal motor asymmetry by neuroleptic medication in schizophrenic patients. *Journal of Neuroscience, 30,* 165–172.

Tomer, R. (1989). Asymmetrical effects of neuroleptics on psychotic patients' performance of a tactile discrimination task. *Journal of Nervous and Mental Disease 177,* 699–700.

Tomer, R., & Flor-Henry, P. (1989). Neuroleptics reverse attention asymmetries in schizophrenic patients. *Biological Psychiatry, 25,* 852–860.

Torrey, E. F. (1980). Neurological abnormalities in schizophrenic patients. *Biological Psychiatry, 15,* 381–388.

Trugman, J. M., & Wooten, G. F. (1986). The effects of L-DOPA on regional cerebral glucose utilization in rats with unilateral lesions of the substantia nigra. *Brain Research, 379,* 264–274.

Weinberger, D. R. (1986). Prefrontal cortex physiological activation: Effect of L-DOPA in Parkinson's disease. *Neurology, 36*(Suppl. 1), 170.

Weisendenger, M. (1981). Organization of sensory motor area of central cortex. In V. Brooks & S. R. Geiger (Eds.), *Handbook of Physiology,* Part 2, Vol. II. (pp. 1121–1147). Baltimore: Williams & Wilkins. Washington, DC: American Physiological Association.

White, N. M. (1986). Control of sensorimotor function by dopaminergic nigrostriatal neurons: Influence on eating and drinking. *Neuroscience and Biobehavioral Reviews, 10,* 15–36.

Wong, D. F., Wagner, H. N., Tune, L. E., Dannals, R. F., Pearlson, G. D., Links, J. M., Tamminga, C. A., Broussolle, P., Ravert, H. T., Wilson, A. A., Toung, J. K. T., Malat, J., Williams, J. A., O'Tauma, L. A., Snyder, S. H., Kuhar, M. J., & Gjedde, A. (1986). Positron emission tomography reveals elevated D2 dopamine receptors in drug-naive schizophrenics. *Science, 234,* 1558–1563.

Wooten, G. F., & Collins, R. C. (1981). Metabolic effects of unilateral lesion of the substantia nigra. *Journal of Neuroscience 1,* 285–291.

Wooten, G. F., & Collins, R. C. (1983). Effects of dopaminergic stimulation on functional brain metabolism in rats with unilateral substantia nigra lesions. *Brain Research, 263,* 267–275.

Wurtz, R. H., Goldberg, E., & Robinson, D. L. (1980). Behavioral modulation of visual response in the monkey: Stimulus selection for attention and movement. *Progress in Psychiatry, Biology, and Physiological Psychology, 9,* 43–83.

3

Dopamine-Initiated Disturbances of Thalamic Information Processing in Schizophrenia?

ARVIN F. OKE
LARRY A. CARVER
RALPH N. ADAMS

We must recollect that all our provisional ideas in psychology will presumably one day be based on an organic substrate.

Sigmund Freud, *On Narcissism*

BACKGROUND OF CLINICAL OBSERVATIONS

The symptom complex we term "schizophrenia" has been known for at least 3,400 years (Lehmann, 1967). The circumstances that are believed to be the etiology of this ailment are consistent with the philosophy and thinking of the time. Therefore, for thousands of years, mystical and supernatural events were believed to produce the dark nights of the soul.

The onset of modern science and psychology in the late 19th century brought along the concept of a possible biological basis for the cause of schizophrenia. J. L. W. Thudichum published his *Treatise on the Chemical Constitution of the Brain* in 1884 and suggested that "insanity" might be the result of poisons influencing the brain (Kety, 1970). One possible antidote to these poisons came in the early 1950s. It was at this time that psychopharmacology came to life with the use of chlorpromazine, and a new era in the treatment and understanding of psychopathology was ushered in. The use of chlorpromazine and other antipsychotic medications produced dramatic changes in

the treatment and care of individuals suffering from schizophrenia. Active treatment took the place of custodial care, patients were released from hospitals, relapses decreased, and the number of hospital beds for the mentally ill were reduced (Davis, Barter, & Kane, 1989).

Possibly of greater significance than the direct clinical effect of these new medications was the change in attitude about psychopathology. If a chemical given to an individual suffering from paranoia, hallucinations, and scattered thoughts could reduce or eliminate these symptoms, just possibly it was some form of aberrant chemical reaction that was creating these disabling symptoms. Thus, the search for an understanding of the chemistry of the brain, especially in those individuals suffering from psychiatric illnesses, was greatly enhanced.

The present state of neurobiological research in schizophrenia offers a rich variety of pathways for investigation—pathways that may eventually merge and work in concert with one another. Genetic research has captured the attention of many (Gottesman & Shields, 1972; Kety, Rosenthal, Wender, Schulsinger, & Jacobson, 1975) and may indeed prove to be the final common pathway of all neurobiological investigations. Findings from computerized tomography (CT) scans and magnetic resonance imaging (MRI) have suggested that individuals suffering from schizophrenia may have enlargement of the third ventricle, widening of cortical sulci, and/or frontal lobe atrophy (Losonczy et al., 1986; MacDonald & Best, 1989; Woods et al., 1990). Cerebral blood flow studies and positron emission tomography (PET) scans have contributed to the concept of hypofrontality in schizophrenia (Buchsbaum et al., 1990; Ingvar & Franzen, 1974; Weinberger, Berman, & Zec, 1986). The fields of virology and immunology have also thrown their hats into the ring (DeLisi & Crow, 1986; Eaves, 1988; Pert, Knight, Laing, & Markwell, 1988).

The area of investigation that appears to have received the most attention, however, is the role of neurotransmitter interactions and the "greatest of these" is the "dopamine theory of schizophrenia." The heightened curiosity about dopamine seems to be the result of two interesting assumptions about the nature of schizophrenia and the human brain. First, most of the present antipsychotic medications on the market are potent antagonists of dopamine. Second, the limbic system, thought to be the source of emotional function in the brain, is richly supplied with dopamine via the mesolimbic and mesocortical tracts. This fascination with dopamine continues unabated to the present.

SIGNS AND SYMPTOMS OF SCHIZOPHRENIA

Looking back at the history and forward to the future of neurobiological research in schizophrenia, investigators are faced with a strange and perplexing problem. When a patient enters a clinic with complaints of bizarre behavior, irrational thoughts, and unfamiliar feelings and beliefs, is he or she suffering from schizophrenia or perhaps the manic phase of a bipolar illness? Or could it be a brief reactive psychosis, paranoia, or a schizotypal personality disorder? Lipkow-

itz and Idupuganti (1983) mailed questionnaires to 1,227 U.S. psychiatrists at the time of the introduction of the *Diagnostic and Statistical Manual of Mental Disorders,* third edition (DSM-III; American Psychiatric Association, 1980) to ascertain their diagnostic approach to schizophrenia. From those forms returned, it was found that only four symptom categories reached a 50% accordance level, and there was little agreement on combinations of signs or symptoms, including those recommended by the DSM-III.

Whatever research diagnostic tool an investigator uses, the bottom line must be: Are the findings consonant in some ways with the signs and symptoms that the clinician sees in his or her office? The standard by which most U.S. clinicians make their diagnoses of schizophrenia is the DSM-III revised edition (DSM-III-R) (American Psychiatric Association, 1987). Probably the most widely accepted scales in research today are the Research Diagnostic Criteria (RDC; Spitzer, Endicott, & Robins, 1975) and the Schedule for Affective Disorders and Schizophrenias (SADS; Endicott & Spitzer, 1978).

The DSM-III-R is quite specific about diagnostic criteria. It lists such factors as time constraints, possible presence of prodromal and/or residual symptoms, and diagnostic exclusions. However, the starting point for such diagnoses must be the presence of positive psychotic symptoms in the overt and active stage. These positive symptoms are *disturbance in thought* and *perceptual disturbance.*

Disturbance in Thought

Disorders of thought might be considered the sine qua non of schizophrenia. They are such a prominent feature that schizophrenia is often referred to as a "thought disorder." Disturbance in thought may be subdivided into disorders in *content* as well as *process and form.* Delusions are possibly the best example of a disorder in content. They may be persecutory, grandiose, religious, or somatic in nature. A delusion may be defined as a false belief. It is as though schizophrenic patients take benign external and/ or internal cues—similar to those that everyone has—and then process this information so that, for them, it becomes highly subjective (*ideas* of *reference*) and grossly inappropriate.

Intrusive thoughts are a prime example of a disorder of process. The patient experiences sudden and unintentional thoughts. Often these are accompanied by the delusional belief that the thoughts are being inserted by others into his or her mind (*thought insertion*). It is as if a neurological gating process has failed to inhibit internal stimuli. The psychoanalyst might describe the process as a failure of the ego to prevent the emergence of unconscious, primitive thoughts into the flow of consciousness.

The problem the clinician or researcher faces here is that disorders in process are subjective in nature and are experienced only by the patient. They can be appreciated or measured by clinicians only insofar as they are demonstrated in the patient's speech. Among the more common speech pathologies (*disorder in form*) are pressured speech, tangentiality or looseness of association, poverty of speech, mutism, neologism, echolalia, or perseveration.

Perceptual Disturbance

Perceptual disturbances are faulty interpretations of sensory functioning. An illusion is a false interpretation of a real perception and appears to be inconsistent with the true meaning of the corresponding external stimuli. A patient may experience a picture in a magazine moving or see the image of the "devil" on the face of a friend.

Hallucinations are experiences of perception in the absence of corresponding external stimuli. They may take the form of auditory, visual, olfactory, tactile, or gustatory sensations. However, auditory hallucinations are by far the most common (50% to 75% of patients; Grebb & Cancro, 1989).

Although auditory hallucinations are sometimes considered to be synonymous with schizophrenia, their origins have indeed been elusive. It can be postulated that hallucinations are the result of some form of dysfunctioning of auditory processing. However, it may be more appropriate to classify them as disorders of thought or speech. Eugen Bleuler (1911/1950), who coined the name schizophrenia, pioneered this concept when he reported patients who described their auditory hallucinations as "audible thoughts" or "soundless voices."

A more contemporary appraisal of auditory hallucinations incorporates the notion of unintended subvocal speech that, when experienced outside of a concurrent plan for verbal discourse, is perceived as alien and nonself (Hoffman, 1986). Attempts at interfering with subvocal speech mechanisms have proved most interesting. Actively hallucinating patients were requested to engage in maneuvers that presumably compete with buccopharyngeal movements involved in subvocalizations. These maneuvers, such as opening the mouth wide (Bick & Kinsbourne, 1987) or softly humming a single note (Green & Kinsbourne, 1989), gave temporary relief from the inner voices. These results support earlier findings of orofacial muscular activation during the process of auditory hallucination (Gould, 1948; Inouye & Shimizu, 1970). The relationship between motoric expressions of covert verbal behavior and inner hallucinatory experiences, although minimally investigated, begins to lend support to the hypothesis that hallucination is an expression of subvocal speech and points to possible sources of this form of perceptual disturbance.

One of the difficult challenges in schizophrenia research has been to generate scientifically valid strategies that can be related to the highly subjective clinical features of schizophrenia. Despite the difficulties of diagnostic uncertainties and clinical inferences, the clinician–patient interactions and their reports constitute one of the most fundamental segments of understanding the "real life" of schizophrenic existence. Valuable neurobiological studies on the nature and possible causes of the disease presumably must attempt to include significant correlations with clinical behavior. With the present limited understanding in the neurosciences, no one can actually bridge the gaps between brain functioning and mental activity. So, neurobiological views of schizophrenia are, at best, limited hypotheses, educated guesses, or what hard physical scientists call "hand waving"—depending on one's viewpoint.

Our objective in this sense is to describe neurochemical abnormalities associated with subcortical brain regions (particularly the thalamus) in postmortem brains from schizophrenic patients. We wish to suggest ways in which these abnormalities can be looked at as congruent with some of the clinical manifestations of schizophrenia. In one major area, that of perceptual distortions, there are ample congruencies of neurochemical abnormalities with breakdowns in information processing from neurophysiological studies (Adler, Waldo, & Freedman, 1985; Adler et al., 1982; Freedman et al., 1987; Geyer & Braff, 1987; Saccuzzo & Braff, 1986). Concepts of thought disorder, and especially disorders of process, reside predominantly within the subjective experience of the patient, and they are very difficult to pin down in measurable terms. Thus, we suggest that examples of more quantifiable speech aberrations in neurological pathology seem to have congruence with neurochemical findings in the thalamus. These more definitive neurological data deserve further attention with regard to their overlap and commonality as possible indicators of disordered thought processes in schizophrenia.

THALAMUS AND SPEECH PRODUCTION

Speech Disorders and Thalamic Lesions

Neural areas responsible for language production have, for the past century, been considered to be located exclusively in the neocortex of the dominant hemisphere. From the early observations of Broca and Wernicke, discrete lesions in the posteroinferior portion of the third frontal convolution (Broca's area) and the parietal–temporal junction (Wernicke's area), as well as the supplementary motor cortex, resulted in dysfunctional language, whereas lesions in other cortical regions did not. This classical view of language localization generally has not included subcortical structure but only cortical gray matter and the transcortical white fibers immediately beneath. Deeper structures in the diencephalon, especially the thalamus and adjacent formations, have been generally ignored. The last 25 years have witnessed a growing body of data supporting aphasia following dominant hemisphere thalamic injury—a view not completely free from doubters (Botez & Barbeau, 1971). Aphasias following insult to the thalamus of the dominant hemisphere have been reported for tumor, hemorrhage, infarction, and stereotaxic surgery (for reviews, see Crosson, 1984). Despite problems of experimental interpretation such as precise neuroanatomical localization, consistently replicated observations of disturbances of language in the left thalamus have emerged.

Symptomatologies include a paucity of spontaneous speech and a poverty of speech content, yet with preserved comprehension. The patient typically speaks only in response to direct questioning and quickly terminates with a brief reply. Voice volume is diminished and becomes progressively lessened if speaking is continued. Rate and rhythm often are disturbed. Although syntax is usually preserved, sentences are often fragmented and filled with perseverative intrusions of unrelated words or phrases. Some patients show perseveration by answering successive questions with the same word. Finding the right word or naming the correct object is difficult for most patients. Paraphasias of the semantic type (i.e., the substitution for one word of another that bears a relationship in meaning to the intended word) are most common. Jargon words are also present in some patients and frequently occur in bursts intermixed with normal speech. In some instances there is an apparent lack of awareness on the part of the patients that they are speaking jargon.

When greater verbal demands are required of the patient, disturbances of speech become more obvious, with a seeming inability to suppress incorrect, even outrageous, words to the point where conversation becomes incoherent. A patient asked to relate the story of Little Red Riding Hood proceeded:

Little Red Riding Hood . . . she went to see her grandmother . . . to take her out with her grandmother, the bread, the butter . . . and then she said to her: grandmother, look out, don't go, don't go, silly things, oh!, that . . . then she decided one day to turn back and see what had happened to her, but Little Red Riding Hood got herself eaten by the wolf . . . and the wolf was very cross. (Cambier & Graveleau, 1985)

(for reviews see Cambier & Graveleau, 1985; Crosson, 1984; Jonas, 1982).

Speech Functions and Thalamic Stimulation

Stimulation of the ventrolateral tier of the dominant thalamus is often a prelude for surgical treatment for dyskinesias. In an extended series of studies, Ojemann has stimulated various sites in the ventrobasal thalamus while patients are engaged in a verbal performance task (Ojemann, 1977). Differential errors were evoked by stimulation within a core of thalamic tissue beginning rostrally at the most lateral aspect of the ventroanterior nucleus, through the medial central portion of the ventrolateral nucleus, and extending caudally to the anterior superior lateral pulvinar. Although spread of effect is always of concern in stimulation studies, evidence of discrete localization of language function was noted for different locations along this neural axis. In the anterior superior lateral pulvinar region, errors were largely of the anomic type. The patient retained the ability to speak, but erred in the correct naming of an object presented in picture form only during the period of stimulation. Errors in this region were of two forms: omissions and misnamings. It is not clear whether the misnamings were paraphasic or jargonaphasic in nature or both.

Stimulation of the medial central portion

of the ventrolateral nucleus evoked errors of what Ojemann labeled the "perseverative" type. These errors were repetitions of the first syllable of the correct object name lasting the duration of stimulation. Stimulation of the lateral aspect of the ventroanterior nucleus resulted in errors that produced a specific incorrect word on each occasion during stimulation when naming was required. Most consistently, that wrong word was the last object correctly named. On other occasions, stimulation of this neural region evoked spontaneous speech. The verbal intrusion, noted by other investigators as well (Schaltenbrand, 1975), may be a single word or phrase and is at present unique to the thalamus. No cortical stimulation in recognized language areas has yet produced spontaneous speech (Ojemann, 1983). Stimulus-linked words of intrusion may interrupt a number counting task, which continues as if without incident when stimulation terminates. At other times the forced intrusions become expressed even when the patient is instructed to remain silent.

Results from the investigations mentioned above, together with similar studies from ventrolateral thalamic stimulations during memory storage or memory retrieval, suggested a specific alerting response role for the thalamus in language production (Ojemann, 1988). Accordingly, Ojemann views the thalamus as a gate controlling access to or from short-term memory storage for the elements of speech production. When the patient is focused on memory units associated with external environmental objects, the thalamus normally blocks the retrieval of already internalized information in memory. Consequently, stimulations during the process of retrieval theoretically open the gate to internalized memory stores, thus eliciting irrelevant or vaguely related words (Ojemann, 1988).

Speech Disorders in Schizophrenia

In his original conceptualization of dementia praecox, Emil Kraepelin (1896) noted distorted words, unusual phrases and expressions, and other forms of pathological speech. He considered the origins of these to be most probably a process occurring in the brain. Some years later, Karl Kleist (1930), also from the Leipzig school, recognized the high degree of similarity between certain schizophrenic disorders of speech and speech disorders in patients with left temporal lobe injury. Despite these early recognitions and a wealth of subsequent clinical descriptions of neologisms, paraphasias, jargonisms, word salads, and other phonological disorders in schizophrenic literature, there are few quantifiable linguistic measurements of schizophrenic utterances. From the perspective of a linguist, Chaika (1974, 1977) initiated a structure analysis of schizophrenic speech from taped interviews. Recognizing that such analysis fails to account for disorganized speech occurring outside the limited contextual framework of the selected portion of the interview, she nevertheless found schizophrenics to demonstrate intermittent aphasia.

Transcribed interviews often contain subtle material that unwittingly informs the evaluator of patient group identification. When cues containing possible biasing information were edited from the transcribed material, schizophrenic patients with a formal thought disorder were found to demonstrate more aphasic abnormalities than did those without a thought disorder (Farber & Reichstein, 1981). In a follow-up study, five specialists blindly assessed interview transcripts of schizophrenic patients having a formal thought disorder and neurologically impaired patients with an aphasia (Farber et al., 1983). Discrimination between the two groups was poor, suggesting the presence of shared language abnormalities between patients with either schizophrenia or aphasia. Similarities between the two syndromes are still quite controversial, with some disclaiming in different degrees any close relationship (DiSimoni, Darley, & Aronson, 1977; Gerson, Benson, & Frazier, 1977; Halpern & McCartin-Clark, 1984; Rausch, Prescott, & DeWolfe, 1980).

A more rigorous attempt at quantification of schizophrenic speech disorders was developed by Andreasen (1979a). Using this new Scale for the Assessment of Thought, Language and Communication, she (Andreasen, 1979b), as well as others using the same scale (Oltmanns, Murphy, Berenbaum, & Dunlop, 1985), cautioned against the notion of widespread disorganized speech in schizophrenia. According to these workers, manifestations of disordered language such as neologisms, perseveration, and echolalia—linguistic features so prevalent in aphasia—are less common than perhaps previously supposed. Their occurrence most probably represents a subtype of schizophrenia (Andreasen, 1982). More prevalent to the schizophrenic patient, in Andreasen's evaluation, is poverty of speech and poverty of speech content—both acknowledged symptoms in thalamic aphasia.

It is not the implied intention here to confirm or confute the debated similarities between the speech of schizophrenics and aphasics, nor is this an attempt to present thalamic aphasia as more reasonable than the classical forms of aphasia when trying to establish a closeness-of-fit to that seen in schizophrenia. Instead, the primary consideration is to focus on the thalamus as a viable neuroanatomical substrate, the disturbed functionalities of which might be responsible for some of the problematic symptoms of schizophrenia, although not necessarily pathognomonic of it.

Mere coincidence may not sufficiently explain common conclusions arrived at by such seemingly disparate investigators as a neurosurgeon electrically stimulating the thalamus of awake patients and a linguist studying the lexical structure of schizophrenic speech from transcribed interviews. In the former, Ojemann (1988) hypothesized the thalamus as a gate blocking access to cortical memory stores of irrelevant information or previously accessed stores. Aberrancies of function, simulated by electrical stimulation, result in language intrusions or perseverations. In the latter, Chaika (1982), after reviewing schizophrenic language samples from a variety of investigators, concluded:

closer inspection suggests that the deviations (neologisms, gibberish, opposite speech, glosso-mania, rhyming, intrusive errors, perseveration) may actually be different manifestations of two underlying dysfunctions: inappropriate persev-erations combined with lack of control over se-lection of linguistic material. (p. 167)

CHEMICAL NEUROANATOMICAL STUDIES OF THE THALAMUS

Our laboratory has for the last few years been carrying out three-dimensional map-ping of the concentration patterns of neuro-transmitters and related substances in post-mortem human brains. Much of this work has concentrated on the catecholamines and related substances in the thalamus. The locus ceruleus–norepinephrine neurotrans-mitter system is known to influence atten-tional and information-processing opera-tions in the brain (Aston-Jones, 1988). Hence, we wished to know whether the nor-epinephrine terminal field projections in the (dorsal) thalamus had any unusual concen-trations, distribution patterns, metabolite abnormalities, or the like in the thalami from schizophrenic subjects as compared to those of normal subjects (persons with no known history of neurological or psychiat-ric illnesses). This original premise proved to be unfounded; the pattern and content of norepinephrine in thalami from schizo-phrenics are essentially indistinguishable from those of normal subjects. However, these studies revealed an unexpected result: There are abnormal amounts of dopamine in thalami from schizophrenic subjects.

Before pursuing the relationship between such results and their possible involvement in the psychopathology of the schizophren-ias, it is important to examine the informa-tion contained in these neurochemical stud-ies. Detailed mapping of the distribution of neurotransmitters has not been used previ-ously in postmortem neurochemical studies of schizophrenia, and it is pertinent to evaluate the potential significance and shortcomings of this approach.

Briefly, human brains were obtained at routine autopsy and frozen to −70°C as soon as possible after removal. For analy-ses, the brain was sliced into 3-mm coronal sections on a mechanical slicer with a smooth blade to minimize local heating. The procedures have been described in detail (Oke, Moghaddam, Ayetey, & Adams, 1987). A 3×3-mm grid was marked on the surface of each slice over regions of interest and the resulting tissue cubes were individ-ually dissected out and refrozen until ana-lyzed. The individual samples were ana-lyzed for catecholamines (dopamine and norepinephrine), indoleamines, and metab-olites by high-performance liquid chroma-tography (HPLC) with electrochemical de-tection, an established procedure for such analyses. The chemical data, such as neuro-transmitter concentrations and ratios, can be combined into computer- or hand-drawn three-dimensional maps of brain regions.

Norepinephrine and Dopamine Patterns in Normal Thalami

Seven normal thalami have been analyzed by the complete grid-mapping procedure described above. Figure 3.1 shows a com-posite of the norepinephrine patterns from these thalami. Although the norepinephrine concentration pattern can hardly be called a chemical fingerprint, its general features are present in every thalamus examined thus far. Consistently, the highest levels of norepinephrine (approximately 100 to 400 ng/g) are in a cylindrically shaped antero-posterior core that decreases rather abruptly at about the beginning of the pulvi-nar, an area that remains uniformly low in norepinephrine. The approximate axis of this core is such that, overall, the elevated norepinephrine density is seen primarily in the lower half of the thalamus. Although these results are not intended to describe norepinephrine concentrations in individual thalamic nuclei, it is clear from Figure 3.1 that the higher norepinephrine levels appear in those subdivisions near the midline and basilar portions (e.g., the center median, parafasicular, and lower portions of the me-

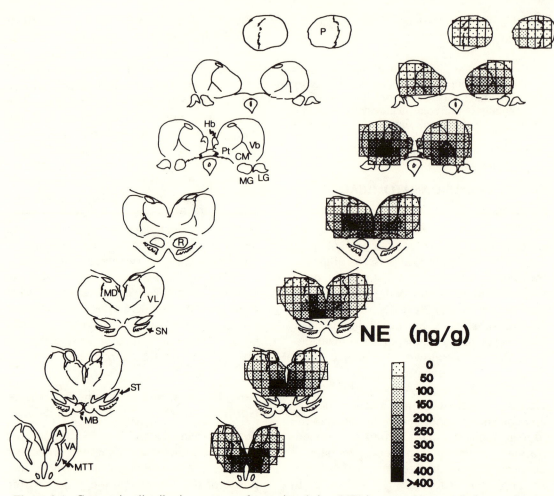

Figure 3.1. Composite distribution pattern of norepinephrine (NE) in normal human thalamus. (Neuro-anatomical designations: MTT, mamillothalamic tract; VA, ventral anterior nucleus; A, anterior nucleus; MB, mammillary body; ST, subthalamic nucleus; SN, substantia nigra; MD, mediodorsal nucleus; VL, ventrolateral nucleus; R, red nucleus; MG, medial geniculate body; LC, lateral geniculate body; CM, centrum medianum; Pf, parafasicular nucleus; Vb, ventrobasal complex; Hb, habenular nucleus; P, pulvinar. These designations also apply, where applicable, in Figures 3.2 and 3.3.)

dial dorsal nucleus). In the middle third of thalamus, high norepinephrine concentrations sometimes extend slightly more laterally to include parts of the ventrolateral nucleus and the so-called ventrobasal complex. The most lateral outer shell, which includes the thalamic reticular nucleus, contains only minimal amounts of norepinephrine. A qualitatively similar picture of norepinephrine distribution was obtained earlier using individual punches instead of grid mapping (Oke, Keller, Mefford, & Adams, 1978).

The patterns shown are essentially inde-

pendent of age, sex, time from death to autopsy, or cause of death. Whereas the *absolute amounts of thalamic norepinephrine vary considerably in different specimens, the pattern of its distribution does not.* For example, one can calculate the average thalamic norepinephrine content over all slices in a given brain (one can exclude the pulvinar region, which has such low norepinephrine). This "average" norepinephrine value is meaningless because of the marked spatial distributions shown in Figure 3.1, but it provides a useful comparison of overall concentrations in different brains. These averages for thalami range from 111 to 196 ng/g. For some reason not apparently correlated with age or time from death to autopsy, the same average of norepinephrine in one case is only 42 ng/g (i.e., only about 25% of that of the other thalami). Still, when normalized for plotting purposes, the distribution pattern of this thalamus is not observably different from the others and matches overall the composite diagram. When one considers the lack of experimental control in dealing with postmortem brains, the consistency of the norepinephrine patterns is quite remarkable.

The dopamine concentration in normal thalami is uniformly low, no more than 15% to 20% of the endogenous norepinephrine. In large portions of the midline central thalamic area the dopamine concentration may be less than the reportable detection limit for these analyses—5 ng/g wet tissue. Thus, unlike norepinephrine, no meaningful distribution pattern exists for dopamine in normal thalami.

Norepinephrine and Dopamine Patterns in Schizophrenic Thalami

Thalami from the brains of schizophrenic patients (as identified by DSM-III or RDC criteria; Oke, Adams, Winblad, & von Knorring, 1988), reasonably matched for both age and time from death to autopsy, show little difference from those of normal patients in norepinephrine distribution patterns. Absolute levels of norepinephrine in schizophrenic thalami show the same kinds of variation as seen in normal thalami, with no discernible relationship to age or time from death to autopsy.

There are very marked increases in dopamine concentration in schizophrenic thalami compared to that of normal thalami. Thus, the results are best presented in terms of the distribution pattern for the ratio or percentage of dopamine to norepinephrine (DA/NE ratio). As mentioned earlier, this ratio for normal thalami rarely exceeds 15% to 20%. This is always so except in the outermost areas, where parts of the thalamus are closest to other brain nuclei with very high dopamine content (e.g., near the tail of the caudate nucleus or in the most ventral aspects where the substantia nigra lies nearby). In these areas samples with a higher DA/NE ratio are occasionally found. However, in thalami from schizophrenic patients, much higher DA/NE ratios, in many cases exceeding 100% to 200%, are found dispersed throughout the thalamus. In individual brains, these DA/NE "hot regions" lie in different thalamic areas—interspersed among regions that may have ratios comparable to those of normal brains (Oke & Adams, 1987). In several schizophrenic thalami examined thus far, the high DA/NE ratios are so pervasive that even values averaged over the entire thalamus demonstrate the abnormality. In other cases, however, an average analysis of, perhaps, the posterior third of the thalamus might show only a minor elevation of dopamine or the DA/NE ratio. Thus, the total distribution patterns developed by the grid-mapping procedure are particularly significant. These patterns have been given earlier (Oke & Adams, 1987), and Figure 3.2 illustrates another comparison of normal versus schizophrenic DA/NE ratios not previously reported. Indeed, in eight of nine thalami from schizophrenic patients, extremely high DA/NE ratio patterns similar to those of Figure 3.2 have been found. *No such abnormalities have ever been seen in 14 normal thalami.* We are convinced that this is a very robust and repeatable finding, but one that ordinarily cannot be evaluated without complete grid mapping of the thalamus.

The grid mapping also allows one to make comparisons of neurotransmitter distribution patterns with literature data that discuss specific brain functionalities. For example, as discussed earlier, speech regions of the thalamus whose output can be altered by electrical stimulation have been delineated in precise anatomical detail by Ojemann (1976, 1977, 1983). From these publications one can identify language distribution areas that match regions of the chemical analyses in the present work. Figure 3.3 is an illustration of the matching of these recognized speech location areas with our tis-

POSTERIOR

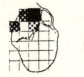

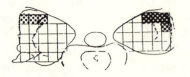

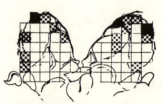

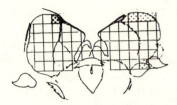

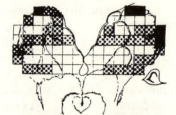

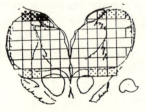

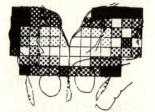

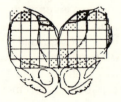

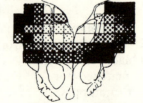

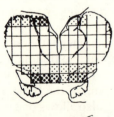

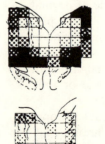

DA/NE X 100

0
25
50
75
100
125
150
175
>175

ANTERIOR

Normal   Schiz

Figure 3.2. Comparison of dopamine/norepinephrine (DA/NE) ratios in thalami from normal and schizophrenic subjects.

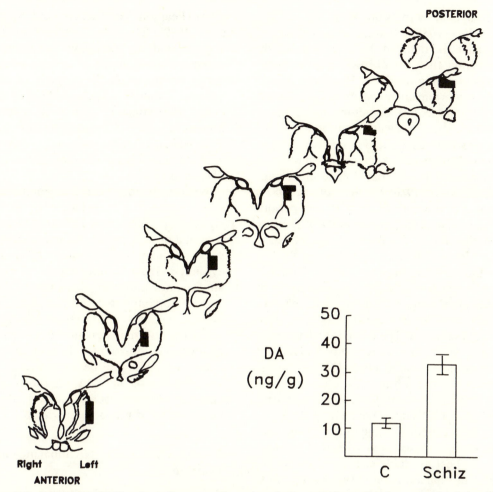

Figure 3.3. Dopamine (DA) values from samples taken from speech production areas in thalami from control and schizophrenic subjects. Shaded regions designate thalamic areas stimulated by Ojemann (see text). Statistical analysis by Student's *t* test; *t* = 4.68; *df* = 271; *p*>.001.

sue analysis scheme for thalami from normal and schizophrenic brains. Speech regions critical for language production are found only within the left or dominant thalamus; only rarely—in certain left-handed individuals—do they involve the right thalamus. Thus, the matching was restricted to left thalamus data. The mean absolute dopamine values for the pooled grid sections were 11.9 ± 1.8 (SEM) and 33.7 ± 3.1 ng/g for normal individuals and schizophrenics, respectively. This approximately threefold difference is significant at the *p*<.001 level. Absolute dopamine rather than DA/NE ratio values are used in this analysis. The heterogeneity of dopamine distribution usu-

ally seen in a whole thalamus slice was not evident in just the medial central core of the ventrolateral thalamus and did not overshadow the variability of dopamine content between brains or between the two groups. This comparison illustrates that schizophrenic subjects may have excessive dopamine in known speech production regions of the thalamus.

Why elevated dopamine is found in the thalami from schizophrenic subjects is not yet known. There is no reason to believe it is due to improper chemical analysis or procedural artifacts such as slicing "carryover" from dopamine-rich areas of the brain (e.g., it is never seen in normal brains sliced in exactly the same way) (Oke et al., 1987). It is possible that the excess thalamic dopamine is induced by the neuroleptic medication that all schizophrenic subjects in this sampling received. However, previous postmortem chemical analyses have not shown endogenous dopamine to be influenced by such medication, although these analyses were conducted in normally dopamine-rich areas such as caudate and nucleus accumbens (Crow, Cross, Johnstone, Longden, & Ridley, 1980; MacKay et al., 1982). Chronic treatment of rats with haloperidol has not induced any change in DA/NE ratios in rat thalami (A. F. Oke et al., unpublished data). In an effort to substantiate further that the results are not medication induced, we have preliminary data on thalami from Huntington's chorea patients who had received considerable dosages of neuroleptics. These data will be presented in the near future, but to date there is no evidence of aberrant dopamine levels or DA/NE ratios. Although the Huntington's chorea model may not be the best for comparison with schizophrenic thalami because of the basal ganglia degeneration and other tissue volume changes associated with that disease, it is the best available at present in the absence of thalami from drug-naive cases. Taken together, the above data strongly suggest that the excessive dopamine in schizophrenic thalami is not medication induced.

We have also carried out complete grid mapping in selected slices that include the thalamus and extend peripherally through the internal capsule into the putamen and toward other dopamine-rich areas such as the tail of the caudate and substantia nigra. In schizophrenic brains one finds gradients of dopamine concentrations that extend, for example, from the putamen across the internal capsule and well into the thalamus. Such gradients rarely invade the thalamus in normal brains and are of considerably lesser concentrations. The internal capsule contains a major portion of tyrosine hydroxylase immunoreactive fibers, many presumably dopaminergic, ascending to both striatal structures and cortical forebrain re-

gions (Pearson, Halliday, Sakamoto, & Michel, 1990). Thus, the present indications suggest that the excessive dopamine may come from misplaced or aberrant dopaminergic terminals in the thalami of schizophrenic subjects. Such patterning might come from some fault in programming of dopamine terminal projections during early neuronal development—a view consistent with developmental theories of the causes of schizophrenia.

We have begun specific dopamine uptake site labeling to examine whether there are significant differences in actual dopamine terminal projections in thalami from normal versus schizophrenic brains. All available evidence from neuroanatomical tracing studies indicates that there are no known major dopaminergic projections to the human thalamus, and the present work confirms that normal thalami have very little endogenous dopamine. If real dopamine nerve terminals can be shown to coincide with regions of high DA/NE ratios in thalami from schizophrenic subjects, this will be a finding of major significance.

Possible Effect of DA/NE Imbalance in Thalamus

We suggest that the findings of an aberrant neurotransmitter discussed above could presumably alter thalamic activity. A rational possibility is that the DA/NE imbalance, interacting with the other neurotransmitter systems of the thalamus, can produce distorted firing patterns of neuronal assemblies that could globally alter normal brain functioning. Alternately, more circumscribed dysfunctions could be produced, varying in individual cases, according to the distribution of the excess dopamine. The caveat underlying this hypothesis is that the excess dopamine is not "just there." It must be assumed to be interactive in the neurotransmitter sense. It should somehow alter the usual functionality of norepinephrine in its interplay with the excitatory glutamate and acetylcholinergic inputs to the thalamus and inhibitory γ-aminobutyric acid from interneurons. Unfortunately, there is as yet no proof for this assertion—*the data from the present studies only verify the chemical presence of excess dopamine, not its functional properties*. However, if for purposes of discussion one grants that the excess dopamine has the potential transmitter-like properties outlined above, the arguments to suggest dysfunctional thalamic operation are evident.

Every bit of information from the outside world, except for olfactory inputs, passes through the dorsal thalamus before being transmitted to the cortex. The thalamus often has been considered a gate, filter, or integrator of this afferent input, but modern studies have proposed that its functionalities are much higher. In many ways it can be considered as the controlling gate of the modes of cortical information processing. This comes about by unique properties of thalamic neurons that have been elucidated by Jahnsen and Llinás (1984a, 1984b). Thalamic relay neurons (which transmit sensory data directly to the cortex), and probably most other neurons of the thalamus, operate in two very distinct firing patterns whose limiting outputs are: (a) a bursting mode in which a packet of fast action potentials is intermittently transmitted, and (b) the single spike or transfer mode. The bursting action is synonymous with rhythmic activity in the cortical electroencephalogram (i.e., the resting, nonattentive brain, characterized in the extreme by slow wave sleep). The transfer mode, in contrast, passes on single action potentials to the cortex in response to incoming sensory afferents and thus provides high-fidelity information to the cortex regarding events in the outside world. It characterizes the attentive brain interacting with the external environment. These unique neuronal activities of the thalamus depend on intrinsic electrophysiological properties of the neurons, their interneuron connections (especially with the thalamic reticular nucleus), and the ascending monoamine and cholinergic systems of the brainstem (Aston-Jones, 1988; Jahnsen & Llinás, 1984a, 1984b; McCormick, 1989; McCormick & Prince, 1988; Shosaku, Kayama, Sumitomo, Sugitani, & Iwama, 1989; Steri-

ade & Deschênes, 1984; Steriade & Llinás, 1988).

Indeed, it is the influence of the monoamine systems, particularly norepinephrine, that is of greatest interest to the present discussion. Animal studies have demonstrated clearly that iontophoretic application of norepinephrine to thalamic relay neurons (acting in concert with other neurotransmitter systems as described above) shifts their firing patterns from the bursting to the transfer mode. It has been postulated that activation of the norepinephrine–locus ceruleus system can shift, via norepinephrine release, the activity of thalamic neuronal assemblies that facilitate the faithful transfer of sensory inputs from the outside world to the cerebral cortex (McCormick, 1989; McCormick & Prince, 1988). In essence, the norepinephrine system in the thalamus is cast as a major influence on proper processing of sensory information by the brain.

It is the thesis of the present arguments that, because the normal human thalamus has negligible levels of dopamine and there are no known major dopaminergic pathways to the human thalamus, dopamine apparently has an insignificant role. In thalami from schizophrenic subjects, the high levels of dopamine may distort the influence of norepinephrine on thalamic activity, possibly resulting in alterations of any continuum between bursting and transfer modes of the neuronal assemblies. Only in the transfer mode is information passed correctly to the cortex—in the partial bursting mode, information transfer could be fragmentary or distorted. Furthermore, every bit of information passed by relay neurons to the cortex returns almost immediately via corticothalamic pathways. All back-and-forth traffic between sensory afferents, thalamus, and cortex passes through the envelope of the thalamic reticular nucleus, with its corresponding inputs to each of the sensory nuclei of the thalamus itself. It can be noted that elevated dopamine is often seen in regions corresponding to the reticular nucleus (see, e.g., Figure 3.2). Temporal disruption, even in a minor way, of this continuously recurrent updating of the cortex with regard to external events could have widespread deleterious effects (Crick, 1984). In thalami from schizophrenic subjects, the elevated dopamine is heterogeneously distributed and, in general, the positions of the "hot spots" vary between individual brains. This variable distribution is certainly consistent with the possibilities of distorted processing in multiple output domains (e.g., perceptual, somatic, and motor behavior, influenced by separate thalamic regions). The abnormal influence of dopamine on thalamic activity might produce the hyperattentiveness and fragmented sensory integration so commonly noted by schizophrenic patients (Mendel, 1989; Torrey, 1988). We have suggested herein that neurological findings indicate that thalamic stimulations and lesions can produce speech alterations with some commonality to schizophrenic behavior. Similar effects might be produced by abnormal DA/NE modulation in the ventrolateral tier of the thalamus as discussed above.

There is very little information at present on an effect of dopamine on thalamic neurons comparable to that of norepinephrine. Because dopamine is not expected to be, and is not normally, found in seemingly important amounts in mammalian thalami, there presumably has been little impetus to study such interactions. Earlier, before the present understanding of thalamic modal activity, dopamine was reported to depress the firing of thalamic relay neurons, and this influence had a more rapid time course than that of norepinephrine (Phillis and Tebêcis, 1967; Tebêcis, 1974). Further substantiation of the possible role(s) of dopamine in thalamic neuronal functioning suggested herein must await more modern electrophysiological studies, as well as proof of the neurotransmitter functionality of the excess dopamine in schizophrenic thalami.

ACKNOWLEDGMENTS

We are much indebted to C. Putz for excellent technical assistance in the brain analyses and to N. Harmony and C. Howard for manuscript preparation. This work was supported by the National Institutes of Health via Grant NS-08740 and in part by Psychiatric Centers of America. The generous assistance of the Kansas AMI group is especially appreciated.

REFERENCES

Adler, L. E., Pachtman, E., Franks, R. D., Pocevich, M., Waldo, M. C., & Freedman, R. (1982). Neurophysiological evidence for a defect in neuronal mechanisms involved in sensory gating in schizophrenia. *Biological Psychiatry, 17*, 639.

Adler, L. E., Waldo, M. C., & Freedman, R. (1985). Neurophysiologic studies of sensory gating in schizophrenia: Comparison of auditory and visual responses. *Biological Psychiatry, 20*, 1284.

American Psychiatric Association. (1980). *Diagnostic and statistical manual of mental disorders* (3rd ed.). Washington, DC: American Psychiatric Press, Inc.

American Psychiatric Association. (1987). *Diagnostic and statistical manual of mental disorders* (3rd ed., rev.). Washington, DC: American Psychiatric Press, Inc.

Andreasen, N. C. (1979a). Thought, language, and communication disorders: I. Clinical assessment, definition of terms, and evaluation of their reliability. *Archives of General Psychiatry, 36*, 1315.

Andreasen, N. C. (1979b). Thought, language, and communication disorders: II. Diagnostic significance. *Archives of General Psychiatry, 36*, 1325.

Andreasen, N. C. (1982). The relationship between schizophrenic language and the aphasias. In F. A. Henn & H. A. Nasrallah (Eds.), *Schizophrenia as a brain disease* (p. 109). Oxford, England: Oxford University Press.

Aston-Jones, G. (1988). Cellular attributes of locus coeruleus: Implications for attentional processes. In M. Sandler, A. Dahlström, & R. Belmaker (Eds.), *Neurology and neurobiology, Vol. 42B, Progress in catecholamine research, Part B: Central aspects* (pp. 133–142). New York: Alan R. Liss.

Bick, P. A., & Kinsbourne, M. (1987). Auditory hallucinations and subvocal speech in schizophrenic patients. *American Journal of Psychiatry, 144*, 222.

Bleuler, E. (1950). *Dementia praecox or the group of schizophrenias* (J. Zinkin, Trans.). New York: International Universities Press. (Original work published 1911)

Botez, M. I., & Barbeau, A. (1971). Role of subcortical structures and particularly of the thalamus in the mechanisms of speech and language. *International Journal of Neurology, 8,* 300.

Buchsbaum, M. S., Nuechterlein, K. H., Haier, R. J., Wu, J., Sicotte, N., Hazlett, E., Asarnow, R., Potkin, S., & Guich, S. (1990). Glucose metabolic rate in normals and schizophrenics during the continuous performance test assessed by positron emission tomography. *British Journal of Psychiatry, 156,* 216.

Cambier, J., & Graveleau, P. (1985). Thalamic syndromes. In *Handbook of clinical neurology, Vol. 45, Clinical neuropsychology* (pp. 87–98). New York: Elsevier.

Chaika, E. (1974). A linguist looks at schizophrenic language. *Brain and Language, 1,* 257.

Chaika, E. (1977). Schizophrenic speech, slips of the tongue and jargonaphasia: A reply to Fromkin and to Lecours and Vaniers-Clement. *Brain and Language, 4,* 464.

Chaika, E. (1982). A unified explanation for the diverse structural deviations reported for adult schizophrenics with disrupted speech. *Journal of Communication Disorders, 15,* 167.

Crick, F. (1984). Function of the thalamic reticular nucleus: The searchlight hypothesis. *Proceedings of the National Academy of Sciences (U.S.A.), 81,* 4586.

Crosson, B. (1984). Role of the dominant thalamus in language: A review. *Psychological Bulletin, 96,* 491.

Crow, T. J., Cross, A. J., Johnstone, E. C., Longden, A., & Ridley, R. M. (1980). Time course of the antipsychotic effect in schizophrenia and some changes in postmortem brain and their relation to neuroleptic medication. *Advances in Biochemical Psychopharmacology, 24,* 495.

Davis, J. M., Barter, J. T., & Kane, J. M. (1989). Antipsychotic drugs. In H. I. Kaplan & B. J. Saddock (Eds.), *Comprehensive textbook of psychiatry IV* (pp. 1591–1626). Baltimore: Williams & Wilkins.

DeLisi, L. E., & Crow, T. J. (1986). Is schizophrenia a viral or immunologic disorder? *Psychiatric Clinics of North America, 9,* 155.

DiSimoni, F. G., Darley, F. L., & Aronson, A. E. (1977). Patterns of dysfunction in schizophrenic patients on an aphasic test battery. *Journal of Speech and Hearing Disorders, 42,* 498.

Eaves, L. (1988). Genetics, immunology and virology. *Schizophrenia Bulletin, 14,* 365.

Endicott, J., & Spitzer, R. L. (1978). A diagnostic interview: The Schedule for Affective Disorders and Schizophrenia. *Archives of General Psychiatry, 35,* 837.

Farber, R., Abrams, R., Taylor, M. A., Kasprison, A., Morris C., & Weisz, R. (1983). Comparison of schizophrenic patients with formal thought disorder and neurologically impaired patients with aphasia. *American Journal of Psychiatry, 140,* 1348.

Farber, R., & Reichstein, M. B. (1981). Language dysfunction in schizophrenia. *British Journal of Psychiatry, 139,* 519.

Freedman, R., Adler, L. E., Gerhardt, G. A., Waldo, M., Baker, N., Rose, G. M., Dreburg, C., Nagamoto, H., Bickford-Wimmer, P., & Franks, R. (1987). Neurobiological studies of sensory gating in schizophrenia. *Schizophrenia Bulletin, 13,* 669.

Gerson, S. N., Benson, D. F., & Frazier, S. H. (1977). Diagnosis: Schizophrenia versus posterior aphasia. *American Journal of Psychiatry, 134,* 966.

Geyer, M. A., & Braff, D. L. (1987). Startle habituation and sensorimotor gating in schizophrenia and related animal models. *Schizophrenia Bulletin, 13,* 643.

Gottesman, I. I., & Shields, J. (1972). *Schizophrenia and genetics: A twin study vantage point.* New York: Academic Press.

Gould, L. N. (1948). Verbal hallucinations and activity of vocal musculature: An electromyographic study. *American Journal of Psychiatry, 105,* 367.

Grebb, J. A., & Cancro, R. (1989). Schizophrenia: Clinical factors. In H. I. Kaplan & B. J. Saddock (Eds.), *Comprehensive textbook of psychiatry IV* (pp. 757–777). Baltimore: Williams & Wilkins.

Green, M. F., & Kinsbourne, M. (1989). Auditory hallucinations in schizophrenia: Does humming help? *Biological Psychiatry, 25,* 630.

Halpern, H., & McCartin-Clark, M. (1984). Differential language characteristics in adult aphasic and schizophrenic subjects. *Journal of Communication Disorders, 17,* 289.

Hoffman, R. E. (1986). Verbal hallucinations and language production processes in schizophrenia. *Behavioral Brain Sciences, 9,* 503.

Ingvar, D. H., & Franzen, G. (1974). Abnormalities of cerebral blood flow distribution in patients with chronic schizophrenia. *Acta Psychiatrica Scandinavica, 50,* 425.

Inouye, T., & Shimizu, A. (1970). The electromyographic study of verbal hallucination. *Journal of Nervous and Mental Disease, 151,* 415.

Jahnsen, H., & Llinás, R. (1984a). Electrophysiological properties of guinea-pig thalamic neurons: An *in vitro* study. *Journal of Physiology (London), 349,* 205.

Jahnsen, H., & Llinás, R. (1984b). Ionic basis

for the electro-responsiveness and oscillatory properties of guinea-pig thalamic neurones *in vitro. Journal of Physiology (London), 349,* 227.

Jonas, S. (1982). The thalamus and aphasia, including transcortical aphasia: A review. *Journal of Communication Disorders, 15,* 31.

Kety, S. S. (1970). Introduction. In H. E. Himwich (Ed.), *Biochemistry, schizophrenias and affective illnesses* (pp. xi–xiv). Baltimore: Williams & Wilkins.

Kety, S. S., Rosenthal, D., Wender, P. D., Schulsinger, F., & Jacobson, B. (1975). Mental illness in the biological and adoptive families of adopted individuals who have become schizophrenic: A preliminary report based upon psychiatric interviews. In R. Fieve, D. Rosenthal, & H. Brill (Eds.), *Genetic research in psychiatry* (pp. 112–116). Baltimore: Johns Hopkins University Press.

Kleist, K. (1930). Alogical thought disorder: An organic manifestation of the schizophrenic psychological deficit. In J. Cutting & M. Shepherd (Eds.), *The clinical roots of the schizophrenia concept: Translations of seminal European contributions on schizophrenia* (pp. 75–76). Cambridge, England: Cambridge University Press.

Kraepelin, E. (1896). Dementia praecox. In J. Cutting & M. Shepherd (Eds.), *The clinical roots of the schizophrenia concept: Translations of seminal European contributions on schizophrenia* (pp. 13–24). Cambridge, England: Cambridge University Press.

Lehmann, H. E. (1967). Schizophrenia I: Introduction and history. In A. M. Freedman & H. I. Kaplan (Eds.), *Comprehensive textbook of psychiatry* (pp. 593–598). Baltimore: Williams & Wilkins.

Lipkowitz, M. A., & Idupuganti, S. (1983). Diagnosing schizophrenia in 1980: A survey of U.S. psychiatrists. *American Journal of Psychiatry, 140,* 52.

Losonczy, M. F., Song, I. S., Mohs, R. C., Mathe, A. A., Davidson, M., Davis, B. M., & Davis, K. L. (1986). Correlates of lateral ventricular size in chronic schizophrenia, II: Biological measures. *American Journal of Psychiatry, 143,* 1113.

MacDonald, H. L., & Best, J. J. K. (1989). The Scottish first episode schizophrenia study VI. Computerized tomography brain scans in patients and controls. *British Journal of Psychiatry, 154,* 492.

Mackay, A. V. P., Iversen, L. L., Rosser, M., Spokes, E., Bird, E. D., Arrequi, A., Creese, I., & Snyder, S. H. (1982). Increased brain dopamine and dopamine receptors in schizophrenia. *Archives of General Psychiatry, 39,* 991.

McCormick, D. A. (1989). Cholinergic and noradrenergic modulation of thalamocortical processing. *Trends in Neurosciences, 12,* 215.

McCormick, D. A., & Prince, D. A. (1988). Noradrenergic modulation of firing pattern in guinea pig and cat thalamic neurons *in vitro. Journal of Neurophysiology, 59,* 978.

Mendel, W. M. (1989). *Treating schizophrenia* (pp. 1–71). San Francisco: Jossey-Bass.

Ojemann, G. A. (1976). Subcortical language mechanisms. In H. Whitaker & H. A. Whitaker (Eds.), *Studies in neurolinguistics* (pp. 103–138). New York: Academic Press.

Ojemann, G. A. (1977). Asymmetric function of the thalamus in man. *Annals of the New York Academy of Sciences, 299,* 380.

Ojemann, G. A. (1983). Brain organization for language from the perspective of electrical stimulation mapping. *Behavioral Brain Sciences, 2,* 189.

Ojemann, G. A. (1988). Effects of cortical and subcortical stimulation on human language and verbal memory. In F. Plum (Ed.), *Language, communication and the brain* (pp. 101–115). New York: Raven Press.

Oke, A. F., & Adams, R. N. (1987). Elevated thalamic dopamine: Possible link to sensory dysfunctions in schizophrenia. *Schizophrenia Bulletin, 13,* 589.

Oke, A. F., Adams, R. N., Winblad, B., & von Knorring, L. (1988). Elevated dopamine/norepinephrine ratios in thalami of schizophrenic brains. *Biological Psychiatry, 24,* 79.

Oke, A. F., Keller, R., Mefford, I., & Adams, R. N. (1978). Lateralization of norepinephrine in human thalamus. *Science, 200,* 1411.

Oke, A. F., Moghaddam, M., Ayetey, W. E. A., & Adams, R. N. (1987). Mechanical slicing of frozen brain tissue: A reappraisal of catecholamine loss. *Journal of Neuroscience Methods, 22,* 41.

Oltmanns, T. F., Murphy, R., Berenbaum, H., & Dunlop, S. R. (1985). Rating verbal communication impairment in schizophrenia and affective disorders. *Schizophrenia Bulletin, 11,* 292.

Pearson, J., Halliday, G., Sakamoto, N., & Michel, J.-P. (1990). Catecholamine neurons. In G. Paxinos (Ed.), *The human nervous system* (chap. 31). New York: Academic Press.

Pert, C., Knight, J. G., Laing, P., & Markwell, M. A. K. (1988). Scenarios for a viral etiology of schizophrenia. *Schizophrenia Bulletin, 14,* 243.

Phillis, J. W., & Tebêcis, A. K. (1967). The responses of thalamic neurons to iontophoretically applied monoamines. *Journal of Physiology (London), 192,* 715.

Rausch, M. A., Prescott, T. E., & DeWolfe, A. S. (1980). Schizophrenic and aphasic language: Discriminable or not? *Journal of Consulting and Clinical Psychology, 48,* 63.

Saccuzzo, D. P., & Braff, D. L. (1986). Information processing abnormalities: Trait- and state-dependent components. *Schizophrenia Bulletin, 12,* 447.

Schaltenbrand, G. (1975). The effects on speech and language of stereotactical stimulation in thalamus and corpus callosum. *Brain and Language, 2,* 70.

Shosaku, A., Kayama, Y., Sumitomo, I., Sugitani, M., & Iwama, K. (1989). Analysis of recurrent inhibitory circuit in rat thalamus: Neurophysiology of the thalamic reticular nucleus. *Progress in Neurobiology, 32,* 77.

Spitzer, R. L., Endicott, J., & Robins, E. (1975). Research diagnostic criteria (RDC). *Psychopharmacology Bulletin, 11,* 22.

Steriade, M., & Deschênes, M. (1984). The thalamus as a neuronal oscillator. *Brain Research Reviews, 8,* 1.

Steriade, M., and Llinás, R. (1988). The functional states of the thalamus and the associated neuronal interplay. *Physiological Reviews, 68,* 649.

Tebêcis, A. K. (1974). *Transmitters and identified neurons in the mammalian central nervous system* (p. 129). Bristol, England: Scientechna.

Torrey, E. F. (1988). *Surviving schizophrenia* (pp. 16–72). New York: Harper & Row.

Weinberger, D. R., Berman, K. F., & Zee, R. F. (1986). Physiological dysfunction of dorsolateral prefrontal cortex in schizophrenia, I: Regional blood flow evidence. *Archives of General Psychiatry, 43,* 114.

Woods, B. T., Yurgelum-Todd, D., Benes, F. M., Frankenburg, F. R., Pope, H. G., Jr., & McSparren, J. (1990). Progressive ventricular enlargement in schizophrenia: Comparisons to bipolar affective disorder and correlation with clinical course. *Biological Psychiatry, 27,* 341.

Part II

GENETIC STRATEGIES AND RESEARCH

4

Schizophrenia Research: Things To Do Before the Geneticist Arrives

RUE L. CROMWELL

At this point in time it is useful heuristically to assume that no evidence exists for a genetic contribution to schizophrenia. The twin, family, and adoptee studies provide evidence that schizophrenia runs in families—*some* families. In particular, adoptee studies provide evidence that a perinatal or prebirth factor contributes to schizophrenia. Among the various possible prebirth factors is the genetic one. Investigators, even those who filed earlier positive reports about genetic linkage, agree that no linkage evidence yet exists for schizophrenia.[1] Therefore, the genetic contribution to schizophrenia remains only a reasonable and compelling hypothesis.

It is also useful to assume that no evidence exists for a genetic contribution that is specific to schizophrenia. Whatever genetic contribution exists might also contribute to other pathologies, forms of thought disorder, susceptibility to tardive dyskinesia, impairment with aging, or other factors. Likewise, it is useful to assume that no evidence exists for schizophrenia to be a single entity from a genetic standpoint. Genetic factors may exist that relate to independent subtypes of schizophrenia.

Certainly, no evidence exists that the genetic contribution to schizophrenia has the same base rate in the population as the base rate for clinically diagnosed schizophrenia itself. The estimates for clinically diagnosed schizophrenia center around 1%. In a model in which the genetic factor combines additively to stress or other environmental factors, the populational base rate of the genetic contribution may be less than 1%. In a model in which specific genetic factors must occur in combination with (i.e., interact with) specific environmental variance, the base rate of the genetic contribution in sum would likely be above 1%. If more than one specific genetic factor must be present to interact with specific environmental variance, again, the base rate of each genetic contributor is likely above 1%. In fact, one or more of such interactive genetic factors could have a high base rate (e.g., near or over 50%) in the general population. Mathematically, it is necessary only that the probabilities for these various requisite environmental and genetic factors multiply out to the expected 1% for the manifest pathology.

Even if genetic factors for schizophrenia are identified, they may be "schizophrenia-

1. Summary comment of Eliot Gershon from a conference program on genetic linkage at the American Psychopathological Association meetings, New York City, March 4–8, 1992.

This chapter is based on the inaugural address for the M. Erik Wright Distinguished Professorship in Clinical Psychology at the University of Kansas, January 21, 1988, and on an invited address at the third annual meeting of the Society for Research in Psychopathology, Harvard University, November 11, 1988. It was partially supported by NIMH Grant MH-34114 and the Graduate Research Fund of the University of Kansas.

related" rather than "schizophrenia" factors. That is, each factor may have phenotypic features of its own that bear no resemblance to specific symptoms in the final clinical syndrome. In the next section, such a possibility is presented.

Finally, it is useful to assume that no evidence exists that conclusively supports one single genetic (or genetic–environmental) model of schizophrenia over others. Among the various possible models, polygenic ones may be either (a) specific to schizophrenia or (b) contributive to lowered functioning in general. Of the latter, schizophrenia would be one alternative outcome of lowered functioning. Likewise, the environmental variance associated with schizophrenia may be specific to schizophrenia or may subsume schizophrenia along with other types of lowered functioning. In other words, it is not clear which, the genetic or the environmental factors (or both in particular combination), sets the boundary of the disorder.

An oligogenic model would hold that two or very few genetic loci are involved in schizophrenia. A single-locus (including monogenic) model, by definition, implies that only one genetic factor is necessary for an individual to become vulnerable to schizophrenia. It represents the "holy grail" for which so many have sought for so long with so little success. Later in this chapter minor evidence is presented that suggests that the single-factor model (whether monogenic or environmental) is not likely to explain schizophrenia.

As already may be surmised, the foregoing assumptions are not restrictive. Indeed, they are enabling. One may proceed from them to pursue any number of alternative genetic hypotheses.

THE SCHIZOPHRENIA-RELATED VARIANTS MODEL

Following from the preceding assumptions, the concept of schizophrenia-related variants (SRVs) is presented as one possible formulation to describe the genetic contribution to schizophrenia. This formulation seems as likely—no more or no less—as

any other. The term "marker" (also "genetic marker") is avoided here because different researchers define a marker in very different ways. For example, a genetic marker could be defined as a measure of a phenotype associated with known chromosomal origin and approximate chromosomal locus. No SRV presently has this status of genetic definition.

Instead, an SRV may be viewed as a measurable variable that has an earlier and relatively closer relationship to specific genes than does clinical schizophrenia itself (see Figure 4.1). Then, combined with requisite environmental variance, the SRVs will lead alternatively to schizophrenia or to other denotable types of functioning in those particular family members who inherit them. In family members who do not receive these specific genetic and environmental contributors, the vulnerability to schizophrenia is not just subthreshold; instead, it is essentially nil.

The SRV model of ontogeny of schizophrenia may be compared and contrasted with the "latent trait" model (Holzman, Kringlen, & Matthysse, 1988), in which phenotypic measures such as eye tracking (and possibly other measures) are viewed as coordinate with the overt schizophrenia phenotype. In other words, no assumption of antecedent–consequent relationship seems necessary in the "latent trait" model, and no assumption appears evident that overt schizophrenia has more variance shared with environmental factors than the eye tracking (or other) traits.

Given these background comments, an SRV would be defined operationally as a variable whose deviance is (a) empirically

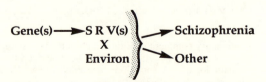

Figure 4.1. A simple model of the relationship among genes, schizophrenia-related variants (SRVs), and environment as necessary antecedents to schizophrenia and alternative levels of functioning.

associated with schizophrenia; (b) present before and after, if not also during, episodes of schizophrenic psychosis; and (c) present among some (but not necessarily all) first-degree relatives of schizophrenics. At least three deductions about this SRV framework should be apparent:

1. The base rate for these deviant SRVs in the general population should exceed the base rate for schizophrenia itself. That is, not all individuals with the requisite SRVs would have the requisite environmental factors.

2. Although one could not conceivably expect a mendelian distribution for clinically defined schizophrenia, the SRV, relatively more under genetic control, may have distributions more closely approximating a mendelian one. The pedigree distribution of schizophrenia itself would be more sparse. The occurrence of schizophrenia in the pedigree would depend directly on which family members with SRV(s) also received the requisite environmental influence.

3. Stated somewhat differently, one cannot argue backward from the familial distribution characteristics of clinical schizophrenia to draw conclusions about the distribution characteristics of SRVs. Instead, one must observe.

For genetic inferences the measurement of an SRV must be separated from the effects of both the acute episode and the subsequent generalized deficit during the chronic phase. Both are well known to be associated with overt schizophrenic disorder. The magnitude of SRVs is often found to be enhanced during episodes of overt schizophrenic illness. (This observation is akin to Nuechterlein's [personal communication] observation concerning "mediated vulnerability variables.") Then, as people continue into chronic illness, they tend to decline along numerous dimensions of be-

havioral and cognitive function. This is commonly referred to as generalized deficit. Because the genetic structure has obviously not changed from the premorbid to the acute to the chronic state, it is clear that the measured increase in SRV magnitudes is not related to genetic variance.

In addition to the possibility that the active psychotic state amplifies the SRV, it should be acknowledged that in other cases it may obscure (i.e., prevent) certain SRVs from being detectable. For these reasons, SRVs are often assumed to be more reliably and validly measured among healthy first-degree relatives and during the period prior to succumbing to schizophrenic illness.

REACTION TIME CROSSOVER

With these foregoing assumptions and definitions, a number of questions are now presented about SRVs. If these questions are answered by behavioral scientists (before the geneticist arrives), the design, analysis, and understanding of genetic investigations may be facilitated. As each question is asked, reaction time crossover (RTX; redundancy deficit) is used as an illustrative SRV example.

RTX is defined here as the progressive slowing of simple motor reaction time when trials shift from irregular to regular preparatory intervals (forewarning periods). Depending on contextual factors, this slowing must usually be measured at or above a 7-second preparatory interval level. The typical measure (Bellissimo & Steffy, 1972) involves the extent to which samples of trials for a regular series exceed that for an irregular series. This RTX measure meets the aforestated criteria for an SRV, and it tends to be independent of the individual's mean reaction time.

Rodnick and Shakow (1940) first identified RTX in the 1930s. Bellissimo and Steffy (1972) developed a more efficient procedure of measurement, as illustrated in Table 4.1, and found that the phenomenon could be assessed from embedded isotemporal trial sets with only four trials per set. Spohn and Coyne (Chapter 16, this volume; 1989; see

Table 4.1. An Illustration of Preparatory Intervals (PIs; in Seconds) on a Sample of Successive Reaction Time Trials[a]

. . . 1 3 7 10 6 4 7 7 7 7 9 . . .
. . .   I   I R R R   . . .

[a] I, irregular trial (preceded by PI of different length); R, regular trial (preceded by PI of same length); RTX = mean R minus mean I across all trials of 7-inch PI.

also Spohn & Coyne, in press; Spohn & Strauss, 1989) have recently verified that the phenomenon is stable and not responsive to neuroleptic drugs.

NINE QUESTIONS TO ASK ABOUT AN SRV

Question 1: What is the base rate of the deviant SRV among schizophrenics (or a specifically defined subgroup or variation thereof)?

Before discussing this question, a prefatory comment is appropriate. The parenthetical insertion in the preceding question represents a reminder that formal clinical nosology (e.g., that of the *Diagnostic and Statistical Manual of Mental Disorders,* third edition, revised [DSM-III-R; American Psychiatric Association, 1987]) need not be viewed as the standard most closely aligned with the genetic variance (see McGuffin & O'Donovan, Chapter 5, this volume). In fact, to use formal clinical nosology alone may dilute or obscure the predictive value of the SRV phenotype. For example, to predict RTX among relatives of schizophrenics, it may be necessary to exclude as genetically irrelevant those cases of DSM-III-R–diagnosed schizophrenia who are not of process type and who do not show some minimal level of RTX. Such a selective process was performed by De Amicis and Cromwell (1979), although no attempt was made to test the superiority of the selective procedure. Actually, only successive studies with varied proband group definitions would eventually yield the definition most closely associated with the genetic variance. Since the DSM-III-R classification series was not built with genetic criteria in

mind, it is unlikely that it alone will depict the most genetically relevant grouping.

The next preliminary issue in addressing the aforestated question concerns the cutoff point for the SRV. In other words, how deviant must the SRV be (as a continuous variable) in order for it to be called deviant? One alternative answer is to use the point of maximal discrimination (i.e., the point at which percentile values between genetically positive and negative groups is maximally disparate). In the case of RTX with process schizophrenics, this point of maximal discrimination between schizophrenic and control groups was found to be at +25 ms RTX (De Amicis & Cromwell, 1979). Independently examined, the point of maximal discrimination between the first-degree relatives of this proband schizophrenia group and the control group was also found to be +25 ms RTX. Thus, this cutoff point appears uniformly useful.

When this cutoff point is used, a total of 47% of the schizophrenic proband group, so defined, was at or above this value. (If a more lenient cutoff score is used [e.g., 0.00 ms], the base rate for RTX in schizophrenia is increased, but the base rate for RTX in the general population is also increased.)

The reasons for asking this first question are several. Obviously, if any given SRV accounted for all the genetic variance in schizophrenia, its base rate should approach 100%. Thus, one should ask: Why not 100%? Is it not 100% because of the unreliability of the SRV measure? Is it because of the unreliability in the diagnostic criteria to define the proband group? Is it because the SRV is relevant to only a subset of the schizophrenic group? Is it because the clinical symptoms and other variables associated with the psychosis (e.g., generalized deficit) blur or mask out the SRV in many proband cases? If the SRV is a deficit measure (which may not always be the case), the generalized deficit hypothesis is always a possibility. One must keep in mind that the variance associated with the genetic contribution is at question, not the variance secondary to clinical symptoms or generalized deficit.

Question 2: What is the base rate of the SRV among healthy first-degree relatives of schizophrenics?

Using the cutoff point and data described above, the base rate for the first-degree relatives of the schizophrenic proband group was found to be 17%. In other words, 17% of the first-degree relatives are above the critical value of +25 ms RTX.

This question is important because it should approximate roughly what percentage of these relatives have the alleged genetic factor. Also, it should reveal the SRV under conditions independent of the generalized deficit. Finally, the characteristics of SRV-positive and SRV-negative relatives might provide clues about what additional environmental or genetic factors must occur in combination with the SRV in question in order to precipitate the overt schizophrenia. Or, contrarily, clues may be offered as to what must occur to protect against the overt psychosis.

One should also ascertain whether this base rate applies to first-degree relatives in general or whether it is age dependent (i.e., more true for parents than for offspring, more true for older than for younger siblings). Finally, the dropoff in base rate from first-degree to second-degree and other relatives is mathematically different in poly-, oligo-, and monogenic models. Thus, this base rate figure may eventually provide clues about the model of genetic transmission.

Question 3: What is the base rate of the SRV for the general population (randomly sampled control subjects)?

When control subjects from several Waterloo studies of RTX were combined ($N = 126$), the base rate for RTX was found to be 8% R. A. Steffy, personal communication). Of interest, these data also had a +25-ms point of maximal discrimination between the combined schizophrenia and combined control groups. Steffy's value is within 1% of the value found in a smaller data set from our laboratory. Of interest, it also compares

with estimates of base rate of eye tracking deficit in the general population (Holzman, 8%; Iacono, 5%; from Iacono, 1991).

The significance of this question concerns the degree to which the particular SRV in question is present in the general population. Although measurement error can distort the estimate, it would appear that the base rate for these SRVs is, as expected, greater than that for clinically defined schizophrenia. One possible explanation for this would be an oligogenic multiplicative (interactive) model in which a small number of genetic and/or environmental factors are required in combination in order to produce the 1% base rate in manifest schizophrenia.

Question 4: What is the base rate of the SRV in a screened control group?

A "screened control group" refers to control subjects who have been psychodiagnostically interviewed and who reveal a history of neither (a) personal psychiatric disturbance nor (b) psychiatric disturbance among their known blood relatives. In the case of RTX, the base rate for a sample of 48 screened control subjects was 0% (De Amicis & Cromwell, 1979).

The significance of this question is that, with large sample size, the base rate of an SRV for screened controls should be lower than that for the population in general. In constituting our screened control group, 5 among 53 subjects were rejected for personal psychiatric history or because they were on neuroleptic medication. Ordinarily in other studies, about 1 in 20 subjects tend to be rejected for having a blood relative with one or more psychiatric hospitalizations. Again, this rate of rejection, in the long run, should relate roughly to the base rate of a given SRV in the general population.

Question 5: Is the magnitude of the SRV in schizophrenic patients correlated with the mean magnitude among their first-degree relatives?

In the case of RTX, this correlation is, as expected, both significant and low in magnitude (r = .27; De Amicis, Huntzinger, & Cromwell, 1981). The relevance of this correlation concerns familiality in intensity of expression. Does intense expression of the SRV in the patient relate to intense expression of it in the relative? One would not expect a high degree of correlation unless the SRV is fully distributed among all the relatives. If only a few relatives are expected to carry the genetic contribution (i.e., if the base rate is low), one would expect relatives not carrying the SRV to detract from the magnitude of the correlation.

Question 6: Does the magnitude of the SRV in the schizophrenic correlate with the number of his or her relatives known to have been psychiatrically hospitalized?

This correlation between the patient's magnitude of RTX and the number of his or her first-degree relatives hospitalized (r = .20) was significant. Also, the correlation between patient RTX and the number of more remote relatives hospitalized (r = .21) was significant.

The answer to this question is important primarily because it provides a rough assurance that the SRV of interest has at least some tie to clinical symptoms. (Remember, if the SRV is examined as a phenotype, a risk exists of erroneously pursuing a phenotype that is valid genetically but has nothing to do with schizophrenia!) However, the variable, "known relatives with psychiatric hospitalization," is notoriously vulnerable to criticism. Both patients and relatives will vary in the number of known relatives, in their knowledge of their relatives' psychiatric hospitalizations, in their willingness to divulge this information, in their memory, and in actual family size. Certainly, almost no relative or patient can be relied on to report accurately the psychiatric diagnosis. Yet, with these built-in shortcomings, one can cross-check, as was done here, by computing the correlation separately for immediate (first-degree) and extended family members.

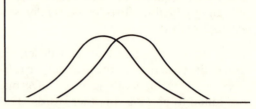

Figure 4.2. A uniformly distributed effect.

Question 7: What is the distribution of the SRV among the first-degree relatives?

Often behavioral scientists think only in terms of effects that are uniformly distributed (see Figure 4.2). When an effect is uniformly distributed, all members of the affected population are equally influenced in the way they differ from the control population. Only the means of the two populations are displaced from each other.

Consider, in contrast, the possibility of an SRV in which only a minority of relatives are affected. In other words, some relatives have inherited the trait and some have not (as might be more likely the cases of monogenic or oligogenic transmission). In such instances, those relatives *without* the SRV deviance would be no different from the control distribution. Those *with* the SRV would aggregate at one end of the distribution. Such a distribution is illustrated in Figure 4.3.

To answer Question 7 with respect to RTX as an SRV candidate, the data are presented in graphic form in Figure 4.4. In the upper graph is the frequency distribution of screened control subjects and first-degree relatives for magnitude of RTX. As may be seen, the curves are astonishingly identical except for the shank (or bulge) that occurs

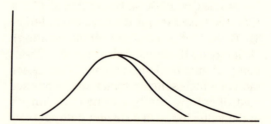

Figure 4.3. A selectively distributed effect.

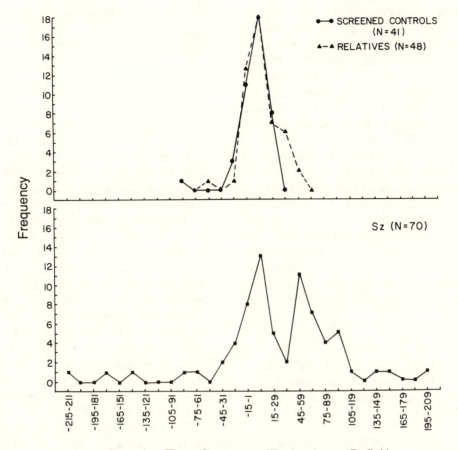

Figure 4.4. Frequency of cases (first-degree relatives and screened controls in upper graph; process schizophrenics in the lower graph) as a function of magnitude of RTX.

on the right side. This bulge essentially contains the 17% subset of first-degree relatives who have the critically high RTX scores. As may be seen, they solely account for the significance of difference between the relatives and screened controls. Because their scores are far from the mean, fewer cases are necessary to yield a significant difference.

The lower graph portrays the RTX distribution of schizophrenics. As Shakow so often noted, the variability of schizophrenics is much greater. These data, perhaps, help attest to the importance of pursuing SRV research among relatives rather than among actively disturbed patients. In the case of RTX, not only is the variance smaller among both relatives and controls, but the variability of the schizophrenics extends below as well as above the normal distribution. In other words, with sufficient sample size, an RTX value for schizophrenia could be identified that is critically low, as well as the +25-ms value, which is critically high. More study is clearly needed to establish commingling and distributional differences for SRVs, including RTX. This visual illustration, however, suggests the importance of asking whether an SRV deviance is diffusely (uniformly) or selectively distributed among relatives. If selectively distributed, the possibility may be strengthened that the variable may segregate across generations as a genetic trait. At least, it would be compatible with a mono- or oligogenic model of transmission. If uniformly distributed, the data would be compatible with a polygenic model of transmission.

Another implication of commingling within the relatives group concerns familial vulnerability and genetic counseling. Currently, first-degree relatives of a schizophrenic proband are viewed as having a 12% to 15% vulnerability for the disorder. If this percentage value is the result of two (or more) commingled distributions, one of which is no different from the control distribution, the possibility exists that a large subset of first-degree relatives of schizophrenics have essentially no vulnerability to the disorder. By contrast, the members of the other distribution may have a much greater than 12% to 15% vulnerability. Such a subgroup could potentially be targeted for prophylactic treatment and special study. Only when the two distributions are commingled would the 12% to 15% value be found.

Question 8: How does the SRV relate to general or socioeconomic functioning among the healthy (nonsymptomatic) relatives?

Behavioral scientists, geneticists, and even family members of schizophrenics may erroneously draw the conclusion that SRVs are always deficits (i.e., factors that impair or lower the level of functioning). In other words, the relative who possesses the genetic contribution to schizophrenia is assumed to be somewhat lowered in functioning or else vulnerable to lowered functioning. In light of findings such as those of McNeil (1971) and Heston (1966) on creative and high-level occupations, respectively, this "flawed gene" notion, as a universal assumption, may be inaccurate. Thus, it is important to examine the level of functioning of the healthy (nonsymptomatic) relatives to see if the presence of the deviant SRV is associated with the general level of functioning.

In our data (De Amicis, Wagstaff, & Cromwell, 1986) the magnitude of RTX was examined in relation to socioeconomic status (SES; years of education and level of occupation). The results are shown in Table

Table 4.2. Correlations between RTX and SES

Group	r
Relatives	.35
Controls	$-.57$
Schizophrenics	NS

4.2. As might be expected, no relationship emerged among schizophrenics. Depending on the age of the schizophrenic and whether he or she was living at home, SES may be pegged to the parents' level or to the "drifted" level the patient has achieved as an independent adult. With such discrepancies, SES is not a highly reliable metric with patients, and any interpretation of relationship among the schizophrenics would be ambiguous. Of greater importance, therefore, are the correlations among screened controls and among relatives. As may be seen, RTX was associated with lowered SES among the controls ($p<.05$). However, it was associated significantly in the opposite direction among relatives ($p<.05$). Relatives with greater RTX tended to have higher, not lower, SES.

No single interpretation can be made of this reversal in RTX–SES relationship from healthy controls to healthy relatives. However, it might usefully be discussed within the context of three models of gene–environment effects offered by Kendler and Eaves (1986).

The first model, already mentioned, is the "flawed gene" notion. This model indeed implies that, if the relevant gene is expressed, the phenotypic evidence will be revealed by impaired functioning. This would suggest a consistent negative relationship between RTX and SES.

The second model concerns *environmental selection*. For example, a genetic factor determining preference for particular environments, such as for the taste of tobacco or for sensation seeking, may place the individual more often in certain environments. From there, environmental variance may account for 100% of the trait. Yet, this trait, although environmentally controlled, will run in the family. This model could apply to genetic attraction to environmental toxins as well as genetic attraction to psychologically disadvantageous environments. The model does not appear to have relevance to the RTX–SES relationship.

The third model concerns genetic differences in "environmental sensitivity." For example, a genetic factor may determine a general supersensitivity to the environment. Then, a second factor interacts with it to determine the direction of functioning. In Kendler and Eaves' (1986) example this second factor is an environmental one. If the environment is favorable, the individual endowed with the extra sensitivity will be above the norm in functioning. If the environment is unfavorable, the endowed individual may deteriorate into a schizophrenic psychosis. Thus, a singular genetic contribution of supersensitivity could potentially be the substrate for either schizophrenia or superior functioning, depending on the second factor. If one views the second factor as a continuous variable (e.g., favorable versus unfavorable environment), the first factor merely determines steepness of slope when level of functioning is plotted as a function of the second factor. This third model would be compatible with the observed reversal of relationship between RTX and SES when relatives are compared with controls.

An important additional comment is necessary about this third model of Kendler and Eaves (1986). The second factor involved need not be environmental. It may be a second *genetic* factor that determines the direction of life functioning when, and only when, the first factor is in place. If such is the case, an oligogenic model of transmission would fit the data. However, if the second factor is purely environmental, a monogenic model would be compatible. In any case these findings about superior or creative relatives of schizophrenics (De Amicis et al., 1986; Heston, 1966; McNeil, 1971) require a multifactorial (at least two-factor) explanation.

The significance of this eighth question is to emphasize that neither SRVs nor genes associated with them need necessarily reflect deficits. A deficit may occur in some family members, but superior functioning may occur in others. Within the oligogenic or monogenic model still other relatives would not inherit the relevant gene and there would be no effect at all. (Note that, although controls had a negative correlation between RTX and SES, no control subject scored in the deviant RTX range.) Because this model appears to fit the RTX data, it would be an important candidate to be examined in other SRV investigations.

The second implication is that RTX cannot be viewed as a singular antecedent of schizophrenia. If it relates to superior functioning among healthy adult relatives who have it, at least one other factor must be present to determine the direction of some toward schizophrenia. This may indeed be a second (or more) genetic factor(s). If so, a monogenic model would not fit the data.

Question 9: Are various SRVs intercorrelated?

One possible interpretation when two SRVs are highly correlated is that they share a single underlying genotype. Alternative interpretations of correlation between SRVs are also possible. Two genetic factors may be closely linked on the same chromosome, so that they co-occur across generations or even within the general population. Also, some nongenetic factor(s) may account for the shared variance between the two SRV measures. In contrast, if no significant correlation exists between two (or more) SRVs, the possibility exists that more than one independent genetic contribution to schizophrenia may be expressed by the respective SRVs.

Because the origins of schizophrenia are not yet clear, the presence and interpretation of intercorrelation among SRVs is of major importance. Unfortunately, most psychopathology laboratories focus only on one or a very few SRVs. Therefore, findings have been sparse in this much-needed area of research.

As has already been implied, it is hazardous to interpret significant interrelations among SRVs in active schizophrenics as being attributable to shared genetic variance. Generalized deficit (which often advances with the course of illness) and other nongenetic extraneous variables may account for correlations among SRVs. SRV intercorrelations among the healthy relatives of schizophrenics more likely reflect genetic variance, because at least some of these irrelevant factors can be ruled out.

Spohn (Chapter 16, this volume) and Spohn and Coyne (1989) have emphasized that method variance and other extraneous variance are so great that multivariate analysis may be necessary to identify latent structure. Some of these latent variables may be hypothesized to be even more closely associated with the genetic variance than the individual SRVs. Other latent variables may be primarily of nongenetic origin. Accordingly, this latent structure analysis may often identify dysfunctional traits. Of these, some may be pathogenic traits, whether genetic or nongenetic. Even here, however, Spohn and Coyne caution that the latent factors (components) identified may be neither patho- nor -genic. Such assertions must await the empirical examination of their predictive utility.

As an illustration of their latent variable approach, Spohn and Coyne (1989) have found that both (a) skin conductance orienting response (SCOR) and (b) RTX are correlated significantly with (c) eye tracking deficit. Yet, the correlation between SCOR and RTX is essentially nil. These data would suggest that eye tracking is not a monolithic variable. Instead, it has two orthogonal components (identified so far). If each component has a genetic substrate, the eye tracking measure cannot be viewed as a single genetic factor.

CONCLUSION

In spite of the fact that the genetic riddle in schizophrenia is fascinating to many researchers, the status of knowledge about schizophrenia genetics is precarious. This precarious state is implied in part by the "no evidence" assumptions stated at the beginning of this chapter.

Perhaps the major unanswered question in schizophrenia genetics is whether the clinical definition, admitted to have environmental influence, represents the most appropriate phenotype for genetic research. If it is indeed the most appropriate, research on the genetics of schizophrenia is on track. However, if other phenotypic indicators, possibly separate from the final clinical syndrome, are indeed more closely associated with the genetic variance, past and present research has been greatly misdirected. This chapter presents a discussion of the phenotypic alternative of schizophrenia-related variants, which can be measured before the clinical syndrome occurs and in healthy biological relatives.

Another remaining unanswered question is whether a monogenic, oligogenic, or polygenic model is the most appropriate fit for the schizophrenia data. The data discussed here suggest that a single-factor explanation is insufficient to explain them. Among the multifactorial models (with genetic and/or environmental factors), the possibility of an oligogenic model (two or a small number of genetic contributors) looms as an attractive hypothesis. The data discussed here offer compatible, but not conclusive, support for such a model.

Even if the oligogenic model proves useful, other crucial questions must be answered. These concern whether the oligogenic model is additive or interactive. That is, do the respective genetic and/or environmental factors simply add until they reach the critical threshold for schizophrenia, or must specific combinations of factors be in place before schizophrenia is precipitated? If the latter is the case, the possibility exists that one (or more) of these factors is highly prevalent in the general population and one (or more) is rare. Only when the factors occur in their requisite combination does the expected 1% of the population precipitate with overt schizophrenia. The data discussed here are compatible with such an interactive model but are insufficient to confirm either it or an alternative model.

Given the current lack of data and theoretical interpretation thereof, the major purpose of this chapter is to argue that the right questions should be asked before genetic linkage and DNA probe methodologies are initiated.

REFERENCES

American Psychiatric Association. (1987). *Diagnostic and statistical manual of mental disorders* (3rd ed., rev.). Washington, DC: American Psychiatric Press, Inc.

Bellissimo, A., & Steffy, R. A. (1972). Redundancy-associated deficit in schizophrenic reaction time performance. *Journal of Abnormal Psychology, 80,* 299–307.

De Amicis, L. A., & Cromwell, R. L. (1979). Reaction time crossover in process schizophrenic patients, their relatives, and control subjects. *Journal of Nervous and Mental Disease, 167,* 593–600.

De Amicis, L. A., Huntzinger, R. S., & Cromwell, R. L. (1981). Magnitude of reaction time crossover in process schizophrenics patients in relation to first-degree relatives. *Journal of Nervous and Mental Disease, 169,* 64–65.

De Amicis, D. A., Wagstaff, D., & Cromwell, R. L. (1986). Reaction time crossover as a marker of schizophrenia and of higher functioning. *Journal of Nervous and Mental Disease, 174,* 177–179.

Heston, L. L. (1966). Psychiatric disorders in foster home reared children of schizophrenic mothers. *British Journal of Psychiatry, 112,* 819–825.

Holzman, P. S., Kringlen, E., & Matthysse, S. (1988). A single dominant gene can account for eye tracking dysfunction and schizophrenia in offspring of discordant twins. *Archives of General Psychiatry, 45,* 641–650.

Iacono, W. G. (1991). Research on eye tracking. Paper presented at the Society for Research in Psychopathology meetings. Cambridge, Massachusetts, December, 1991.

Kendler, K. S., & Eaves, L. J. (1986). Models for the joint effect of genotype and environment on liability to psychiatric illness. *American Journal of Psychiatry, 143,* 279–289.

McNeil, T. F. (1971). Prebirth and postbirth influence on the relationship between creative ability and recorded mental illness. *Journal of Personality, 39,* 391–406.

Rodnick, E. H., & Shakow, D. (1940). Set in the schizophrenic as measured by a composite reaction time index. *American Journal of Psychiatry, 97,* 214–225.

Spohn, H. E., & Coyne, L. (1989). *Pathogenic traits in schizophrenia: A proposal for the conceptualization, identification, and research utilization.* Unpublished manuscript, Menninger Clinic, Topeka, KS.

Spohn, H. E., & Coyne, L. (in press). Attention/information processing impairment, neuroleptics, and tardive dyskinesia in chronic schizophrenics. *Brain and Cognition.*

Spohn, H. E., & Strauss, M. E. (1989). Relation of neuroleptic and anticholinergic medication to cognitive functions in schizophrenia. *Journal of Abnormal Psychology, 98,* 267–380.

5

Modern Diagnostic Criteria and Models of Transmission of Schizophrenia

PETER McGUFFIN
MICHAEL C. O'DONOVAN

SCHIZOPHRENIA: WORKING HYPOTHESIS

Since the mid-1970s the science of genetics has gone through a remarkably sustained phase of revolutionary change brought about by discoveries in the "new genetics" of recombinant DNA technology (Weatherall, 1985). For much of this period, the progress report on the genetics of schizophrenia has been one of "modest gains while playing for time" (Gottesman, McGuffin, & Farmer, 1987). Recently, however, more dramatic claims have been made, with two groups of workers (Collinge et al., 1989; Sherrington et al., 1988) reporting potentially major steps forward, by finding linkage between DNA markers and two putative major gene loci for schizophrenia. Before we can consider these findings, they must be placed in the context of developments of "normal science" (Kuhn, 1962) taking place in the previous decade or so.

It is probably best to begin with the remembrance of Luxenburger's statement, quoted by Jaspers (1962), that, for the purposes of genetic research, "schizophrenia" is no more than a working hypothesis. (Indeed, for some, this may not be a remembrance but rather a complete new discovery in itself.) The fact that the hypothesis has survived the 60 years since Luxenburger put forward this skeptical notion attests to

its usefulness, but the fact that modern interpretations and refinements of the hypothesis are still much at variance with one another warns us to adhere to a similar level of skepticism.

In this chapter we therefore begin by reconsidering the classical methods of psychiatric genetics, family, twin, and adoption studies in the light of modern definitions of schizophrenia, and then consider the problem of determining the mode of transmission. We then explore what modern perspectives on clinical heterogeneity can tell us about etiological heterogeneity before concluding with a review of linkage marker strategies and applications of molecular genetics.

MODERN DIAGNOSTIC CRITERIA

Many different operational definitions of schizophrenia have now been put forward. They vary considerably in their constituent items, their combinatorial rules, and the amount of emphasis placed on cross-sectional descriptions of psychopathology as opposed to longitudinal features such as premorbid features, course, duration, and outcome (Berner, Gabriel, Katsching, Kieffer, Kuhler, Leng, et al., 1983). The feature that nearly all modern definitions have in common is that they purport to be explicit and attempt to provide an operational definition of the disorder in the sense that the term "operational" has been used by Hempel (1961). Such an approach has been seen by many authorities as the remedy for diagnostic confusion in schizophrenia (Kendell, 1975). Operational definitions undoubtedly enhance reliability, but this alone does not ensure validity. Therefore, it must be remembered that competing definitions of schizophrenia are at best alternative conventions or alternative formulations of the working hypothesis. Hence, although one particular definition may have become adopted as the nationally approved set of instructions for diagnosis (American Psychiatric Association, 1980, 1987), this does not, in the absence of any other validating evidence, ensure that it is correct.

At best we can judge which definition of schizophrenia is most useful for a particular purpose. Recognizing this, various authors have attempted outcome studies using a number of competing operational definitions in order to discover which has the best predictive utility (Bland & Orne, 1979; Brockington, Kendall, & Leff, 1978; Stephens, Astrup, Carpenter, Schaffer, & Goldberg, 1982). It may be equally important to ask which definition best predicts response to treatment (Crow, 1980; Murray & Murphy, 1978) or which best delineates a disorder with a high degree of genetic determination (Gottesman & Shields, 1972; Robins & Guze, 1970).

Here we are chiefly concerned with the use of genetic heritability as a potential means of validating definitions of schizophrenia. Table 5.1 shows a summary of the results of many studies carried out before the modern era of operational definitions showing the morbid risk of schizophrenia in various classes of relatives of schizophrenic probands (Gottesman & Shields, 1982). Although some of these classical studies might be criticized as lacking the rigor of modern methodology (e.g., Kallmann, 1938), others have been scrupulous in their systematic ascertainment of probands, their detailed description of case material, and their use of consensus ratings of blinded assessors (Gottesman & Shields, 1972). It is therefore surprising, in the face of such evidence, that some workers have questioned whether any results obtained before the recent introduction of operational criteria are reliable.

Table 5.1. Expectancy of Schizophrenia in the Relatives of Schizophrenics

Relationships	Percentage schizophrenic
Monozygotic twins	46
Dizygotic twins	14
Parent	6
Sibling (when one parent also affected)	10
Children	17
Children (both parents affected)	13
Uncles/aunts/nephews/nieces	46
Grandchildren	4
Unrelated	1

Source: Data compiled by Gottesman and Shields (1982).

Thus, instead of asking the vital question of whether enhancement of reliability is accompanied by validity, some workers (Abrams & Taylor, 1983; Pope, Jonas, Cohen, & Lipinski, 1983) have turned the question on its head and asked whether schizophrenia is really a familial condition once it has been defined using a new diagnostic convention. Pope et al. reported that none of 199 first-degree relatives of schizophrenics had an illness fulfilling the *Diagnostic and Statistical Manual of Mental Disorders,* third edition (DSM-III; American Psychiatric Association, 1980) criteria for schizophrenia, whereas Abrams and Taylor (1983) applied their own criteria to a sample of 128 first-degree relatives of schizophrenics and claimed that only 2 were affected, giving a lifetime prevalence of 1.6%. Neither group of workers had a control sample or independent estimate of population frequency with the new definition of schizophrenia, but it is now known that the risk of the restrictively redefined DSM-III form of schizophrenia can be as low as 0.2% in studies of subjects who are not relatives of schizophrenics (Kendler, Gruenberg, & Tsuang, 1985). Therefore the sample size required to confidently reject the hypothesis that schizophrenia is familial would need to be substantially higher than either of the two negative studies, and it seems likely that a combination of methods of low sensitivity (case record assessment rather than interviews), small sample size, and narrow criteria combined to produce negative results.

This conclusion is supported by the results of other investigations in which more satisfactory methods have been used with larger sample sizes. Thus studies using modified St. Louis criteria (Feighner et al., 1972) or DSM-III definitions have shown convincingly that schizophrenia does not cease to be familial once a modern, explicit definition is applied (Baron, Gruen, Kane, & Asnis, 1985; Guze, Cloninger, Martin, & Clayton, 1983; Kendler et al., 1985).

It cannot be overstressed that familial transmission does not necessarily mean genetic transmission. For many, the most compelling evidence that schizophrenia has an important genetic contribution comes from the natural experiment of adoption studies. Although there is a large study currently in progress in Finland, only preliminary results have so far been published (Tienari, Sorri, Lahte, Naarla, Wahlberg, Moring, et al., 1987), and this is the only study in which the use of operational criteria has been part of the original design. All the best known adoption work predated the use of operational research definitions. Fortunately an updating of the Copenhagen sample of the Danish adoption material collected by Kety, Rosenthal, Wender, Schulsinger, and Jacobsen (1976) provided adequate clinical details for Kendler and Gruenberg (1984) to carry out a reassessment applying DSM-III definitions. Inevitably these proved to be more restrictive than the criteria adopted by the original researchers, so that only 19 out of 34 original index adoptees returned a diagnosis within the schizophrenia "spectrum." This was redefined to include DSM-III–diagnosed schizophrenia and schizotypal personality disorder. A further five of the original index adoptees were diagnosed as having schizophreniform disorder. This tightening of criteria had the result of increasing the apparent magnitude of the genetic effect, because 22% of 69 biological relatives of index adoptees now received a diagnosis of schiz-

ophrenia spectrum disorder compared with 2% of 137 control adoptees. This use of blinded reassessment applying a narrowed definition actually resulted in a more striking difference than that reported earlier in the absence of explicit criteria (Kety et al., 1976).

Twins and the Heritability of Modern Definitions

Recent reports based on twin data also suggest that the DSM-III and some of its predecessors perform well when judged by their ability to define a highly heritable syndrome (Farmer, Jackson, McGuffin, & Storey, 1987; McGuffin, Farmer, Gottesman, Murray, & Reveley, 1984). Unfortunately, there are again no purpose-built data sets, no large twin studies that have specifically set out to apply DSM-III or other modern definitions of schizophrenia. However, one of the larger series from the preoperational era (Gottesman & Shields, 1972) has been sufficiently detailed and robust to allow a recycling exercise. Researchers therefore applied a variety of operational diagnostic criteria to the detailed case abstracts on a series consisting of 22 monozygotic (MZ) twin pairs (26 probands) and 32 dizygotic (DZ) pairs (34 probands). The assessment was carried out blindly so that abstracts were identified only by a code number and the zygosity and identity of the co-twin were unknown. In a data analysis the multifactorial/threshold model was assumed (Reich, James, & Morris, 1972; Smith, 1974) and heritability, the proportion of phenotypic variance contributed by added gene effects, was calculated. Some of the more noteworthy results are summarized in Table 5.2.

Thus the DSM-III and its predecessors, the criteria of Feighner et al. (1972) and Spitzer, Endicott, and Robins (1978), defined highly heritable syndromes. Somewhat surprisingly, a definition based on Schneider's (1959) first-rank symptoms gave a heritability estimate of zero. It is also worth noting that all of the definitions provided in the table gave highly satisfactory interrater reliability, and, using Schneider's

Table 5.2. Twin Concordance and Heritabilities of Operational Criteria for Schizophrenia

	MZ twins			DZ twins			
Criteria	No. of probands	Concordance[a] (%)	r[b]	No. of probands	Concordance (%)	r	h^2 ($\pm$ S.E.)[c]
Spitzer et al. (1978)							
Broad	22	45.5	0.86	23	8.7	0.45	0.83 $\pm$ 0.4
Narrow	19	52.6	0.90	21	9.5	0.48	0.83 $\pm$ 0.4
Feighner et al. (1972)							
Probable	21	47.6	0.88	22	9.1	0.46	0.84 $\pm$ 0.4
Definite	19	47.4	0.88	18	11.1	0.52	0.72 $\pm$ 0.
DSM-III (APA, 1980)	21	47.6	0.87	21	9.5	0.44	0.85 $\pm$ 0.4
Schneider (1959)	9	22.2	0.74	4	50.0	0.91	0 $\pm$ 0.59

[a] Concordance is expressed proband-wise.
[b] r = correlation in liability.
[c] h^2 = approximate broad heritability.
Source: Farmer et al. (1987) and McGuffin et al. (1984).

definition, two raters achieved perfect agreement. The fact that, in this instance, Schneider's definition appears to be of low utility and validity is a pointed reminder that we cannot put our faith in reliability alone.

It must also be pointed out that the results summarized in Table 5.2 derive from studies with a number of shortcomings. The original case abstracts were not specifically designed for this type of use, and, because they were not originally prepared by "Schneider-oriented" researchers, Schneider's definition may have been most adversely affected. The reassessment was carried out by blinded investigators rating conservatively to achieve the goal of high agreement, but possibly they did so at the expense of sensitivity. The resultant sample sizes were small, with consequent high standard errors for the heritability estimates. Furthermore, because the estimates of heritability are effectively the results of repeated measures on the same subjects, there is no simple way of testing whether they differ significantly.

Despite these caveats, it is reasonable to conclude that current North American criteria all provide satisfactory definitions of the schizophrenic phenotype, whereas Schneider's first-rank symptoms, from the point of view of genetic studies, may be less useful. Furthermore, although outcome validity and etiological validity need not necessarily be equated (Kendell, 1982), it is of interest that the definitions that prove most useful in this genetic study are also those that appear to be most useful in studies that have sought to predict outcome (Brockington et al., 1978; Helzer, Brockington, & Kendell, 1981; Stephens et al., 1982). These results are encouraging, but it would be a mistake to assume that the work of defining the phenotype at the clinical level is complete. This appears to be also the view of the authors of the DSM-III, who have continued to revise their definitions of psychiatric disorders in the light of new knowledge (American Psychiatric Association, 1987). Investigation of concordance in twins can be unshackled from the prescribed DSM-III categories and used in an exploratory way to attempt to discover if repositioning the boundaries of phenotype alters the results.

In scrutinizing the validity of the DSM-III definition of schizophrenia, Farmer et al. (1987) followed the precedent of Gottesman and Shields (1972), who first demonstrated that an overstrict or an overgenerous definition of schizophrenia lowered the MZ/DZ concordance ratio and that the "most genetic" definition occurred in the middle range of diagnostic stringency. Therefore, Farmer et al. broadened the definition of schizophrenia to include not only schizotypal personality disorder and atypical psychosis but also affective disorder with mood-incongruent delusions. In doing so, they produced a proband-wise MZ concordance of 59%, a DZ concordance of 7.7%, and a MZ/DZ ratio of 7.7. This compares favorably with the DSM-III definition of schizophrenia alone, which gives an MZ concordance of 47.6%, a DZ concordance of 9.5%, and a MZ/DZ ratio of 5. By contrast, broadening the definition further resulted in a drop in the MZ/DZ concordance ratio. For example, broadening to include any Axis I DSM-III diagnosis in the co-twin reduced proband-wise concordances of 70.4% in MZ twins and 29.4% in DZ twins, giving a concordance ratio of 2.4.

It is once again important to bear in mind the limitations of this approach, and to point out that the MZ/DZ concordance ratio is but a crude index. Nevertheless, there is some suggestion that, from the genetic viewpoint, the DSM-III definition of schizophrenia could be somewhat improved by being broadened slightly.

MODELS OF TRANSMISSION

Throughout the preceding section we have made the implicit assumption that the transmission of schizophrenia can be formulated in terms of a liability/threshold model in which a variable termed ''liability to develop the disorder'' is continuously distributed in the population but only those individuals whose liability at some stage exceeds a certain threshold manifest the disorder. We have also assumed that liability is multifactorial and receives contributions from genes and the environment. However, it is now important to consider these assumptions more closely and critically. It is clear that in studying schizophrenia we are not dealing with a disorder that has a simple mendelian mode of transmission. As with other common familial diseases, the concepts of liability and threshold provide the most useful framework for understanding the mode of transmission. This is quite widely accepted, and the only real controversy concerns the main sources of contribution to liability. Nevertheless, this controversy is a major one, and one that has major implications for current molecular genetic research strategies.

The simplest hypothesis is that the only source of resemblance between relatives regarding liability to schizophrenia is a major gene. The generalized single major locus model is shown schematically in Figure 5.1. Here a single locus with two alleles (A_1 and A_2) is postulated. There are therefore three genotypes—A_1A_1, A_1A_2, and A_2A_2—with differing means on the liability scales. The model allows that, within each genotype, there will be variations in liability that depend on nonfamilial environmental factors. In the figure, for the purposes of illustration, a substantial proportion of those with the genotype A_2A_2 and a small proportion of those with the genotype A_1A_2 lie beyond the threshold and are less effective. However, the model is perfectly general, so that the three genotypes have penetrances of f_1, f_2, and f_3, respectively, where penetrance is the probability of manifesting the trait given the genotype. For example, therefore, in a classical dominant condition where there were no sporadic cases, penetrance $f_1 = 0$ and $f_2 = f_3 = 1$. For classical mendelian

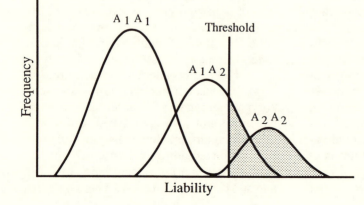

Figure 5.1. The general two-allele single major locus model. Only individuals beyond the threshold (*shaded area*) exhibit the trait.

autosomal recessive disorders, $f_1 = f_2 = 0$ and $f_3 = 1$. However, for disorders such as schizophrenia, which do not conform to mendelian segregation ratios, it is necessary to propose general single major locus (SML) solutions wherein penetrances differ from the necessary mendelian values of 0 and 1. Based on published family data, solutions have been proposed in which all A_2A_2 homozygotes are affected ($f_3 = 1$), there are no sporadics ($f_1 = 0$), and there is a low penetrance (f_2) of under 20% of heterozygotes (Elston & Campbell, 1970; Slater & Cowie, 1971). Unfortunately, published data are almost always given in the form of incidence data (i.e., morbid risks of schizophrenia in various classes of relatives of schizophrenics) (e.g., Table 5.1).

It can be shown that, having estimated the population frequency of a trait (K_p), observations on pairs of relatives can provide estimates of two further parameters, the variance due to additive gene effects (V_A) and the variance due to dominance (V_D). Expressions can be derived relating K_P, V_A, and V_D to the four parameters of the general SML model, the gene frequency q, and the penetrances f_1, f_2, and f_3. Unfortunately, we then have three known values and four unknowns, so that it is impossible to arrive at a unique solution. James (1971) pointed out that there is no single correct answer when SML models are thus applied, so that statistical goodness-of-fit tests may be misleading. A way of dealing with this difficulty was proposed by Suarez, Reich, and Trost (1976), who showed that, if SML model parameters were all constrained within biologically meaningful limits (i.e., between 0 and 1), the area of fit of the model could be graphically delineated so that it may be possible to exclude SML inheritance. An application of this method to all available published data demonstrated that the findings were *mathematically* incompatible with SML inheritance (O'Rourke, Gottesman, Suarez, Rice, & Reich, 1982). Subsequently, McGue, Gottesman, and Rao (1985) attempted to fit an SML model to a similar combined data set and showed that the data were *statistically* incompatible with pure single gene inheritance.

A polygenic liability threshold model was first put forward by Gottesman and Shields (1967) based on the approach of Falconer (1965). Here it was assumed that liability was contributed by many genes each of comparatively small effect at multiple loci, combining together in a predominantly additive fashion. Gottesman and Shields pointed out that a polygenic model, in the straightforward way in which they apply it, had certain drawbacks. For example, some published data sets resulted in calculations of heritability that were too high (i.e., over 100%). Nevertheless, a polygenic model has appeal for a number of reasons. If clinical severity can be equated with severity on a liability scale, the polygenic model might explain why concordance in twins or first-degree relatives increases with severity of illness in the proband. Similarly, it would explain why the risk of schizophrenia increases with the number of affected relatives. Furthermore, persistence of schizophrenia in the population, despite the selective disadvantage of the disorder (i.e., the probability of producing children is reduced by as much as one half) is more easily explicable in terms of polygenic than of SML transmission.

McGue et al. (1985) have shown that a simple polygenic model can adequately explain published data, but it could be argued that a more complex model is more realistic. Thus we might consider multifactorial models in which familial liability is contributed by cultural transmission as well as polygenes, and in which other factors such as positive correlation and liability between spouses (assortative mating) and shared environmental factors specific to twins can be incorporated. Using data points from pooled West European family and twin studies, McGue et al. estimated that genetic heritability of schizophrenia was substantial at 63%, with cultural transmission accounting for a further 29% of the variance. However, on fitting reduced models, only two factors appeared to be significant, polygenic transmission and special environmental effects due to twinning. Interestingly, McGue et al. applied a similar analysis to twin and family data on tuberculosis as a precaution against misleading results of the modeling procedure itself. Here it was found that the overwhelming component was cultural transmission. It accounted for 62% of the variance in liability, whereas genetic heritability was only 6%.

So far we can conclude that pure SML inheritance of schizophrenia is unlikely. That is, we are effectively excluding a major locus that is the sole source of resemblance between relatives regarding liability to schizophrenia. However, in concluding in favor of multifactorial inheritance, we must allow that either a polygenic multifactorial model or a major gene operating against a multifactorial background could probably explain the findings equally well. The "mixed" model of a major gene effect on a multifactorial background is shown in Figure 5.2 (Morton, 1982). The parameters of this model are the multifactorial heritability, H, (i.e., the proportion of the variance in liability due to polygenic and family environmental factors); q, the gene frequency of A_2; t, the difference in standard deviations between the mean liabilities of homozygotes A_1A_1 and A_2A_2; and dt, the difference in mean liability between A_1A_1 and A_1A_2.

Rather than analyzing incidence data on pairs of relatives, complex segregation analysis is carried out in which information from entire pedigrees is utilized. The procedure is to test a full mixed model against reduced models that form its subsets. A computer program (Lalouel, Rao, Morton, & Elston, 1983) uses an iterative optimization routine to arrive at the best fit for each model, in which the likelihood that the hypothesis is correct, given the observed data, is maximized. Hypotheses can be paired directly using a likelihood ratio test, which depends on the fact that twice the difference in log likelihoods approximates asymptotically to a chi-square distribution.

Complex segregation analysis using the mixed model has proved useful in resolving the mode of inheritance of several complex traits but has so far given disappointing, inconclusive results in schizophrenia. One problem is that, despite its sophistication, the method lacks power to distinguish between models when dealing with dichotomous traits (i.e., affected/unaffected) in nuclear families (Carter & Chung, 1980; Risch & Baron, 1984). Data on the extended pedigrees may help provide a more satisfactory resolution on major gene effects, but so also could measures that are strongly correlated with liability. For example, if some reliable

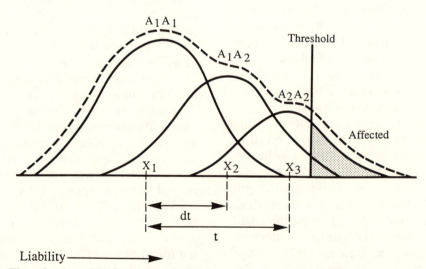

Figure 5.2. The mixed model of a major two-allele gene effect on a multifactorial background. Only individuals beyond the threshold (*shaded area*) exhibit the trait. X_1, X_2, X_3 are the main liabilities of the 3 major genotypes.

and continuous measure of schizotypia could be devised, this might lend itself to a mixed-model analysis of segregation within pedigrees. Unfortunately, devising a scale that successfully captures the essence of schizotypal traits and reliably differentiates between the nonschizophrenic relatives of the patients and control populations has proven remarkably difficult (Gottesman, 1987).

HETEROGENEITY

Few would argue with the idea that schizophrenia is clinically heterogeneous, but is it correct to consider that this is a reflection of underlying heterogeneity? In considering models of transmission of schizophrenia, most workers, recognizing that they are already faced with a difficult problem, have begun with the simplifying assumption that schizophrenia is a single condition. However, more than 40 years ago Slater (1947) pointed out that there is a statistically significant tendency for clinical subtypes to breed true in parent–offspring pairs where both are schizophrenic. More recently, researchers have produced evidence that subtypes such as hebephrenic and paranoid schizophrenia show a tendency toward homotypia in the first-degree relatives (Scharfetter & Nusperli, 1980; Tsuang, Fowler, Cadoret, & Monnelly, 1974).

One problem with diagnostic subtypes is that they have proven unstable and difficult to define. Adopting operational definitions can again help overcome this. Tsuang and Winokur (1974) have produced operational definitions of hebephrenic and paranoid subtypes that can be applied with high reliability (McGuffin, Farmer, & Gottesman, 1987). Other subtypes derived by multivariate statistical methods can also be reliably defined and show some resemblance to traditional subcategories, for example, two such subtypes have been called H type (hebephrenic like) and P type (paranoid like) (Farmer, McGuffin, & Gottesman, 1984).

A rather different approach to subtyping has been taken by Crow (1980, 1985), who has proposed that type I schizophrenia is

characterized by prominent positive symptoms and a good response to neuroleptics. The computerized tomographic (CT) brain scan appearance is usually normal and there is an absence of negative symptoms and cognitive impairment. A type II disorder is associated with negative symptoms, poor response to neuroleptics, and a tendency to show enlarged lateral cerebral ventricles on CT scan. It is allowed that these categories may overlap to a considerable extent so that, in practice, mixed forms also will occur.

Table 5.3 summarizes the results obtained when three reliable methods of subtyping (Crow, 1980; Farmer et al., 1984; Tsuang & Winokur, 1974) are applied to MZ twin data. It can be seen that hebephrenic, H type, and type II/mixed schizophrenia all provide higher concordances than paranoid, P type, and type I schizophrenia, respectively. However, it has also been shown that there is poor separation of subtypes in identical twin pairs, so that for all three subtyping systems it is possible to identify some probands with one type of schizophrenia and co-twins with another (McGuffin et al., 1987). These findings lead us to conclude that there might be a quantitative rather than a qualitative difference between subtypes in all three methods of classification. A multiple threshold liability–continuum model offers an explanation (Reich, Cloninger, Wette, & James, 1979; Reich et al., 1972). Thus we could propose that we are merely separating forms of schizophrenia

Table 5.3. Concordance for Schizophrenia in Monozygotic Co-twins According to Subtype of Proband

Subtypes	Concordance (%)
Tsuang and Winokur (1974)	
Paranoid	40
Hebephrenic	62
Crow (1980)	
Type I	53
Type II/mixed	64
Farmer et al. (1984, 1987)	
P type	33
H type	79

Source: McGuffin et al. (1987).

that have a high liability loading from those that have a low liability. High-liability schizophrenics will inevitably show higher concordance in relatives than low-liability cases. The twin data are too scant to allow adequate testing of a two-threshold model, but if we take material from Kallmann's (1938) family study (still one of the largest data sets available and the one used by Slater to demonstrate homotypia), we can propose that so-called nuclear schizophrenia (hebephrenic and catatonic types) lies beyond the more extreme threshold of severity than "peripheral" schizophrenia (simple and paranoid forms). It has been shown that, on applying such a two-threshold hypothesis, an excellent fit is obtained (McGuffin et al., 1987).

The data therefore support the possible existence of "more genetic" and "less genetic" forms of schizophrenia that differ in terms of their relative positions on the continuum of liability. An older, and more clear-cut view, that schizophrenia can be usefully separated into genetic and nongenetic varieties has been reintroduced by Murray, Lewis, and Reveley (1985). These authors suggested that a substantial proportion of schizophrenics who are "family history negative" have an environmental cause of illness that in the majority of cases is undetected but that may be reflected in such findings as a greater frequency of abnormality seen on CT brain scan. Although this proposition has a certain appeal, there is unfortunately little empirical support. Obvious organic brain disease accounts for only a tiny minority of psychotic patients (Johnstone, Crow, Johnstone, & McMillan, 1986), and there is no consistent relationship between CT brain scan findings, such as enlarged lateral cerebral ventricles, and absence of familial predisposition (McGuffin et al., 1987).

Fundamental to the hypothesis of nongenetic schizophrenia has been the well-documented presence of discordant MZ twins. Generally speaking, two alternative hypotheses have been forwarded to explain this phenomenon. First, discordance could arise if the schizophrenia gene(s) show re-

duced penetrance (of nonenvironmental origin) for the affected phenotype. Alternatively, discordant pairs may arise through the influence of relevant environmental factors such as viral infections and obstetric complications that affect only one of the twins. These hypotheses can be explored by studying the offspring of discordant MZ twins. If the first hypothesis is correct, the children of the unaffected twin will have the same increased risk for schizophrenia as those of the affected twin, and this risk will be equal to that in the offspring of schizophrenic parents in general. If the nongenetic phenocopy hypothesis is correct, the children of the nonaffected co-twin should be affected at a rate equal to that of the general population. However, the children of the proband (the affected twin) should either be affected at a rate similar to the offspring of schizophrenics in general (if the etiological factor is familial but nongenetic) or at the general population rate (if the etiological factor is neither familial nor genetic).

Using this methodology, Gottesman and Bertelsen (1989) found the morbid risk for schizophrenia and related disorders in the offspring of schizophrenic MZ twins to be 16.8% compared with 17.4% in the offspring of unaffected co-twins. The risks for the offspring of DZ twins were 17.4% and 2.1%, respectively. These results are precisely as predicted by the hypothesis that explains discordance by nonpenetrance rather than by nongenetic phenocopies. A study published at the same time (Kringlen & Cramer, 1989), although tending to support the second hypothesis, was unable to reject the first hypothesis. In summary, therefore, the limited data available provide encouragement to the genetic investigator by suggesting that nongenetic phenocopies (at least in twin studies) are not common and therefore are unlikely to have a seriously distorting impact on the linkage studies described below.

MOLECULAR BIOLOGY OF SCHIZOPHRENIA

Genetic marker studies can greatly improve the prospect of detecting major gene effects and resolving heterogeneity in schizophrenia. Given that we have no clear answer concerning the mode of transmission or whether one, several, or many genes are involved, a key question is: How large an effect must a gene have in order for it to be detectable using marker strategies? At present, there is no definite answer. However, it is probable that genes that play a comparatively modest role can be detected, and it is possible that several loci affecting a single trait may be identifiable. Studies of other diseases can shed some light on this issue. For example, numerous publications have confirmed the finding that blood group O is associated with an increased liability to duodenal ulcer, but it has been calculated that the ABO type accounts for only about 1% of the variance in liability (Edwards, 1965). More recently, work on human leukocyte antigens (HLA) and multiple sclerosis suggests that an affected sibling method of linkage analysis can detect linkage with genes of only modest effect that account for only about 3% of the variance (Suarez, O'Rourke, & Van Eerdwegh, 1982).

Current attention is focused most closely on family linkage strategies rather than population association studies. In linkage analysis it is considered that schizophrenia or some subforms of schizophrenia have major locus inheritance. The cosegregation of the disorder and genetic markers is studied within pedigrees containing multiple affected individuals. A genetic marker, strictly defined, is a reliably detectable character that has a known simple mode of inheritance and is polymorphic (i.e., there exist two or more alleles with a gene frequency of at least 1%). Prior to the advent of recombinant DNA technology, several types of marker were available, and these are now often referred to as "classical" markers. They include red cell antigens (ABO, rhesus, MN, etc.), HLA, red cell enzymes, serum protein polymorphisms, and chromosomal banding polymorphisms. Regrettably, even with excellent laboratory facilities, it is not usually possible to study more than about 30 different classical marker loci, altogether covering only a fraction of the human genome map. Therefore, it is perhaps not surprising that the yield of positive results from studies of classical markers in schizophrenia has been quite meager (McGuffin & Sturt, 1986). The only well-replicated finding has been a weak association between paranoid schizophrenia and HLA-A9, but, using the method developed by Edwards (1965), it has been calculated that the HLA locus contributes only a little over 1% of the variance to the liability to paranoid schizophrenia.

Fortunately, the techniques of molecular genetics have brought forth a new generation of markers called restriction fragment length polymorphisms (RFLPs). These exist because of individual differences in DNA base sequences and consequent variations in the positions of the sites at which bacterial enzymes called restriction endonucleases will cleave the DNA molecule. Particular RLFPs can be identified using a probe made from radiolabeled complementary DNA in conjunction with an electrophoretic technique called the Southern blot method. This method means that vastly more markers can be available in the search for disease genes, and a virtually complete human genetic linkage map has now been published (Donis-Keller, Green, Helms, Cartinhour, Weiffenbach, Stephens, et al., 1987). Consequently, the search is now on in a number of laboratories for a DNA polymorphism that consistently segregates with the schizophrenic phenotype within families and that can be inferred to occupy a locus in close proximity to a major gene for schizophrenia.

A preliminary clue has come from a report of a family containing an uncle and nephew pair both affected by schizophrenia and both showing a translocation involving chromosome 5. No other individuals in the pedigree were affected, but the mother of the index case was shown to have a balanced "carrier" karyotype (Bassett, Jones, McGillivray, & Pantzar, 1988). Subsequently, Sherrington et al. (1988) studied several moderately large Icelandic and British pedigrees and demonstrated consistent evidence within their sample of linkage between a putative schizophrenia gene and a chromosome 5 marker.

Relevant to our earlier discussion on the boundaries of schizophrenia, the strongest evidence of linkage was found when the phenotype included a very wide spectrum of disorders, including some generally not thought to be schizophrenia spectrum disorders. Unfortunately, however, workers from other centers have been unable to replicate this finding in Swedish (Kennedy, Giuffra, Moises, Pakstis, Kidd, Castiglione, et al., 1988), Scottish (St. Clair, Blackwood, Muir, Baillie, Hubbard, Wright, et al., 1989), North American (Detera-Wadleigh, Goldin, Sherrington, Encio, de Miguel, Barrettini, et al., 1989), and Welsh (McGuffin et al., 1990) pedigrees. McGuffin et al. have also combined all the published data and have convincingly rejected the hypothesis of a schizophrenia locus in this particular region of chromosome 5. However, considering the studies individually, it is still conceivable, if genetic heterogeneity is postulated, that Sherrington et al. (1988) fortuitously sampled pedigrees in both Britain and Sweden that coincidentally shared a mutation in chromosome 5 and all the other investigators by chance did not include such pedigrees. Although possible, the presence of such an alleged schizophrenia gene in both Sweden and Britain but not elsewhere seems highly improbable. The most likely explanation, therefore, is that the finding of linkage to the 5q region of chromosome 5 is due to chance. This contention cannot be proven but awaits rejection by independent replication of the finding.

In contrast to the studies mentioned above, which have focused on the autosomes, one group has proposed that a gene for schizophrenia is located in the pseudoautosomal region of the sex chromosomes (Crow, 1988). Such pseudoautosomal genes are not inherited as classical sex-linked genes because recombination takes place between the X and Y chromosomes. The predicted pattern of inheritance for a disease the gene for which is so located is that the disease, when transmitted from the pa-ternal side, will occur more often than by chance in same-sexed siblings (if the disease allele is on his X chromosome, the affected individuals are most likely to be female; if the allele is on the Y chromosome, they are most likely to be male). If, in contrast, transmission is through the maternal side, pairs of affected sibs are as likely to be mixed as same sexed. Crow, DeLisi, and Johnstone (1989), in an analysis of sib-pair concordance by sex, have offered supportive evidence. However, after their own re-analysis in response to criticism, the case seems less strong (Crow, DeLisi, & Johnstone, 1990). Nevertheless, in further support of the hypothesis, linkage between Research Diagnostic Criteria–diagnosed schizophrenia or schizoaffective disorder and pseudoautosomal polymorphic DNA markers has been found (Collinge et al., 1989), albeit at a level of statistical significance ($p < .01$) that may not be sufficiently rigorous for a study of this type (Ott, 1985). Thus, although it provides an interesting twist to the pursuit of genes for schizophrenia, the pseudoautosomal hypothesis lacks clear-cut support, and attempts to find linkage by other groups have so far proved negative (Asherson et al., 1992).

CONCLUSION

The past 10 years or so have seen the working hypothesis of schizophrenia modestly refined and improved from the perspective of the genetic investigator. The status of the disorder as having an important genetic etiology has been strengthened, although the mode of inheritance and the interplay of environmental factors are no better understood. The new tools generated by the growth of molecular biology, although offering the hope of major gains to come, have yet to provide more than argument and unconfirmed reports of (as yet) doubtful significance. With the promise of extensive collaborative projects in Europe and the United States, this period of "playing for time" may be coming to an end.

REFERENCES

Abrams, R., & Taylor, M. A. (1983). The genetics of schizophrenia: A reassessment using modern criteria. *American Journal of Psychiatry, 140,* 171–175.

American Psychiatric Association. (1980). *Diagnostic and statistical manual of mental disorders* (3rd ed.). Washington, DC: American Psychiatric Press, Inc.

American Psychiatric Association. (1987). *Diagnostic and statistical manual of mental disorders* (3rd ed., rev.). Washington DC: American Psychiatric Press, Inc.

Asherson, P., Parfitt, E., Sargeant, M., Tidmarsh, L. S., Buckland, P., Taylor, C., Clements, A., Gill, M., McGuffin, P. & Owen, M. J. (1992). No evidence for a pseudo-autosomal locus for schizophrenia from linkage analysis of multiply affected families. *British Journal of Psychiatry 161,* 63–68.

Baron, M., Gruen, R., Kane, J., & Asnis, L. (1985). Modern research criteria and the genetics of schizophrenia. *American Journal of Psychiatry, 142,* 297–301.

Bassett, A. S., Jones, B. D., McGillivray, B. C., & Pantzar, J. T. (1988). Partial trisomy chromosome 5 cosegregating with schizophrenia. *Lancet, 1,* 799–801.

Berner, P., Gabriel, E., Katschnig, A., Kieffer, W., Kohler, K., Leng, G., & Simhandel, H. (1983). *Diagnostic criteria for schizophrenia and affective psychoses* (World Psychiatric Association). Washington, DC: American Psychiatric Press, Inc.

Bland, R. C., & Orn, H. (1979). Diagnostic criteria and outcome. *British Journal of Psychiatry, 134,* 34.

Brockington, I. F., Kendell, R. E., & Leff, J. P. (1978). Definitions of schizophrenia: Concordance and prediction of outcome. *Psychological Medicine, 8,* 387–398.

Carter, C. L., & Chung, C. S. (1980). Segregation analysis of schizophrenia under a mixed model. *Human Heredity, 30,* 350–356.

Collinge, J., Boccio, A., DeLisi, L., Johnstone, E., Lofthouse, R., Owen, F., Poulter, M., Risby, D., Shah, T., & Crow, T. J. (1989). Evidence for a psuedoautosomal locus for schizophrenia. *Cytogenetics and Cell Genetics, 51,* 978.

Crow, T. J. (1980). The molecular pathology of schizophrenia: More than one disease process? *British Medical Journal, 280,* 66–68.

Crow, T. J. (1985). The two syndrome concept: Origins and current states. *Schizophrenia Bulletin, 11,* 471–476.

Crow, T. J. (1988). Sex chromosomes and psychosis: The case for a pseudoautosomal locus. *British Journal of Psychiatry, 153,* 675–683.

Crow, T. J., DeLisi, L., & Johnstone, E. C. (1989). Concordance by sex in sibling pairs with schizophrenia is paternally inherited. Evidence for a pseudoautosomal locus. *British Journal of Psychiatry, 155,* 92–97.

Crow, T. J., DeLisi, L. E., & Johnstone, E. C. (1990). In reply. . . . A locus closer to the telomere? *British Journal of Psychiatry, 156,* 416–420.

Detera-Wadleigh, S. D., Goldin, L. R., Sherrington, R., Encio, I., de Miguel, E., Barrettini, W., & Gurling, H. (1989). Exclusion of linkage to 5q11–13 in families with schizophrenia and other psychiatric disorders. *Nature, 339,* 391–393.

Donis-Keller, H., Green, P., Helms, P., Cartinhour, S., Weiffenbach, B., Stephens, K., Keith, T. P., Bowden, D. W., et al. (1987). A genetic linkage map of the human genome. *Cell, 51,* 319–337.

Edwards, J. H. (1965). Association between blood groups and disease. *Annals of Human Genetics, 29,* 77–83.

Elston, R. C., & Campbell, A. A. (1970). Schizophrenia, evidence for a major gene hypothesis. *Behavioural Genetics, 1,* 101–106.

Falconer, D. S. (1965). The inheritance of liability to certain disease, estimated from the incidence among relatives. *Annals of Human Genetics, 29,* 51–76.

Farmer, A. E., Jackson, R., McGuffin, P., & Storey, P. (1987). Cerebral ventricular enlargement in schizophrenia: Consistencies and contradictions. *British Journal of Psychiatry, 150,* 324–330.

Farmer, A. E., McGuffin, P., & Gottesman, I. I. (1984). Searching for the split in schizophrenia: A twin study perspective. *Psychiatry Research, 13,* 109–118.

Farmer, A. E., Jackson, R., McGuffin, P., & Storey, P. (1987). Cerebral ventricular enlargement in schizophrenia: Consistencies and contradictions. *British Journal of Psychiatry, 4,* 541–545.

Feighner, J. P., Robins, E., Guze, S. B., Woodruffe, R. A., Winokur, G., & Munoz, R. (1972). Diagnostic criteria for use in psychiatric research. *Archives of General Psychiatry, 26,* 57–63.

Gottesman, I. I. (1987). The borderlands of psychosis or the fringes of lunacy. *British Medical Bulletin, 43,* 557–569.

Gottesman, I. I., & Bertelsen, A. (1989). Confirming unexpressed for schizophrenia. Risks in the offspring of Fischer's Danish identical and fraternal discordant twins. *Archives of General Psychiatry, 46,* 867–872.

Gottesman, I. I., McGuffin, P., & Farmer, A. E. (1987). Clinical genetics as clues to the 'real' genetics of schizophrenia. (A decade of modest gains while playing for time.) *Schizophrenia Bulletin, 13,* 23–48.

Gottesman, I. I., & Shields, J. (1967). A polygenic theory of schizophrenia. *Proceedings of the National Academy of Sciences (U.S.A.), 58,* 199–205.

Gottesman, I. I., & Shields, J. (1972). *Schizophrenia and genetics: A twin study vantage point.* London: Academic Press.

Gottesman, I. I., & Shields, J. (1982). *Schizophrenia, the epigenetic puzzle.* Cambridge, England: Cambridge University Press.

Guze, S. B., Cloninger, C. R., Martin, R. L., & Clayton, P. J. (1983). A follow-up and family study of schizophrenia. *Archives of General Psychiatry, 40,* 1273–1276.

Helzer, J. E., Brockington, I. F., & Kendell, R. E. (1981). Predictive validity of DSM-III and Feighner definitions of schizophrenia: A comparison with research Diagnostic Criteria and CATEGO. *Archives of General Psychiatry, 38,* 791–797.

Hempel, C. G. (1961). Introduction to problems of taxonomy. In J. Zubin (Ed.), *Field studies in the mental disorders* (pp. 3–22). New York: Grune & Stratton.

James, J. (1971). Frequency in relatives for an all-or-none trait. *Annals of Human Genetics, 35,* 47–49.

Jaspers, K. (1963). *General psychopathology* (M. W. Hamilton & J. Hoenig, Trans.). Manchester, England: Manchester University Press. (Original work published 1913).

Johnstone, E. C., Crow, T. J., Johnstone, A. L., & McMillan, A. F. (1986). The Northwick Park Study of First Episodes of Schizophrenia: Presentation of the illness and problems relating to admission. *British Journal of Psychiatry, 148,* 115–120.

Kallmann, F. J. (1938). *The genetics of schizophrenia.* New York: J. J. Augustus.

Kendell, R. E. (1975). Schizophrenia: The remedy for diagnostic comparison. In T. Silverstone & B. Barraclough (Eds.), *Contemporary psychiatry.* British Journal of Psychiatry Special Publication No. 9 (pp. 11–17). Ashford, Kent, England, Headley Brothers.

Kendell, R. E. (1982). The choice of diagnostic criteria for biological research. *Archives of General Psychiatry, 39,* 1334–1339.

Kendler, K. S., & Gruenberg, A. M. (1984). An independent analysis of the Copenhagen sample of the Danish Adoption Study of schizophrenia, VI. The relationship between psychiatric disorders as defined by DSM-III in relatives and adoptees. *Archives of General Psychiatry, 41,* 555–564.

Kendler, K. S., Gruenberg, A. M., & Tsuang, M. T. (1985). Psychiatric illness in first degree relatives of schizophrenics and surgical control patients. A family study using DSM-III criteria. *Archives of General Psychiatry, 42,* 770–779.

Kennedy, J. L., Giuffra, L. A., Moises, H. W., Pakstis, A. J., Kidd, J. R., Castiglione, C. M., Sjogren, B., Wetterberg, L., & Kidd, K. K. (1988). Evidence against linkage of schizophrenia to markers on chromosome 5 in a northern Swedish pedigree. *Nature, 336,* 167–169.

Kety, S. S., Rosenthal, D., Wender, P. H., Schulsinger, F., & Jacobsen, B. (1976). Mental illness in the biological and adoptive families of individuals who have become schizophrenic. *Behavioural Genetics, 6,* 219–225.

Kringlen, E., & Cramer, G. (1989). Offspring of monozygotic twins discordant for schizophrenia. *Archives of General Psychiatry, 46,* 873–877.

Kuhn, T. S. (1962). *The structure of scientific revolutions.* Chicago: University of Chicago Press.

Lalouel, J. M., Rao, D. C., Morton, M. E., & Elston, R. L. (1983). A unified model for complex segregation analysis. *Journal of Human Genetics, 35,* 816–826.

McGue, M., Gottesman, I. I., & Rao, D. C. (1985). Resolving genetic models for the transmission of schizophrenia. *Genetic Epidemiology, 2,* 99–110.

McGuffin, P., Farmer, A. E., & Gottesman, I. I. (1987). Is there really a split in schizophrenia? The genetic evidence. *British Journal of Psychiatry, 150,* 581–592.

McGuffin, P., Farmer, A. E., Gottesman, I. I., Murray, R. M., & Reveley, A. (1984). Twin concordance for operationally defined schizophrenia. Confirmation of familiality and heritability. *Archives of General Psychiatry, 41,* 541–545.

McGuffin, P., Sargeant, M., Hett, G., Tidmarsh, S., Whatley, S., & Marchbanks, R. M. (1990). Exclusion of a schizophrenia susceptibility gene from the chromosome 5q11-q13 region: New data and a reanalysis of previous reports. *American Journal of Human Genetics, 47,* 529–535.

McGuffin, P., & Sturt, E. (1986). Genetic markers in schizophrenia. *Human Heredity, 36,* 65–88.

Morton, N. E. (1982). *Outline of genetic epidemiology.* Basel, Karger.

Murray, R. M., Lewis, S., & Reveley, A. M. (1985). Towards an aetiological classification of schizophrenia. *Lancet; 1,* 1023–1026.

Murray, R. M., & Murphy, D. L. (1978). Drug response and psychiatric nosology. *Psychological Medicine, 7,* 667–681.

O'Rourke, D. H., Gottesman, I. I., Suarez, B. K., Rice, J., & Reich, T. (1982). Refutation of the single locus model in the aetiology of schizophrenia. *American Journal of Human Genetics, 33,* 630–649.

Ott, J. (1985). *Analysis of human genetic linkage.* Baltimore: John Hopkins University Press.

Pope, H. G., Jonas, J., Cohen, B. A., & Lipinki, J. F. (1983). Heritability of schizophrenia. *American Journal of Psychiatry, 140,* 132–133.

Reich, T., Cloninger, C. R., Wette, R., & James, J. (1979). The use of multiple thresholds and segregation analysis in analysing the phenotypic heterogeneity of multifactorial traits. *Annals of Human Genetics, 42,* 371.

Reich, T., James, J. W., & Morris, C. A. (1972). The use of multiple thresholds in determining the mode of transmission of semi-continuous traits. *Annals of Human Genetics, 36,* 163–184.

Risch, N., & Baron, M. (1984). Segregation analysis of schizophrenia and related disorders. *American Journal of Human Genetics, 36,* 1039–1059.

Robins, E., & Guze, S. B. (1970). Establishment of diagnostic validity in psychiatric illness: Its application to schizophrenia. *American Journal of Psychiatry, 126,* 983–987.

Scharfetter, C., & Nusperli, M. (1980). The group of schizophrenias, schizoaffective psychoses and affective disorders. *Schizophrenia Bulletin, 6,* 586–591.

Schneider, K. (1959). *Clinical psychopathology* (M. W. Hamilton, Trans.). London: Grune & Stratton.

Sherrington, R., Brynjolfsson, J., Petursson, H., Potter, M., Dudleston, K., Barraclough, B., Wasmuth, J., Dobbs, M., & Gurling, H. (1988). Localization of a susceptibility locus for schizophrenia on chromosome 5. *Nature, 336,* 164–170.

Slater, E. (1947). Genetical causes of schizophrenia symptoms. *Monatsschrift fur Psychiatrie und Neurologie, 113,* 50–58. (Reprinted in Shields, J., & Gottesman, I. I. [Eds.]. [1971]. *Man, mind and heredity.* Baltimore: Johns Hopkins Press.

Slater, E., & Cowie, V. (1971). *The genetics of mental disorder.* Oxford, England: Oxford University Press.

Smith, C. (1974). Concordance in twins: Methods and interpretation. *American Journal of Human Genetics, 26,* 454–466.

Spitzer, R. L., Endicott, J., & Robins, E. (1978). *Research diagnostic criteria. Instrument No. 58.* New York: New York State Psychiatric Institute.

St. Clair, D., Blackwood, D., Muir, W., Baillie, D., Hubbard, S., Wright, A., & Evans, H. J. (1992). Absence of linkage of chromosome 5q11-q13 markers to schizophrenics in Scottish families. *Nature, 339,* 305–309.

Stephens, J. H., Astrup, C., Carpenter, W. T., Schaffer, J. W., & Goldberg, J. (1982). A comparison of nine systems to diagnose schizophrenia. *Psychiatry Research, 6,* 127–143.

Suarez, B. K., O'Rourke, D., & Van Eerdwegh, P. (1982). Power of the affected sib pair method to detect disease susceptibility loci of small effect: An application to multiple sclerosis. *American Journal of Medical Genetics, 12,* 309–326.

Suarez, B. K., Reich, T., & Trost, J. (1976). Limits of the genetic two allele single major locus model with incomplete penetrance. *Annals of Human Genetics, 40,* 231–244.

Tienari, P., Sorri, A., Lahti, J., Naarla, M., Walberg, K. E., Moring, J., Pahjola, J., & Wynn, L. C. (1987). Interaction of genetic and psychosocial factors in schizophrenia. *Schizophrenia Bulletin, 13,* 477–484.

Tsuang, M. T., Fowler, R. C., Cadoret, R. J., & Monnelly, E. (1974). Schizophrenia among first degree relatives of paranoid and non paranoid schizophrenics. *Comprehensive Psychiatry, 15,* 295–302.

Tsuang, M. T., & Winokur, G. (1974). Criteria for sub-typing schizophrenia. *Archives of General Psychiatry, 31,* 43–47.

Weatherall, D. J. (1985). *The new genetics and clinical practice* (2nd ed.). Oxford, England: Oxford University Press.

6

Smooth Pursuit Oculomotor Dysfunction as an Index of Schizotaxia

WILLIAM G. IACONO

At a time when most people thought schizophrenia was the product of an unfortunate environment, Meehl used the occasion of his 1961 presidential address to the American Psychological Association to advance a provocative neurological theory (Meehl, 1962, 1989, 1990). He posited that the complex of interpersonal, cognitive, and soft neurological features that constitute schizophrenia were the product of a "neural integrative defect," christened *schizotaxia*, that was viewed as a ubiquitous aberration in single cell functioning. For the first time, a theory was put forth that focused not on manifest schizophrenia, but on those persons vulnerable to develop the disorder. "Schizotypes," Meehl's term for these individuals, are hypothesized to share in common with schizophrenics a genetic diathesis (inherited as an autosomal dominant gene) expressed as schizotaxia. Depending on perinatal factors, social learning history, and chance events, some schizotypes become schizophrenic whereas others remain compensated despite their neurophysiological defect.

This theory cannot be tested using the extant family and twin studies of schizophrenia, which suggest that a single gene acting alone cannot account for the data (McGue & Gottesman, 1989). This is so because these family and twin investigations focus on clinical phenomenology and, ultimately, the diagnosis of manifest schizophrenia and

related disorders. To paraphrase Meehl (1989), because we are trying to track a putative central nervous system (CNS) deficit, not a clinical disease, even of a borderline character, the challenge to testing this theory is to identify phenotypic indicators or markers of schizotaxia.

Although there are many types of candidate markers for schizophrenia (referred to as schizophrenia-related variants by Cromwell [1984]), Meehl (1989) argued that some are likely to identify compensated schizotypes with greater precision than others. Social, cognitive, and personality indicators, because of their relative remoteness in the long causal chain from genes to learned behaviors, may have less utility than endophenotypic indicators, which do not depend on overt behavioral dispositions. The biochemical/neurophysiological endophenotype, although closer to the gene product, cannot easily be examined in intact humans. Moreover, we have as yet not pinpointed the CNS deficit underlying schizophrenia, thus making the identification of promising biological indicators difficult. By contrast, as Iacono and Ficken (1989) have noted, psychophysiological measures, because of their ability to assess general aspects of CNS functioning, have great potential as endophenotypic indicators. If the integrity of any aspect of brain anatomy or physiology is compromised in schizophrenia, there is good reason to expect that the dysfunction may be tapped using psychophysiological techniques.

In this chapter, my aim in part is to convince the reader that we have psychophysiological measures with the potential to identify schizotypes. In so doing, I have focused on one psychophysiological attribute, eye tracking dysfunction. That deviant smooth pursuit oculomotion may be a schizotaxic sign is supported by an extensive and consistent set of research findings (for recent comprehensive reviews of this literature, see Clementz & Sweeney, 1990; Iacono, 1988). In my effort to highlight the significance of this area of research, I have concentrated especially on recent investigations that I have carried out with my colleagues and students over the last several years.

SMOOTH PURSUIT EYE TRACKING

Smooth pursuit eye movements are generated when the eyes follow a slowly moving (e.g., less that 40°/s) target that is in continuous motion. In the early oculomotor studies of schizophrenia, the pursuit tracking response was evaluated by having subjects watch a swinging pendulum. Because (a) the amplitude of the pendulum swing is attenuated with each oscillation, (b) the determination of oscillation frequency is only approximate, and (c) the pendulum moves through two spatial dimensions as it describes an arc, this target does not provide an ideal stimulus for assessing pursuit function.

Greater flexibility as well as precision over target path, amplitude, and frequency can be achieved by electronically simulating the sinusoidal motion of a pendulum. Besides using electromechanical apparatus to generate targets in sinusoidal motion, it is also possible to produce targets driven by "triangular" waveforms, which, unlike sinusoidal targets, move with constant velocity. The target can be projected on a wall or driven across an oscilloscope or computer screen.

Whatever method is used to generate target motion, it is crucial that the motion be continuous and the background against which the target is displayed be plain and free of distracting stimuli. If these requirements are not met, the visual display may stimulate fixations and saccadic eye movement intrusions and provide an inadequate appraisal of the pursuit system. Discontinuous motion especially can be a problem with computer displays. Careful programming of the computer is required to create the appearance of continuous motion. All the pixels must be used, and the target movement must be synchronized with the refresh rate of the screen. Operating overhead (multitasking) must be minimized to ensure that the computer is not drawn away from the task of creating and moving the target. If these steps are not taken, occasions will be created when the target will disappear or appear to move abruptly.

The neural mechanisms involved in the control of smooth pursuit oculomotion are both extensive and complex. Proficient tracking requires a functional visual system as well as a healthy oculomotor system. Accurate pursuit tracking is thus dependent on the integrity of the retina and optic tract; oculomotor muscles, nerves, and nuclei; the vestibular system; the cerebellum; a host of other brainstem nuclei, including a portion of the reticular formation; and the frontal, occipital, and parietal cortex. If a subtle lesion, neurotransmitter deficit, or other neuroanatomical dysfunction exists in the brain of a human, it is quite likely that the pursuit system will be affected and that eye movement recordings will provide an indication of the consequent deficit.

ASSESSMENT OF SMOOTH PURSUIT EYE TRACKING

Recording Methods

Although there are many methods for recording eye movements, only two are routinely used in oculomotor studies of schizophrenia, in part because these two techniques are generally convenient to apply and they produce satisfactory recordings. The most commonly employed procedure involves recording the electro-ocu-logram (EOG), a measure derived from the potential difference that exists between the cornea and the retina. Because the distribution of electrical charge generated by the ocular globes is altered when the eyes move, it is possible to monitor eye movements from electrodes attached to the skin around the eyes. The other method, infrared (IR) recording, involves projecting an (invisible) infrared light on the eyeball and measuring the amount of light reflected off its surface. This is accomplished by positioning an IR light source less than 1 cm away from the center of one eye and monitoring reflected light from photodetectors positioned on each side of the light. Because the sclera has greater reflectance than the iris and the boundary between the two is sharp, the ratio of reflected light on either side of the limbus can be used to determine eye position.

Because the IR system provides a precise representation of eye movements, whereas the EOG always contains some biopotential noise, it is tempting to argue that IR recording should be the preferred of the two methods. However, it is more accurate to conclude that both measures have advantages and disadvantages. Each is more or less appropriate for certain applications. When only a general index of tracking ability is desired, the two types of recording generate essentially identical results (Iacono & Lykken, 1981). Because the EOG cannot be used reliably in all subjects to record oculomotor events less than 3° in amplitude (Iacono & Koenig, 1983), it is preferable to use IR when a fine-grained analysis of eye movements is desired. However, the latter method has four major disadvantages. First, slight movements of the subject's face or head may require time-consuming repositioning of the IR source and photosensors and their recalibration. Second, eyeglasses cannot be worn by subjects when the IR technique is used. Thus, subjects with limited visual acuity who do not have contact lenses cannot be tested. In pedigree analysis, wherein all relatives are to be tested, the use of IR may make it impossible to assess adequately all of the family members. Third, IR recordings are severely disrupted by eye blinks. Eye blinks occur frequently with this procedure because the IR light source may irritate the eye. Finally, IR recordings can be adversely affected by ambient sources of illumination.

The calibration of EOG recording is more straightforward than that for the IR method. Thus, the former is easier to use with uncooperative subjects and subjects can be tested while wearing corrective lenses, a major advantage. Especially when the electrodes are carefully aligned, EOG recordings are usually unaffected by eye blinks. However, because the EOG electrodes are sensitive to all biopotential signals generated in the head, EOG recordings in some subjects can become contaminated by biopotential artifacts (especially electroencephalographic [EEG]; Iacono & Lykken, 1981). This problem makes it difficult to measure small saccades accurately. Interestingly, subjects whose EOG recordings contain EEG artifact tend to be poor smooth pursuit trackers (Iacono & Koenig, 1983; Iacono & Lykken, 1981), a finding that suggests the artifact is not merely a random intrusion. When only a general indication of tracking proficiency is desired or when it is important to test all subjects, including those who are uncooperative or have poor uncorrected vision, EOG is the method of choice.

Data Quantification

The most common method for quantifying pursuit performance has involved rating tracking proficiency on a dichotomous (e.g., Holzman, Kringlen, Levy, & Haberman, 1980) or multipoint (e.g., Shagass, Amadeo, & Overton, 1974) scale. However, with the proliferation of personal computers and laboratory software, the subjectivity, imprecision, and limited information inherent in ratings easily can be eliminated. Employing electronically controlled stimulus displays, digitizing target motion and the associated eye movement response, and subjecting the digitized record to quantitative analysis are now fully possible. Although there are many ways to quantify such data, several methods have become common.

Signal-to-noise ratio. Lindsey, Holzmann, Haberman, and Yasillo (1978) introduced this measure, which is calculated by performing a Fourier transformation on the subject's eye tracking response. The power associated with target frequency (e.g., usually sinusoidal stimuli oscillating at 0.4 Hz are used) represents the signal (S) and the power in a much broader frequency band that excludes the target frequency (e.g., 1.2 to 20 Hz) defines the noise (N). The natural logarithm of this ratio yields the dependent measure. Although this measure has been found consistently to discriminate schizophrenics and their relatives from normal subjects, it is an odd variable in several respects. It is not evident why it is desirable to take the natural logarithm of the S/N ratio. The S/N distribution tends to be negatively skewed (a low score represents poor performance). Under these circumstances, the logarithmic transform will not correct the skewness and does not seem necessary. In addition, in its application, the criteria for signal and noise bandwidths have varied from study to study without explanation. These varying definitions have made comparisons of ln (S/N) data across studies difficult. An advantage of the S/N score is that, because it is unitless, it can be calculated without knowing how many measurement units correspond to a degree of visual arc. It thus can be used without calibrating the recording system. Also, it can be used when control over target motion is imprecise, as is the case with a pendulum. However, when the system is calibrated and target motion is controlled, both the strength of the signal and the amount of noise are interesting pieces of information. Their meaning is lost when the ratio is calculated.

Root-mean-square error. Iacono and Lykken (1979a, 1979b) were the first to use root-mean-square (RMS) error to quantify pursuit performance. This score is computed by calculating the RMS difference between target and eye movement channels. Conceptually, it represents the degree of fit between the target waveform and the pursuit tracking response. Because the eye lags slightly behind the target when the pursuit system is functioning properly, the RMS error of a good tracker will be inflated by phase differences between the two signals. Iacono and Lykken (1979a, 1979b) corrected for this problem by aligning the two channels for phase differences before calculating RMS error. Other investigators using this measure have sometimes not made this adjustment, thus leaving their operational definition of this variable at variance with that employed by Iacono and his colleagues. Lykken, Iacono and Lykken (1981) have shown that, in theory, RMS scores can be derived from S/N scores, although the mathematical relationship between the two measures is not linear.

Gain. Investigators studying the pursuit system itself, rather than psychopathology, have commonly used gain to quantify pursuit tracking. The gain of the pursuit system can be determined by taking the ratio of eye movement velocity to target velocity. A value of 1.0 indicates a perfect pursuit response; gains of less than 1 are commonly seen in schizophrenics and indicate poor pursuit tracking. Although the definition of gain is straightforward, its calculation is not. The simplest way to calculate gain is to use a constant-velocity target, identify the portions of the eye movement response that clearly show a pursuit response (i.e., by eliminating segments during which blinks, saccades, and fixations occur), and then determine the extent to which pursuit velocity matches target velocity (by computing the gain ratio). Because the eyes slow in anticipation of target reversal, smooth pursuit segments immediately preceding the reversal of target movement probably should not be used in these computations. Otherwise, a target with reversal points that are unpredictable should be used (see Clementz & Sweeney, 1990, for a discussion of the consequences of using predictable targets).

Most pursuit eye tracking studies of

schizophrenia use sinusoidal rather than constant-velocity targets. From sinusoidal data, gain can be calculated by dividing peak eye by peak target velocity. However, peak velocities associated with saccades must be eliminated from this computation, which in the end is based on only a tiny fraction of the available data (peak velocity can be calculated at only two points for each cycle of tracking). All the data can be used if the calculation of gain is based on a Fourier analysis in which the power of the fundamental frequency evident in the tracking response is compared to the power that would derive if the eye tracking were perfect. By carefully calibrating signals, the latter quantity can be obtained from a Fourier analysis of the target waveform.

Either single- or dual-mode gain can be calculated. To estimate single-mode gain, the saccades and blink artifacts must be edited from the data before the Fourier analysis is undertaken. The resulting ratio describes the gain of the pursuit system alone. Dual-mode gain is computed without editing saccades from the data. To the extent that saccades have frequency characteristics that do not overlap with the target frequency, single- and dual-mode calculations based on the same data would yield identical results. They do not in practice, however, because some of the saccadic activity will contribute to power at the fundamental frequency. Thus, although single- and dual-mode gain calculations are likely to yield similar gain estimates (Clementz, Sweeney, Hirt, & Haas, 1991), when the computations are based on the same data, dual-mode calculations should generate somewhat higher values. In addition, dual-mode gain has been found to approximate more closely the theoretical models for how the smooth pursuit system functions (e.g., Bahill, Iandolo, & Troost, 1980).

The calculation of (especially single-mode) gain provides an estimate of how well the pursuit system is tracking the target. Hence, it is unlike the S/N and RMS error measures, which provide a global index of all tracking deviations, including deviations contributed by saccadic intrusions.

Saccadic events. Another way of quantifying disrupted pursuit is to identify the saccades that intrude on pursuit tracking and those that correct for position error. Saccades can be counted and their amplitudes and velocities determined. They can be categorized by various characteristics, such as whether they compensate for pursuit error (by catching up or backing up to the position of the target) or anticipate target movement (see Clementz & Sweeney, 1990, for a full description of various saccade types). The advantage of calculating gain and monitoring saccades over the other methods of quantifying pursuit dysfunction is that it is possible to determine the nature of the deficit that characterizes disrupted pursuit (Abel & Ziegler, 1988).

Evaluation of Measures

Because they seem to characterize the nature of pursuit dysfunction, gain and saccadic measures have great appeal. They are the obvious measures of choice when the research aim is to identify specific neuro-opthalmological anomalies associated with dysfunctional pursuit. Unfortunately, little research has been published that can be used to evaluate these measures for their potential as schizotaxic markers. Moreover, what literature is available has not demonstrated that these measures have an advantage over the more "global" indices for quantifying the pursuit of schizophrenics. In the most thorough application to date of gain and saccadic measures, these variables produced mixed results; for instance, they did not significantly differentiate schizophrenic from normal control subjects (Clementz, Sweeney, Hirt, & Haas, 1990), whereas RMS error did. In addition, the saccadic measures showed relatively low within-session retest reliability compared to RMS error (the reliability of gain was not determined). Ross et al. (1988) also could not successfully differentiate schizophrenic and normal groups using specific saccadic variables or gain. This study used relatively small samples ($n = 30$), but RMS error nevertheless produced a substantial group difference.

Whicker, Abel, and Dell'Osso (1985) posited that anticipatory saccades (those that move the eye ahead of the target) may be a specific oculomotor abnormality in the relatives of schizophrenic patients. However, Clementz, Grove, Iacono, and their colleagues (Clementz, Grove, Iacono, & Sweeney, 1992; Clementz et al., 1991; Grove et al., 1991) have shown that these saccades are not related to schizotypal features in the relatives of schizophrenics, but RMS error and gain are. These neuro-opthalmological measures were thus not superior to RMS error in their potential as schizotaxic markers. Because global measures now have a substantial data base demonstrating excellent reliability, construct validity, heritability, and differentiation of the relatives of schizophrenics from normal subjects, it would be unfortunate to apply the more specific but generally unused measures exclusive of the global ones (see Iacono & Clementz, 1993), for a more thorough evaluation of pursuit tracking measures).

SMOOTH PURSUIT EYE TRACKING AS A PSYCHOPHYSIOLOGICAL MARKER

The qualities a psychophysiological variable should have to qualify as a schizotaxic marker have been comprehensively discussed elsewhere (e.g., Iacono, 1985, 1988; Iacono & Ficken, 1989). The extent to which deviant smooth pursuit ocular motion satisfies these qualities has also been thoroughly reviewed in recent publications (Clementz & Sweeney, 1990; Iacono, 1988). Hence, this topic is only briefly considered here. The interested reader is referred to the cited review papers for a more complete presentation of this material.

If a variable is to have potential as a schizotaxic marker, it should satisfy a number of criteria. Studies both of nonpsychiatric subjects selected from the general population and of psychiatric patients are relevant. In the general population, the putative marker should have a low base rate, be sta-

ble over time, be genetically transmitted, and identify individuals unaffected with schizophrenia but deemed to be at risk for it. Studies of psychiatric patients must indicate that the trait is relatively specific to schizophrenia, appears in patients with schizophrenia in remission, is evident in at least some of the unaffected first-degree relatives of schizophrenic probands, and segregates with schizophrenia and schizophrenia spectrum disorders in families with affected members.

A considerable body of converging evidence indicates that smooth pursuit dysfunction satisfies these requirements. Abnormal eye tracking appears infrequently in normal individuals, with only about 8% showing dysfunctional pursuit according to the reports of Holzman and colleagues (e.g., Holzman, Solomon, Levin, & Waternaux, 1984). Eye tracking performance is stable over intervals as long as 2 years (Iacono & Lykken, 1981), shows a monozygotic–dizygotic twin concordance ratio of approximately 2:1 in both psychiatric (Holzman et al., 1980) and normal (Iacono, 1982) twins, and identifies psychiatrically maladjusted individuals selected from the general population (Siever, Coursey, Alterman, Buchsbaum, & Murphy, 1982, 1984; Seiver et al., 1989). In addition, deficient pursuit tracking has been observed in schizophrenic but not affective patients in remission (Iacono, Peloquin, Lumry, Valentine, & Tuason, 1982; Iacono, Tuason, & Johnson, 1981); in the first-degree relatives of schizophrenic probands (e.g., Holzman et al., 1984; Kuechenmeister, Linton, Mueller, & White; 1977; Mather, 1985; Whicker et al., 1985), and in first-degree relatives with schizophrenia spectrum diagnoses (Clementz et al., 1990), but not in the relatives of affective probands (Holzman et al., 1984; Levy et al., 1983). Poor pursuit tracking performance has also been found in psychiatric patients with schizotypal but not other types of personality disorder (Siever, Keefe, Bernstein, Cocaro, Klar, & Zemishlany, 1990).

Holzman, Matthysse, and their colleagues (Holzman et al., 1988; Matthysse, Holzman, & Lange, 1986) have advanced a genetic model to account for their eye tracking findings. Their model suggests that almost all cases of schizophrenia can be accounted for by a latent trait governed by a nearly completely dominant gene in a two-allele system. The expression of the gene is purported to be pleiotropic, with carriers manifesting either schizophrenia, dysfunctional pursuit eye tracking, or both of these traits. An interesting feature of their model is that it accounts for families in which the schizophrenic proband has normal pursuit performance and a first-degree relative has abnormal oculomotion. Indeed, according to Matthysse et al. (1986), "schizophrenics with good tracking *tend* to have relatives with bad tracking even when these relatives are not schizophrenic" (p. 58, emphasis added). From the Holzman–Matthysse perspective, then, it would be neither necessary nor expected that deviant pursuit segregates with schizophrenia.

RECENT FINDINGS FROM THE UNIVERSITIES OF BRITISH COLUMBIA AND MINNESOTA

Over the past decade I have been conducting a large-scale study of various psychophysiological variables with potential as schizotaxic markers. This research has been carried out with the collaboration of my colleagues (Morley Beiser, Brett Clementz, Jon Fleming, Will Grove, Tsung-Yi Lin, and Margaret Moreau) and students (Anna Cerri, John Ficken, Diane Gooding, Joanna Katsanis, Geoff Smith, and Karen Tallman) in British Columbia and Minnesota. The major thrust of this research is captured by a project that operates under the acronym MAP (for "markers and predictors" of schizophrenia). The MAP project is a large-scale, longitudinal study of individuals experiencing their first episode of psychosis. Our operational definition of "first episode" required that none of the patients had been treated with neuroleptic, antidepressant, or antimanic medications. A primary goal of this investigation was to identify and recruit all individuals in

Vancouver, Canada, and selected suburban communities who made their first lifetime contact with a helping agency or professional because of psychotic symptoms. To accomplish this aim, we established a community-wide network of referral sources. The network was composed of psychiatric hospitals and psychiatric services of general hospitals, university and college counseling centers, community mental health agencies, employment and immigration counseling services, psychiatrists in private practice, and a one-in-six probability sample of general practice physicians. The procedures we used to identify and recruit subjects were very similar to those employed in the recent World Health Organization study of the incidence of schizophrenia (Sartorius et al., 1986). A total of 175 psychotic subjects, 13% of whom were not hospitalized, were entered into the study over a 2.5 year interval spanning 1982 to 1984. These individuals, together with a large normal control group, were reassessed at approximately 9, 18, and 60 months following intake into the study.

Relatives of the study subjects were also recruited and assessed, in part to provide ancillary information on the patients, but also to provide data pertinent to the evaluation of various psychophysiological variables (eye tracking, electrodermal activity, visual evoked potentials, and resting EEG) for their potential as markers of psychosis. In addition to the first-episode patients, a group of 67 patients with chronic schizophrenia was also recruited for comparison purposes for the psychophysiological assessment. Additional specific aims of the project were many. They included examining factors that predict course of disorder (Bieser, Fleming, Iacono, & Lin, 1988; Iacono & Beiser, 1989); the temporal stability of diagnostic assignment (Beiser, Iacono, & Erickson, 1989; Iacono & Beiser, 1989); anomalies in brain morphology and neuropsychology (Iacono, Smith, et al., 1988; Katsanis & Iacono, 1989, 1991; Smith et al., 1988); the effects of social support on short-term outcome (Erickson, Beiser, Iacono,

Fleming, & Lin, 1989); psychometric indicators of risk for schizotypy (Katsanis, Iacono, & Beiser, 1990; Katsanis, Iacono, Beiser, & Lacey, 1992); and labeling by the self and significant others (Beiser et al., 1987). A comprehensive overview of the study subjects and selection criteria can be found in Iacono and Beiser (1989).

Oculomotor Dysfunction and the Frontal Lobes

Levin (1984) hypothesized that, at the cortical level, smooth pursuit dysfunction was likely to be represented in the frontal lobes of the brain. To evaluate this possibility, Katsanis and Iacono (1991) examined the association between neuropsychological test performance and pursuit eye tracking ability in 65 of the chronic schizophrenics who were recruited as a MAP comparison group. Frontal lobe tasks included the Wisconsin card sorting test, finger tapping, the trailmaking test, and verbal fluency. An array of nonfrontal tests was also used, including the full Wechsler Adult Intelligence Scale–Revised, the Benton visual retention test, and the Rey auditory verbal learning test. Scores on the frontal lobe tasks generally were correlated with smooth pursuit performance, whereas scores on the nonfrontal tasks were not.

Katsanis and Iacono evaluated the hypothesis further by conducting a multiple regression analysis with blockwise variable selection in which the neuropsychological variables were entered as a set defined by their tapping frontal or nonfrontal functions. Whether the frontal set was entered into the regression analysis first or last, only these tests accounted for significant eye tracking variance. The two frontal tests that accounted for the most variance were word fluency and perseverative errors from the Wisconsin card sorting task. Katsanis and Iacono also found that negative clinical symptoms, a possible manifestation of frontal lobe dysfunction, were correlated with deficient pursuit tracking. These findings support those of Bartfai, Levender, Ny-

back, Berggren, and Schalling (1985), who also reported an association between performance on frontal lobe tasks and smooth pursuit.

Eye Tracking Dysfunction and Trisomy of Chromosome 5

Many of the eye tracking data from the MAP study have now been analyzed. The first interesting finding came from the discovery by Anne Bassett that one of the index cases had partial trisomy of chromosome 5 (Bassett, McGillivray, Jones, & Panzar, 1988). The proband's maternal uncle had the same chromosomal anomaly and also had schizophrenia. The proband's mother had a balanced translocation in which genetic material deleted from chromosome 5 was inserted into chromosome 1. The different type of karyotypic anomaly possessed by the mother makes her a candidate for meiotically transmitting genetic material shared by the proband and maternal uncle. The mother was otherwise normal. The proband's father, brother, and two other maternal uncles had normal karyotypes and no psychiatric disorder. These findings suggest that genes in the trisomic area of chromosome 5 may play a role in the development of schizophrenia, a hypothesis that was supported by an unreplicated report from Sherrington et al. (1988), who demonstrated linkage between the same region of chromosome 5 and schizophrenia (see McGuffin et al., 1990, for a review of the many failures to replicate Sherrington et al.'s findings).

If we assume that schizophrenia in the proband and uncle arose because they had the chromosomal anomaly, this family is unique in that we know from the karyotypes which members carry schizotaxic genetic material and which ones do not. If eye tracking dysfunction is to serve as a schizotaxic marker, it should be present only in the two individuals with the trisomal chromosomal anomaly. To test this hypothesis, we (Iacono, Bassett, & Jones, 1988, 1989) examined pursuit eye tracking in all the family members residing in Vancouver (the two normal uncles living outside of Canada were not tested). We recorded eye movements using both EOG and IR simultaneously and quantified performance by calculating RMS error. The two methods produced highly correlated results ($r = .96$), indicating that they were essentially interchangeable in this family.

To determine which family members had pursuit tracking dysfunction, we compared the RMS errors of the five available family members to RMS data collected from 24 unrelated schizophrenic patients in remission and 21 normal subjects who were part of an earlier investigation (Iacono et al., 1981). The results showed that the two trisomic schizophrenic family members generated error scores that exceeded the mean and corresponding 95% confidence interval for the remitted schizophrenic patients. The brother, father, and mother produced scores that fell below the mean and 95% confidence interval of the normal subjects. Hence, the eye tracking of the proband and his uncle were clearly abnormal and the pursuit performance of the other family members was slightly better than normal. Samples of the raw eye tracking data from this family are presented in Figure 6.1.

We interpreted the results as consistent with the hypothesis that eye tracking was "marking" the presumed schizophrenia "genotype." For this family, genes within the trisomic region of chromosome 5 may have contributed to both the development of schizophrenia and deviant oculomotion. Of course, we cannot reach firm conclusions from such a case study. The pairing of these traits may reflect coincidence. It could also be due to a neurological dysfunction brought on by the chromosomal anomaly. However, neither of the two affected individuals showed evidence of neurological impairment or mental retardation (in fact, the proband was a university student). Finally, as already noted, it should be stressed that this family is unique. Its uniqueness may mean that our findings have little or no significance for schizophrenia in general.

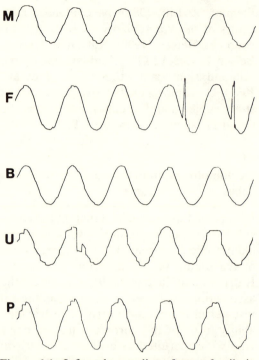

Figure 6.1. Infrared recordings from a family in which the proband (P) and his maternal uncle (U) were found to have both partial trisomy of chromosome 5 and schizophrenia. The proband's mother (M), father (F), and brother (B) had neither trisomy nor schizophrenia. Note that the smooth pursuit of the nonpsychiatric relatives is normal, interrupted only occasionally by small saccades. The proband and his uncle show more frequent and larger saccades than the other family members. The two spikes in the last two cycles of the father's eye tracking are caused by blinks.

An Epidemiological Study of Smooth Pursuit Dysfunction

Because the MAP project was in part an incidence study, it has come as close as possible, given the necessity of procuring informed consent, to obtaining a complete sample of first-episode psychotic subjects. Hence, the sample is epidemiologically based and, therefore, findings derived from the MAP study are probably more broadly generalizable than those derived from the investigation of patients at a single hospital. This feature of the MAP project, together with the comprehensive recruitment of patients with all types of functional psychosis and a large normal control group, affords a heretofore unrealized opportunity to examine the specificity of smooth pursuit tracking dysfunction to schizophrenia and the prevalence of deviant oculomotion in normal subjects.

Ambiguity regarding these issues arises from a lack of systematic study of nonschizophrenic psychiatric patients and the lack of an agreed-on operational definition of what constitutes pursuit impairment. Few studies have included comparison groups of affective disorder or nonschizophrenic patients. Those that have, have used samples too small to generate meaningful prevalence estimates (Holzman et al., 1974; Lipton, Levin, & Holzman, 1980; Shagass et al., 1974); patients who were not acutely ill when tested (Iacono et al., 1982); or subjects who were medicated with drugs that may affect pursuit tracking (Holzman et al., 1984). To the best of my knowledge, there are no studies that have examined the rate of deviant tracking in acutely ill individuals with schizophreniform disorder, psychotic major depression, or other functional psychoses.

The absence of a commonly accepted standard for what constitutes deviant eye tracking also renders difficult the evaluation of the extant prevalence data. In a study of young adult twins, Iacono and Lykken (1979b) reported prevalence rates for abnormal tracking that ranged from 5% to 36% depending on the criteria used to classify pursuit as deviant. Most studies employing psychopathological samples report only group means from which prevalence estimates cannot be derived. Virtually all of the prevalence data come from investigations of Holzman and associates, who rely primarily on ratings to classify tracking performance as good or bad. No empirical data have been presented by this group to identify clearly or justify the cutoff point used to separate normal from deviant performance. Because their ratings depend partly on inexplicit criteria, it is not possible for others to apply unambiguously the same criteria to their samples.

In addition to tackling these concerns, the MAP study provided an opportunity to ex-amine the relatives of types of psychotic patients who have not been studied previously. Hence, this study addresses several of the issues important to the evaluation of eye tracking dysfunction as a schizotaxic marker. Because a detailed presentation of the eye tracking portion of the MAP project is available elsewhere (Iacono, Moreau, Beiser, Fleming, & Lin, 1992), only highlights are presented here.

Pursuit eye tracking was assessed in a total of 482 subjects, including 157 psychotic subjects (schizophrenia, $n = 51$; schizophreniform disorder, $n = 29$; major depression, $n = 25$; bipolar disorder, $n = 37$; and other psychoses, $n = 15$). The patients were diagnosed using criteria from the *Diagnostic and Statistical Manual of Mental Disorders,* third edition (American Psychiatric Association, 1980) following administration of the Present State Exam and a comprehensive case conference in which all the clinical data available on each subject were reviewed. In addition, 158 of their first-degree relatives participated (schizophrenia, $n = 52$; schizophreniform disorder, $n = 30$; major depression, $n = 28$; bipolar disorder, $n = 38$; and other psychoses, $n = 10$). The control group consisted of 119 normal volunteers, recruited from the same communities as the psychiatric patients, and 48 of their first-degree relatives, all screened for psychiatric disorder in themselves and their families. All subjects tracked a sinusoidally driven target traversing 20° of visual arc and oscillating at a frequency of 0.4 Hz. The EOG was recorded and quantified by computing RMS error.

Preliminary analyses indicated that the normal subjects and their relatives generated equivalent RMS distributions, so these two groups were combined to form one large ($n = 167$) normal comparison sample. Because the patients with "other psychoses" represent a small, heterogeneous group, their data are not considered further here.

The primary results are summarized in Figure 6.2. The figure presents plots depicting the percentage of probands and relatives distributed over the range of RMS scores.

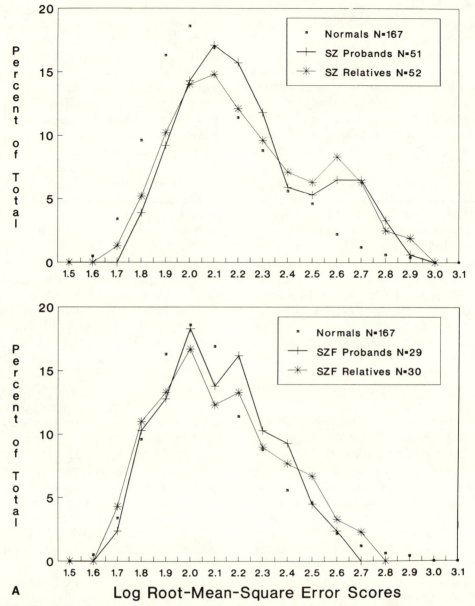

Figure 6.2. Smoothed frequency histograms indicating the percentage of psychotic probands and their relatives across the distribution of log RMS error scores. For each plot, the distribution for the normal subjects is provided for comparison purposes. (*A*), SZ, schizophrenia; SZF, schizophreniform disorder.

The data were subjected to an admixture analysis using the program SKUMIX (MacLean, Morton, Elston, & Yee, 1976; McGue, Gerrard, Lebowitz, & Rao, 1989) to determine if the distribution of eye tracking performance was bimodal and discontinuous. A bimodal phenotypic distribution suggests a discontinuous cause that, if genetic, would ordinarily be attributable to a single gene (see Falconer, 1989). If smooth pursuit dysfunction is determined by at least two alleles, one of which is dominant at a single major locus related to schizophrenia, the RMS error distribution should be bimodal (one mode for each phenotype) for the schizophrenic probands and their relatives. The SKUMIX analysis allowed us to evaluate the hypothesis that each distribution

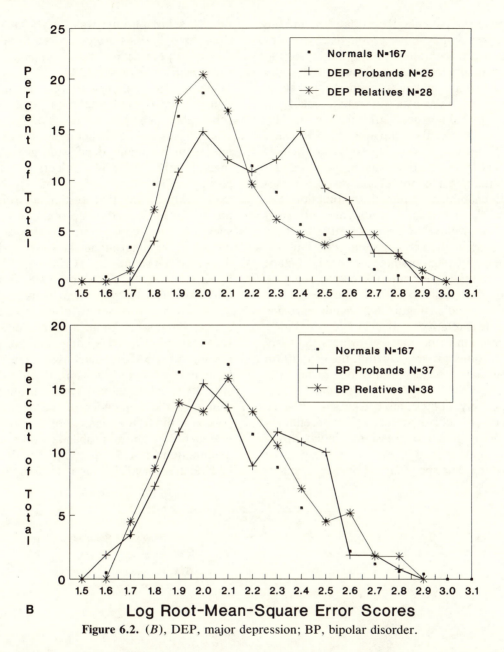

Figure 6.2. (*B*), DEP, major depression; BP, bipolar disorder.

was bimodal against the null hypothesis that the distribution had a single mode.

The results confirmed what is apparent from Figure 6.2: Only the distributions for the schizophrenics and their relatives and the psychotic depressed patients and their relatives showed significant departure from unimodality. For the two schizophrenia groups, the second mode can be identified by an inflection point occurring at a log RMS value of about 2.50. The same point

defines the beginning of the second mode for the depressed probands' relatives. The distribution for the depressed probands is more difficult to characterize. It is apparent that there are a number of depressed probands with RMS scores >2.50, but there is also an apparently deviant group with scores between 2.20 and 2.50. The characteristics of depressed patients whose RMS scores exceed these values are considered below. The distributions for the schizophreniform patients, their relatives, and the relatives of the bipolar probands closely approximate the unimodal distribution of the normal subjects. Although the error distribution of the bipolar probands did not show a significant departure from unimodality, it did show, like the distribution of the depressed probands, a dip at a log RMS value of 2.20, a feature considered further below.

These observations can be quantified by determining the proportion in each group with unambiguous pursuit dysfunction. Essentially identical results are obtained whether we use the point of rarity (log RMS = 2.51) in the schizophrenia distributions or the control group mean plus two standard deviations as the cutoff score to separate good from poor tracking. The results are summarized in Figure 6.3; schizophrenics and their relatives had a significantly larger proportion of deviant performers than any of the other groups. Overall, the proportion of deviant trackers in any one group was small, with 20%, 5%, 13%, 7%, and 5%, respectively, of the combined patient–relative groups of schizophrenic, schizophreniform disorder, major depression, bipolar disorder, and normal subjects showing poor tracking. The specificity of pursuit dysfunc-

tion to schizophrenia was high (.93 when the schizophrenics are compared to all the nonschizophrenic psychotic subjects), but the sensitivity was low (.20).

The major challenge to the conclusion that deviant pursuit tracking is specific to schizophrenia and the relatives of these patients arises with consideration of the findings from the major depression group and their relatives. Could subjects in these groups either have a form of psychotic major depression that resembles schizophrenia or be related to a proband who has such a form of depression? To answer this question, we determined the rate at which Research Diagnostic Criteria (RDC; Spitzer, Endicott, & Robins, 1978) schizoaffective disorder was concurrently diagnosed in the probands (whose assignment to the depressed group was made using DSM-III criteria). We compared the proportion of DSM-III–diagnosed depressed probands who had deviant RMS values (>2.50) or who had relatives with deviant scores to the remainder of the depressed group for the RDC diagnosis of schizoaffective disorder. Of the probands with pursuit dysfunction ($n = 3$) and the probands who had relatives with impaired tracking ($n =$

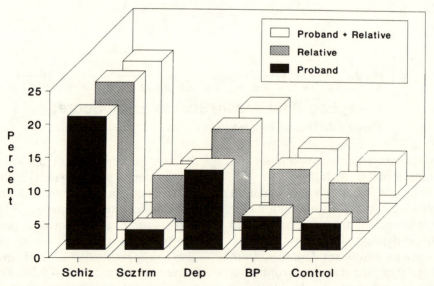

Figure 6.3. Bar graph indicating the percentage of abnormal trackers in each subject group. Schiz, schizophrenia; Sczfrm, schizophreniform disorder; Dep, major depression; BP, bipolar disorder; Control, normal.

4), 71% had RDC-diagnosed schizoaffective disorder. For the remaining 19 families, 26% of the probands had this RDC diagnosis. The difference in proportions was statistically significant and suggests that DSM-III–diagnosed depressed probands who were members of families with impaired smooth pursuit were likely to have schizophrenia-like psychotic features.

For both the bipolar and major depressive probands, there is an inflection point (where log RMS = 2.20) on the descending limb of the leftmost mode that is not seen in the corresponding distributions of their relatives. A substantial number of patients fell to the right of this point, a finding that raises the possibility that there may be something about the clinical condition of the patients who fall beyond the inflection point that affected their performance. To determine if the affected patients falling on either side of this point differed on some important variable, this point was used to divide these patients into two groups and they were compared on a variety of variables, including age, the presence of an Axis II disorder, positive and negative symptoms, premorbid functioning, socioeconomic status, occupational functioning, and medication with lithium carbonate. None of these variables differentiated the patients in these two groups. Hence, it is not evident that this inflection point has any significance in these distributions.

To examine further the possible influence of lithium on eye tracking in the mood disorder subjects, we carried out a number of analyses using a large subset ($n = 57$) of these patients (Gooding, Iacono, Katsanis, Beiser, & Grove, 1993). We compared patients on lithium ($n = 16$) to those not taking this medication ($n = 41$) on RMS error and number of saccadic intrusions. These analyses were repeated using only bipolar patients on ($n = 15$) and off ($n = 16$) lithium. None of the analyses showed a lithium effect. Some of the bipolar patients ($n = 10$) were tested twice, once while receiving lithium and once while almost all the patients were totally drug free and none were receiving lithium. Comparing the eye tracking of these individuals at these two points in time on the same dependent variables again failed to reveal an eye tracking effect. These results are inconsistent with those of Iacono et al. (1982) and Levy et al. (1985), who found that lithium was associated with poor eye tracking performance. The differences in the findings among these studies may be due to our use of first-episode, previously unmedicated subjects, whereas Iacono et al. and Levy et al. studied older, more chronic samples, including subjects with extensive histories of pharmacotherapy. In any event, our present findings indicate that lithium does not necessarily lead to dysfunctional tracking, and we suggest that lithium effects must be evaluated on a study-by-study basis.

If genes influence pursuit tracking performance in schizophrenia, schizophrenic patients with bad tracking should have relatives with the dysfunction and vice versa. Our results (depicted in Figure 6.4) showed that the relatives of schizophrenics with pursuit dysfunction did indeed tend to have dysfunctional pursuit. However, the reverse relationship did not hold: some relatives with dysfunctional tracking were not related to probands with poor pursuit performance. Overall, the schizophrenic probands generated 29 families yielding at least two study participants. Thirty-eight percent of these families contained at least one member whose eye tracking was deviant; 62% of the families did not display evidence of pursuit dysfunction in either the probands or their relatives.

Replication and Extension of MAP Project Findings

Several of the salient MAP findings have been replicated and extended in our most recent work using a combined sample of subjects recruited in New York and Minnesota (Clementz, Grove, Iacono, & Sweeney, 1992). In this study, the eye tracking of 38 probands with DSM-III-R–diagnosed schizophrenia and 99 of their first-degree relatives was examined using an oculomotor protocol similar to that employed

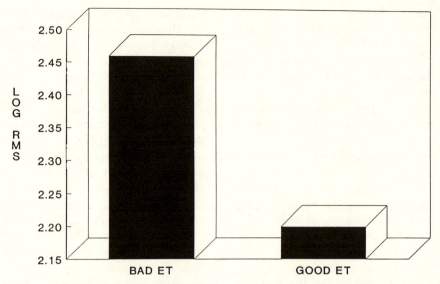

Figure 6.4. Bar graph illustrating the mean RMS error score for the relatives of the schizophrenic patients who had good eye tracking (ET) ($n = 43$) versus those with bad eye tracking ($n = 9$).

in the MAP project, except that the New York sample was evaluated using IR recording only. In addition to RMS error, anticipatory saccades, dual-mode gain, and the S/N ratio were also used to quantify oculomotor performance. Also, all the first-degree relatives were assessed for schizophrenia and schizophrenia spectrum disorders using the Structured Clinical Interview for DSM-III-R (SCID) and the Schedule for Schizotypal Personalities (SSP; Baron, Asnis, & Gruen, 1981).

An admixture analysis of the data was again carried out using SKUMIX for each of the oculomotor variables. The anticipatory saccade data were so severely positively skewed that they did not yield reliable parameter estimates, so these data could not be used in the SKUMIX analysis. Both the RMS error and gain distributions showed significant bimodality, but the S/N ratio did not. The proportion of deviant trackers identified by RMS error was the same for the probands and relatives in this study as it was for the schizophrenic probands and their relatives in Iacono et al. (1992). Interestingly, the proportion of poor trackers identified as falling two standard deviations beyond the normal control mean in the gain distribution was approximately equivalent

to that identified in the MAP study using RMS error (actually, it was the same for relatives but slightly larger for probands).

When correlations were calculated between family members, the sibling–sibling correlation for pursuit performance exceeded the parent–offspring correlation. Nonadditive genetic variance is shared by siblings (on average 25% of the dominance variance) but not by offspring and parents. Both sibling and offspring–parent pairings share 50% of additive genetic variance in common. Hence, this pattern of results suggests that dominant genetic variance contributes to the expression of pursuit tracking ability.

RMS error and gain, but not S/N and the number of anticipatory saccades, were significantly correlated with schizophrenia-related characteristics on the SSP, suggesting that oculomotor dysfunction is associated with manifest schizotypy in the relatives. When the SSP was divided into subscales emphasizing cognitive–perceptual and social–interpersonal items, eye tracking dysfunction was found to correlate significantly with only the social items. The findings from the MAP project indicating that probands with poor eye tracking were likely to have relatives with tracking impairment suggested that pursuit dysfunction may be specific to certain families rather than a general indictor of schizophrenia risk. This supposition was supported by the present study. We identified six large families (in addition to some smaller ones) with no evidence of pursuit dysfunction. These families contain 8 individuals with schizophrenia and a total of 40 members, 38 of whom were tested. None of these individuals was found to have dysfunctional eye tracking (i.e., a gain or RMS score falling more than two standard deviations beyond the nonpsychiatric comparison group mean). We also identified seven family members (five probands and two relatives) with schizophrenia spectrum disorders who did not show tracking impairment, although they were members of families in which at least one individual manifested deviant tracking.

To determine if eye tracking dysfunction was associated with schizotypal characteristics in some families but not others, we divided families into two groups, those with at least one member with pursuit impairment and those composed entirely of individuals with good tracking. The correlations between eye tracking performance and SSP scores were again calculated. These variables were significantly correlated in only the former group of families, again with the social–interpersonal but not the cognitive–perceptual subscale. Because the correlations were calculated using ranked data, this result was not due simply to changes in the range and variance of eye tracking scores that resulted when families were divided into two groups. The finding that social but not cognitive schizotypal features are correlated with eye tracking is consistent with other eye tracking reports (Clementz, et al., 1991; Siever et al., 1989) as well as with other studies suggesting that social characteristics of SSP are more closely related to the genetic predisposition to schizophrenia than are cognitive–perceptual characteristics (Grove et al., 1991; Gunderson & Siever, 1985; Kendler, 1985). Among the families showing eye tracking dysfunction, the sensitivity of oculomotor dysfunction for detecting family members with schizo-

phrenia and schizotypal personality disorder was high (.74 for gain, .76 for RMS error); the same was true for specificity (.67 for gain, .78 for RMS error).

We also explored directly the relationship between gain and RMS error in this study. When a cutoff point two standard deviations above the normal control mean was used to identify deviant tracking, these two measures classified 90% of the total sample ($n = 178$) identically. Seven percent of subjects were identified as deviant using gain but not RMS error; 3% were labeled deviant using RMS error but not gain. Turning to the number of families identified as containing at least one member with oculomotor dysfunction, gain identified 21 such families. RMS error identified 20 of these plus two additional families. The two measures were correlated at .88 in the schizophrenic probands and at .78 in their relatives. Among siblings who were from the families with oculomotor dysfunction, we calculated the genetic cross-correlation between RMS error and gain (indicating the degree to which these measures share genes in common). The resulting correlation was .93. Coupling these findings with the other results from this study, we concluded that dual-mode gain and RMS error are roughly equivalent measures that yield highly similar findings.

CONCLUSIONS

The findings presented in this chapter provide further evidence in support of the hypothesis that deviant pursuit oculomotion may be a schizotaxic marker. Earlier investigations showed that abnormalities in pursuit performance that are independent of clinical state are specific to schizophrenia (Iacono et al., 1981, 1982) and that pursuit dysfunction showed familial specificity (Holzman et al., 1984; Levy et al., 1983). Our current findings suggest that the dysfunction itself is specific to schizophrenia when tracking performance is quantified using RMS error and an empirically derived cutoff score is used to identify deviant tracking. In addition, our data have important implications for understanding the genetics of schizophrenia.

The most intriguing result to emerge from this research was that pursuit eye tracking was quasi-discontinuously distributed in schizophrenics and their relatives, but not in other groups of psychotic patients and their family members (unless the proband was likely to have RDC-diagnosed schizoaffective disorder). This discontinuity was evident in samples of schizophrenics and their relatives from western Canada, Minnesota, and New York. It was present using RMS error as well as dual-mode gain to quantify tracking irregularity, and these two quantitative indices yielded similar results even though they were derived from different samples. Taken together, these findings suggest that the bimodality apparent in the pursuit performance of the schizophrenic probands and their family members is robust and broadly generalizable. The results support the notion that a single gene related to schizophrenia may govern smooth pursuit tracking ability.

However, these results are not entirely consistent with all of the propositions put forth by Holzman, Matthysse, and colleagues (Holzman et al., 1988; Matthysse et al., 1986). Contrary to the assertion of these investigators, it was not the case that the eye tracking performance of probands and their relatives was unrelated. Instead, patients with poor tracking tended to have relatives who tracked poorly. However, as Holzman et al. (1988) have noted, it is the case that some schizophrenics with normal pursuit have relatives with abnormal tracking. These observations leave open the possibility that deviant tracking is one manifestation of a gene with pleiotropic effects. They also raise the possibility that abnormal smooth pursuit is an imperfect measure of the genetic predisposition to schizophrenia. Therefore, it may be useful to combine eye tracking with other putative indicators in studies of schizotaxia. We have recently provided an interesting demonstration of the possible advantage of using multiple indicators of schizotaxia (Grove et al., 1991). We examined pursuit eye tracking together

with personality measures and scores on a continuous performance task in schizophrenics and their relatives. We found that abnormal scores on these measures tend to run together in families, suggesting that a single core dimension contributes to covariation in these measures and that the use of multiple indicators is likely to be more informative than reliance on just one.

The Holzman–Matthysse model also assumes that almost all cases of schizophrenia share the same genetic etiology. Our data suggest that deviant eye tracking not only is not present in many probands with schizophrenia, but it may be absent in up to half of families ascertained through an affected proband. As we have shown elsewhere (Clementz, Grove, Iacono, & Sweeney, 1992), the probability of finding our several large families with no evidence of pursuit dysfunction, given the parameters of the Holzman–Matthysse model, is essentially nil. Our results indicate that schizophrenia may be etiologically heterogeneous, with perhaps more than one genetic etiology or genetic and environmental etiologies. They also suggest that, although smooth pursuit eye movement may be a risk indicator for many cases of schizophrenia, many cases may also be best identified by other (as yet unknown) schizotaxic markers. Again, our results anticipate considerable advantage in the simultaneous study of multiple putative schizotaxic markers to determine if they identify risk in different subsets of patients and relatives.

These findings, coupled with those from our study of the family with the chromosome 5 aberration, suggest that molecular genetic studies of schizophrenia would likely be more profitable if probands were selected because they had both schizophrenia and deviant eye tracking rather than schizophrenia alone. Selecting cases for linkage studies because they have both traits could reduce genetic heterogeneity, which can be a serious problem in such research, and would ensure that the study subjects were likely to be gene carriers.

A second important finding to emerge from our work was that dysfunctional tracking (as assessed by RMS error) was relatively specific to schizophrenics and their relatives, occurring in about 20% to 23% of our Vancouver, Minnesota, and New York schizophrenia samples (total n = 88 probands, 150 relatives) compared to no more than 7% in the bipolar, schizophreniform, and normal proband–relative groups in the MAP study (see Figure 6.2). Thirteen percent of the major depression proband–relative group had oculomotor dysfunction, but if the probands and the relatives of probands with RDC-diagnosed schizoaffective disorder are removed from the group, the proportion with deviant tracking drops to under 5%. These prevalence rates are not consistent with those reported by Holzman et al. (1974, 1980, 1984), who have identified deviant oculomotion in 44% to 86% of schizophrenics, 34% to 54% of their relatives, 41% of bipolar patients, 10% to 13% of their relatives, and 8% of normal subjects. The rates of tracking impairment we identified in the relatives of probands with mood disorders (10% if we combine bipolar and major depressive groups and do not eliminate schizoaffective cases or relatives of schizoaffective probands) and in normal subjects (5%) are roughly equivalent to those found by Holzman and associates. Our prevalence rates are much lower than those of Holzman et al. for schizophrenics and their relatives. Also, unlike Holzman et al. (1984), we found a low rate of tracking dysfunction in probands with affective disorders.

These discrepant findings cannot be explained by our use of a more conservative criterion to identify abnormal eye movements. For this to be the case, our choice of cutoff point should have altered prevalence rates in all groups, but some of our subject groups showed rates of impairment that are similar to those found by the Holzman group. Although we do not know what cutoff point Holzman et al. have used to identify aberrant tracking, we can estimate it by determining the point in our data that would classify the same proportion of schizophrenics as deviant as these investigators have found. Suppose, for example, we were to assume that, on average, 40% of schizo-

phrenics (a low estimate given the reports of Holzman et al.) can be expected to have deviant pursuit. If we identify the cutoff point in the distribution of eye tracking scores for the MAP schizophrenics that defines 40% of the sample as deviant and determine the percentage of subjects in other groups who exceed this value (i.e., have poor tracking), 44% of the probands with affective disorder could be classified as abnormal along with 30% of their relatives and 25% of the normal subjects. Thus, in order to classify 40% of schizophrenics as dysfunctional trackers, the rates of poor tracking in other groups would be unacceptably high.

Why our prevalence rates do not match those of Holzman and colleagues is unclear, but probably stems from methodological differences. The findings of Holzman et al. are derived largely from qualitative ratings and subjective criteria. The exact procedure used to make such ratings is unspecified in the literature. In contrast, our prevalence rates are quantitatively based and derived from a cutoff score that was determined empirically. In addition, they were drawn from a broadly representative and large sample of psychotic patients, and, at least for the schizophrenics and their relatives, have been replicated in three samples from across North America.

Finally, it is worth noting that, despite the limitations inherent to EOG technology and the general nature of RMS error as an index of tracking proficiency, our findings indicate that the EOG and RMS error are suitable for the study of oculomotor functioning in psychotic patients. In the investigation of the family with trisomy of chromosome 5 and in the Minnesota–New York extension of the MAP study, EOG and IR recordings produced the same results. Likewise, RMS error and gain produced virtually identical and discriminating results in our studies, whereas the S/N ratio and the tally of anticipatory saccades did not show promise as methods for identifying schizotaxia. The results with regard to the S/N measure are especially intriguing. This measure is mathematically related to RMS error (Lykken et al., 1981). It distinguishes the eye tracking of schizophrenics and their relatives as abnormal, and it is strongly correlated with RMS error in our data sets ($r = -.75$, $n = 178$). Yet, unlike RMS error, it was not a genetically informative measure. These results indicate that not all measures of eye tracking dysfunction have equivalent utility and that empirical investigations must be carried out to determine the properties and usefulness of each.

ACKNOWLEDGMENTS

The preparation of this chapter was supported by National Institute of Mental Health grant MH 44643. I wish to thank Brett Clementz and William Grove for their helpful comments on an earlier version of this chapter.

REFERENCES

Abel, L. A., & Ziegler, A. S. (1988). Smooth pursuit eye movements in schizophrenics—What constitutes quantitative assessment? *Biological Psychiatry, 24,* 747–762.

American Psychiatric Association. (1980). *Diagnostic and statistical manual of mental disorders* (3rd ed.). Washington, DC: American Psychiatric Press, Inc.

Bahill, A. T., Iandolo, M. J., & Troost, B. T. (1980). Smooth pursuit eye movements in response to unpredictable target waveforms. *Vision Research, 20,* 923–931.

Baron, M., Asnis, L., & Gruen, R. (1981). The Schedule for Schizotypal Personalities (SSP): A diagnostic interview for schizotypal features. *Psychiatry Research, 4,* 213–228.

Bartfai, A., Levander, S. E., Nyback, H., Berggren, B. M., & Schalling, D. (1985). Smooth pursuit eye tracking, neuropsychological test performance, and computed tomography in schizophrenia. *Psychiatry Research, 15,* 49–62.

Bassett, A. S., McGillivray, B. C., Jones, B. D., & Panzar, J. T. (1988). Partial trisomy chromosome 5 cosegregating with schizophrenia. *Lancet, 1,* 799–801.

Beiser, M., Fleming, J. A. E., Iacono, W. G., & Lin, T-Y. (1988). Refining the diagnosis of schizophreniform psychosis. *American Journal of Psychiatry, 145,* 695–700.

Beiser, M., Iacono, W. G., & Erickson, D. (1989). Temporal stability in the major mental disorders. In L. N. Robins & J. E. Barrett (Eds.), *The validity of psychiatric diagnosis* (pp. 77–98). New York: Raven Press.

Beiser, M., Waxler-Morrison, N., Iacono, W. G., Lin, T-Y., Fleming, J. A. E., & Husted, J. (1987). A measure of the "sick" label in psychiatric disorder and physical illness. *Social Science and Medicine, 25,* 251–261.

Clementz, B. A., Grove, W. M., Iacono, W. G., & Sweeney, J. A. (1992). Smooth-pursuit eye movement dysfunction and liability for schizophrenia: Implications for genetic modeling. *Journal of Abnormal Psychology, 101,* 117–129.

Clementz, B. A., & Sweeney, J. A. (1990). Is eye movement dysfunction a biological marker for schizophrenia? A methodological review. *Psychological Bulletin, 108,* 77–92.

Clementz, B. A., Sweeney, J. A., Hirt, M., & Haas, G. (1990). Pursuit gain and saccadic intrusions in first-degree relatives of probands with schizophrenia. *Journal of Abnormal Psychology, 99,* 327–335.

Clementz, B. A., Sweeney, J. A., Hirt, M. & Haas, G. (1991). Phenotypic correlations between oculomotor functioning and schizophrenia-related characteristics in the relatives of schizophrenic probands. *Psychophysiology, 28,* 570–578.

Clementz, B. A., Sweeney, J. A., Hirt, M., & Haas, G. (1992). Phenotypic correlations between oculomotor functioning and schizophrenia-related characteristics in relatives of schizophrenic probands. *Psychophysiology, 28,* 570–578.

Cromwell, R. L. (1983). Preemptive thinking and schizophrenia research. In W. D. Spaulding (Ed.), *Nebraska symposium on motivation, 1983* (pp. 1–46). Lincoln: University of Nebraska Press.

Erickson, D. H., Beiser, M., Iacono, W. G., Fleming, J. A. E., & Lin, T-Y. (1989). The role of social relationships in the course of first episode schizophrenia and affective psychosis. *American Journal of Psychiatry, 146,* 1456–1461.

Falconer, D. S. (1989). *Introduction to quantitative genetics* (3rd ed.). New York: Wiley.

Gooding, D. C., Iacono, W. G., Katsanis, J., Beiser, M., & Grove, W. M. (1993). The association between lithium carbonate and smooth pursuit eye tracking among first-episode patients with psychotic effective disorders. *Psychophysiology, 30,* 3–9.

Grove, W. M., Lebow, B. S., Clementz, B. A., Cerri, A., Medus, C., & Iacono, W. G. (1991). Familial prevalence and co-aggregation of schizotypy indicators: A multitrait family study. *Journal of Abnormal Psychology, 100,* 115–121.

Gunderson, J. G., & Siever, L. J. (1985). Relatedness of schizotypal to schizophrenic disorders: Editors' introduction. *Schizophrenia Bulletin, 11,* 532–537.

Holzman, P. S., Kringlen, E., Levy, D. L., & Haberman, S. J. (1980). Deviant eye tracking in twins discordant for psychosis: A replication. *Archives of General Psychiatry, 37,* 627–631.

Holzman, P. S., Kringlen, E., Matthysse, S., Flanagan, S. D., Lipton, R. B., Cramer, G., Levin, S., Lange, K., & Levy, D. L. (1988). A single dominant gene can account for eye tracking dysfunctions and schizophrenia in offspring of discordant twins. *Archives of General Psychiatry, 45,* 641–647.

Holzman, P. S., Proctor, L. R., Levy, D. L., Yasillo, N. J., Meltzer, H. Y., & Hurt, S. W. (1974). Eye tracking dysfunctions in schizophrenic patients and their relatives. *Archives of General Psychiatry, 31,* 143–151.

Holzman, P. S., Solomon, C. M., Levin, S., & Waternaux, C. S. (1984). Pursuit eye movement dysfunctions in schizophrenic patients and their relatives. *Archives of General Psychiatry, 45,* 1140–1141.

Iacono, W. G. (1982). Eye tracking in normal twins. *Behavior Genetics, 12,* 517–526.

Iacono, W. G. (1985). Psychophysiologic markers of psychopathology: A review. *Canadian Psychology, 26,* 96–112.

Iacono, W. G. (1988). Eye movement abnormalities in schizophrenic and affective disorders. In C. W. Johnston & F. J. Pirozzolo (Eds.), *Neuropsychology of eye movements* (pp. 115–145). Hillsdale, NJ: Lawrence Erlbaum.

Iacono, W. G., Bassett, A. S., & Jones, B. D. (1988). Eye tracking dysfunction is associated with partial trisomy of chromosome 5 and schizophrenia. *Archives of General Psychiatry, 45,* 1140–1141.

Iacono, W. G., Bassett, A. S., & Jones, B. D. (1989). Eye tracking dysfunction is associated with partial trisomy of chromosome 5 and schizophrenia: In reply. *Archives of General Psychiatry, 46,* 757–758.

Iacono, W. G., & Beiser, M. (1989). Age of onset, temporal stability, and eighteen-month course of first episode psychosis. In D. Cicchetti (Ed.), *The emergence of a discipline: Rochester Symposium on Developmental Psychopathology* (Vol. 1, pp. 221–260). Hillsdale, NJ: Lawrence Erlbaum.

Iacono, W. G., & Clementz, B. A. (1993). A strategy for elucidating genetic influences on complex psychopathological syndromes

(with specific reference to oculamotor functioning and schizophrenia). In L. J. Chapman, J. P. Chapman, & D. C. Fowles (Eds.), *Progress in experimental personality and psychopathology research.* (Vol. 16, pp. 11–65). New York: Springer.

Iacono, W. G., & Ficken, J. (1989). Psychophysiological research strategies. In G. Turpin (Ed.), *Handbook of clinical psychophysiology* (pp. 45–70). London: John Wiley & Sons.

Iacono, W. G., & Koenig, W. G. R. (1983). Features that distinguish schizophrenic, affective disorder, and normal smooth-pursuit eye tracking. *Journal of Abnormal Psychology, 92,* 29–41.

Iacono, W. G., & Lykken, D. T. (1979a). Electro-oculographic recording and scoring of smooth-pursuit and saccadic eye tracking: A parametric study using monozygotic twins. *Psychophysiology, 16,* 94–107.

Iacono, W. G., & Lykken, D. T. (1979b). Eye tracking and psychopathology: New procedures applied to a sample of normal monozygotic twins. *Archives of General Psychiatry, 36,* 1361–1369.

Iacono, W. G., & Lykken, D. T. (1981). Two-year retest stability of eye tracking performance and a comparison of electro-oculographic and infrared recording techniques: Evidence for EEG in the electro-oculogram. *Psychophysiology, 18,* 49–55.

Iacono, W. G., Moreau, M., Beiser, M., Fleming, J. A. E., & Lin, T-Y. (1992). Smooth pursuit eye tracking in first-episode psychotic patients and their relatives. *Journal of Abnormal Psychology, 101,* 104–116.

Iacono, W. G., Peloquin, L. J., Lumry, A. E., Valentine, R. H., & Tuason, V. B. (1982). Eye tracking in patients with unipolar and bipolar affective disorders in remission. *Journal of Abnormal Psychology, 91,* 35–44.

Iacono, W. G., Smith, G. N., Moreau, M., Beiser, M., Fleming, J. A. E., Lin, T-Y., & Flak, B. (1988). Ventricular and sulcal size at the onset of psychosis. *American Journal of Psychiatry, 145,* 695–700.

Iacono, W. G., Tuason, V. B., & Johnson, R. A. (1981). Dissociation of smooth-pursuit and saccadic eye tracking in remitted schizophrenics. *Archives of General Psychiatry, 38,* 991–996.

Katsanis, J., & Iacono, W. G. (1989). Association of left-handedness with ventricular size and neuropsychological performance in schizophrenia. *American Journal of Psychiatry, 146,* 1056–1058.

Katsanis, J., & Iacono, W. G. (1991). Clinical, neuropsychological, and brain structural correlates of smooth-pursuit eye tracking performance in chronic schizophrenia. *Journal of Abnormal Psychology, 100,* 526–534.

Katsanis, J., Iacono, W. G., & Beiser, M. (1990). Anhedonic and perceptual aberration in first-episode psychotic patients and their relatives. *Journal of Abnormal Psychology, 99,* 202–206.

Katsanis, J., Iacono, W. G., Beiser, M., & Lacey, L. (1992). Clinical correlates of anhedonia and perceptual aberration in first-episode psychotic patients. *Journal of Abnormal Psychology, 99,* 202–206.

Kendler, K. S. (1985). Diagnostic approaches to schizotypal personality disorder: A historical perspective. *Schizophrenia Bulletin, 11,* 538–553.

Kuechenmeister, C. A., Linton, P. H., Mueller, T. V., & White, H. B. (1977). Eye tracking in relation to age, sex, and illness. *Archives of General Psychiatry, 34,* 578–599.

Levin, S. (1984). Frontal lobe dysfunctions in schizophrenia—I. Eye movement impairments. *Journal of Psychiatric Research, 18,* 27–55.

Levy, D. L., Dorus, E., Shaughnessy, R., Yasillo, N. J., Pandey, G. N., Janicak, P. G., Gibbons, R. D., Gaviria, M., & Davis, J. M. (1985). Pharmacologic evidence for specificity of pursuit to schizophrenia: Lithium carbonate associated with abnormal pursuit. *Archives of General Psychiatry, 42,* 335–341.

Levy, D. L., Yasillo, N. J., Dorus, E., Shaughnessy, R., Gibbons, R. D., Peterson, J., Janicak, P. G., Gaviria, M., & Davis, J. M. (1983). Relatives of unipolar and bipolar patients have normal pursuit. *Psychiatry Research, 10,* 285–293.

Lindsey, D. T., Holzman, P. S., Haberman, S., & Yasillo, N. J. (1978). Smooth-pursuit eye movements: A comparison of two measurement techniques for studying schizophrenia. *Journal of Abnormal Psychology, 87,* 491–496.

Lipton, R. B., Levin, S., & Holzman, P. S. (1980). Horizontal and vertical pursuit eye movements, the oculocephalic reflex, and the functional psychoses. *Psychiatry Research, 3,* 193–203.

Lykken, D. T., Iacono, W. G., & Lykken, J. D. (1981). Measuring deviant eye tracking. *Schizophrenia Bulletin, 7,* 204–205.

MacLean, C. J., Morton, N. E., Elston, R. C., & Yee, S. (1976). Skewness in commingling distributions. *Biometrics, 32,* 695–699.

Mather, J. A. (1985). Eye movements of teenage children of schizophrenics: A possible inherited marker of susceptibility to the disease. *Journal of Psychiatric Research, 19,* 523–532.

Matthysse, S., Holzman, P. S., & Lange, K. (1986). The genetic transmission of schizophrenia: Application of Mendelian latent structure analysis to eye tracking dysfunctions in schizophrenia and affective disorder. *Journal of Psychiatric Research, 20,* 57–76.

McGue, M., Gerrard, J. W., Lebowitz, M. D., & Rao, D. C. (1989). Commingling in the distributions of immunoglobin levels. *Human Heredity, 39,* 196–201.

McGue, M., & Gottesman, I. I. (1989). A single dominant gene still cannot account for the transmission of schizophrenia. *Archives of General Psychiatry, 46,* 478–479.

McGuffin, P., Sargeant, M., Hett, G., Tidmarsh, S., Whartler, S., & Marchbanks, R. M. (1990). Exclusion of a schizophrenic susceptibility gene from the chromosome 5q11-q13 region: New data and a reanalysis of previous reports. *American Journal of Human Genetics, 47,* 524–535.

Meehl, P. E. (1962). Schizotaxia, schizotypy, schizophrenia. *American Psychologist, 17,* 827–838.

Meehl, P. E. (1989). Schizotaxia revisited. *Archives of General Psychiatry, 46,* 935–944.

Meehl, P. E. (1990). Toward an integrated theory of schizotaxia, schizotypy, and schizophrenia. *Journal of Personality Disorders, 4,* 1–99.

Ross, D. E., Ochs, A. L., Hill, M. R., Goldberg, S. C., Pandurangi, A. K., & Winfrey, C. J. (1988). Erratic eye tracking in schizophrenic patients as revealed by high resolution techniques. *Biological Psychiatry, 24,* 675–688.

Sartorius, N., Jablensky, A., Korten, A., Ernberg, G., Anker, M., Cooper, J. E., & Day, R. (1986). Early manifestations and first-contact incidence of schizophrenia in different cultures. *Psychological Medicine, 16,* 909–928.

Shagass, C., Amadeo, M., & Overton, D. A. (1974). Eye-tracking performance in psychiatric patients. *Biological Psychiatry, 9,* 245–260.

Sherrington, R., Brynjolfsson, J., Petursson, H., Potter, M., Dudleston, K., Barraclough, B., Wasmuth, J., Dobbs, M., & Gurling, H. (1988). Localization of a susceptibility locus for schizophrenia on chromosome 5. *Nature, 336,* 164–167.

Siever, L. J., Coursey, R. D., Alterman, I. S., Buchsbaum, M. S., & Murphy, D. L. (1982). Psychological and physiological correlates of variation in smooth pursuit eye movements. In E. Usdin & I. Hanin (Eds.), *Biological markers in psychiatry and neurology* (pp. 359–370). Elmsford, NY: Pergamon.

Siever, L. J., Coursey, R. D., Alterman, I. S., Buchsbaum, M. S., & Murphy, D. L. (1984).

Impaired smooth pursuit eye movement: Vulnerability marker for schizotypal personality disorder in a normal volunteer population. *American Journal of Psychiatry, 141*, 1560–1566.

Siever, L. J., Coursey, R. D., Alterman, I. S., Zahn, T., Brody, L., Bernad, P., Buchsbaum, M., Lake, C. R., & Murphy, D. L. (1989). Clinical, psychophysiological, and neurological characteristics of volunteers with impaired smooth pursuit eye movements. *Biological Psychiatry, 26*, 35–51.

Siever, L. J., Keefe, R., Bernstein, D. P., Cocavo, E. F., Klar, H. M., Zemishlany, Z., Peterson, A. E., Davidson, M., Mahon, T., Horvath, T. & Mohr, R. (1990). Eye tracking impairment in clinically identified patients with schizotypal disorder. *American Journal of Psychiatry, 147*, 740–745.

Smith, G. N., Iacono, W. G., Moreau, M., Tallman, K., Beiser, M., & Flak, B. (1988). Choice of comparison group and computerized tomography findings in schizophrenia. *British Journal of Psychiatry, 153*, 667–674.

Spitzer, R. L., Endicott, J., & Robins, E. (1978). *Research diagnostic criteria (RDC) for a select group of functional disorders* (3rd ed). New York: Biometrics Research Department, New York State Psychiatric Institute.

Whicker, L., Abel, L. A., & Dell'Osso, L. F. (1985). Smooth pursuit eye movements in the parents of schizophrenics. *Neuro-ophthalmology, 5*, 1–8.

Wing, J. K., Cooper, J. E., & Sartorius, N. (1974). *The measurement and classification of psychiatric symptoms*. New York: Cambridge University Press.

7

Schizotaxia and Sensory Gating

ROBERT FREEDMAN
MERILYNE WALDO
LAWRENCE E. ADLER
HERBERT NAGAMOTO
ELLEN CAWTHRA
ALICE MADISON
LEE HOFFER
PAULA BICKFORD-WIMER

The word "schizotaxia" was coined by Paul Meehl in a landmark address to the American Psychological Association (Meehl, 1962). It is a concept closely tied to attempts to understand the genetic basis of schizophrenia. Meehl believed that his colleagues were ignoring important findings on the familial clustering of schizophrenia. He was particularly impressed with the concordance for schizophrenia in monozygotic twins. The high concordance rate led him to conclude that there is a significant genetic component to the illness. The fact that the concordance is not 100% led him to propose that the genes must not code for schizophrenia itself, but rather for some predisposing element that he termed "schizotaxia." He speculated that, at the neurobiological level, this schizotaxia might involve an increased sensitivity of neurons to their synaptic inputs. This theory was based on extensive psychophysiological work showing that schizophrenics are overly sensitive to sensory stimulation (Venables, 1964).

Our work is an attempt to find evidence for the neurobiological basis of schizotaxia. The research efforts have involved studies of schizophrenic patients and their rela-

tives, as well as studies in animal models. Like Meehl, we have hypothesized that there is a defect in the regulation of neuronal responsiveness to synaptic inputs. Because many synaptic pathways transmit sensory information, this regulation of responsiveness might be demonstrated as a defect in the regulation or gating of response to sensory input.

SENSORY GATING IN SCHIZOPHRENIA

A classical method for the assessment of the inhibitory gating function of neuronal circuits is a conditioning–testing paradigm. In this paradigm, stimuli are presented in pairs. The first or conditioning stimulus has two functions. First, it excites the neuronal population under study, which allows the investigator to measure the magnitude of the neurons' initial excitatory response. Second, it activates gating mechanisms, which alter the response to subsequent stimuli. The subsequent or test stimulus is then presented. Change in the magnitude of the response that it evokes is putative evidence for the activity of a gating mechanism. In most cases, repeated stimuli produce smaller neuronal responses. These gating mechanisms allow the brain to alter its sensitivity to stimuli. For example, the brain can be quite alert to the occurrence of some stimuli, such as a baby crying, while tuning out others, such as the hum from an air conditioner. Generally, alertness is increased at the expense of sharpness of discrimination. For example, if you are intently listening for burglars, every creak in the house can sound like a window being forced open.

Schizophrenics describe problems with these sorts of discriminations. They recount how they frequently mistake the squealing of tires in traffic for a person screaming. They are unable to tune into one conversation at large gatherings while ignoring others. They are bothered by background noises, such as the sounds from refrigerators. Venables (1964) calls these problems a defect in the involuntary mechanisms of attention. As one of our patients put it: "Everything has to have my attention."

To understand the neuronal basis of this problem, we used the conditioning–testing paradigm to study the response of schizophrenic patients to auditory stimuli. The stimuli were clicks, and the responses were recorded as averaged evoked potentials using electroencephalographic techniques. The greatest differences between schizophrenics and normal subjects were seen with the P50 wave of the auditory evoked potential, when the stimuli were presented 0.5 seconds apart. As shown in Figure 7.1, normal subjects suppressed most of the P50 response to the second stimulus. Schizophrenic subjects had a normal P50 response to the first stimulus but showed absent or diminished suppression of the P50 response to the second stimulus. Diminished suppression of P50 was present in schizophrenic patients regardless of their clinical status (i.e., whether they were acutely psychotic or in relative remission). It was also not affected by medication (Adler et al., 1982, 1990). Diminished suppression of the

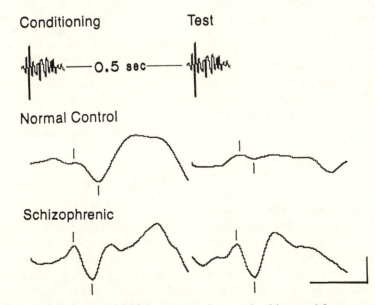

Figure 7.1. Auditory evoked potentials from a normal control subject and from a patient with schizophrenia. The top line shows the auditory stimuli, generated by 0.04-ms pulses, with a peak intensity of 90 dB SPL. The computer-generated tic below each evoked potential tracing marks the P50 wave, whose amplitude the computer algorithim measures relative to the preceding negativity shown by the tic above each tracing. The normal control subject demonstrated suppression of the P50 wave in the conditioning–testing paradigm, whereas the schizophrenic subject, who was on neuroleptic medication and in clinical remission, failed to suppress the response to the test stimulus. The vertical calibration is 2.5 μV, positive down, and the horizontal is 50 ms.

auditory evoked response in the conditioning–testing paradigm would seem to be an electrophysiological manifestation of a defect in sensory gating.

SENSORY GATING DEFECTS IN RELATIVES OF SCHIZOPHRENICS

Using the same recording techniques, we found nonsuppression in approximately half of the first-degree relatives of schizophrenics. The suppression was measured as the ratio of the amplitude of the test response to the conditioning response. A ratio of up to 50%—that is, a test amplitude equal to less than half the conditioning amplitude—was within the 95% confidence interval range of the normal population. Most of the schizophrenics exceeded this value. The relatives appeared to have a bimodal distribution, with one group in the normal range and the other in the range expected for the schizophrenics (Siegel, Waldo, Mizner, Adler, & Freedman, 1984) (Figure 7.2).

Except for schizophrenia, none of the family members with sensory gating defects have had any other major psychiatric disorder. Some of the relatives with defects have been characterized as schizotypal by clinicians or other family members, but they have rarely fulfilled the criteria of the *Diagnostic and Statistical Manual of Mental Disorders*, third edition, revised (American Psychiatric Association, 1987) for schizotypal personality disorder. Many of the relatives were given the Minnesota Multiphasic Personality Inventory. Compared to relatives with normal evoked potentials, relatives with sensory gating defects ranked higher on the Sc subscale, but they were still well within the normal range. Generally, only one parent and half the siblings of the schizophrenic index case had sensory gating defects. The parent with the defect was the one more likely to have a family history of schizophrenia. These findings about schizophrenics and their families suggest that poor suppression of P50 in the conditioning–testing paradigm could be a phenotypic manifestation of a genetically transmitted characteristic that is at least

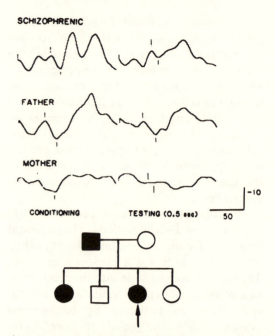

Figure 7.2. Familial distribution of sensory gating deficits in the family of a schizophrenic patient. The traces at the top show the auditory evoked potentials from a schizophrenic patient and her father and mother, recorded as described in Figure 7.1. Like the patient, her father failed to suppress the P50 response to the second stimulus. The mother showed normal suppression. In the genogram below, the father is therefore coded black, as is the patient (*arrow*). The oldest sibling also failed to suppress the response to the second stimulus. The mother and two other siblings are coded white to indicate normal sensory gating.

part of the schizotaxia hypothesized by Meehl.

ANIMAL MODELS OF SENSORY GATING AND ITS DEFECTS

Further understanding of schizotaxia would seem to depend on more precise knowledge of the neurobiology of the sensory gating deficit. Auditory evoked potentials recorded from the skull surface cannot directly identify neuronal mechanisms that are malfunctional in schizophrenia, yet more invasive recording is not generally possible in human subjects. It seemed to us that further progress in the study of schizotaxia might come from modeling one of the defects in a laboratory animal, where its neurobiology could be understood in more detail. There have been other attempts to do such modeling, principally by Braff and Geyer and their colleagues (Braff et al., 1978; Swerdlow, Braff, Geyer, & Koob, 1986). In their paradigm, schizophrenic patients or normal subjects are exposed to two tones. The first tone is a low-volume warning tone, which is followed several hundred milliseconds later by a loud tone. By itself, the loud tone would cause the subject to startle, with contraction of the muscles of the head and neck. However, most normal subjects suppress the startle response when the low-volume tone precedes the louder tone; this behavior is called prepulse inhibition. Schizophrenics fail to show such prepulse inhibition. This defect and the diminished gating of P50 in the conditioning–testing paradigm would seem to be similar. Both paradigms are suitable for animal modeling because they involve very simple responses that do not require language or complex motor responses.

Previous research on animal modeling of schizophrenia has concentrated primarily on psychotomimetic drugs, drugs that cause psychoses in humans that resemble schizophrenia, and antipsychotic drugs, drugs that ameliorate schizophrenia. Studies of both classes of drugs have pointed to the catecholamines dopamine and norepinephrine as being involved in schizophrenia. However, studies of dopamine and norepinephrine metabolism in schizophrenic subjects have shown that these neurotransmitters are more likely to be responsible for acute psychotic episodes than for the chronic features of the illness, at least as judged by the changes in the levels of metabolites during various periods of illness (Pickar et al., 1984). Abnormalities in catecholamine metabolism do not seem to account for the more chronic features of schizophrenia.

Startle is mediated by neurons in the nuclei pontis oralis and pontis caudalis of the brainstem reticular formation (Davis, Gendleman, Tischler, & Gendleman, 1982). These neurons are classically known to exhibit rapidly habituating responses (i.e., they show diminshed response to repeated stimuli). However, prepulse inhibition of startle may also involve forebrain control of this mechanism. Several limbic structures have been proposed to provide this modulation. Braff et al. (1978) have been most interested in the nucleus accumbens, in the ventral basal forebrain. They have shown that drugs such as apomorphine, which mimics dopaminergic neurotransmission in the nucleus accumbens, can diminish prepulse inhibition of startle.

The relationship between the reticular formation and the limbic system interested us, and our efforts began with attempts to model the P50 wave and its behavior in the conditioning–testing paradigm. We found that a wave recorded at the skull surface in the rat, N40, also exhibited suppression in the conditioning–testing paradigm. Depth recording with macroelectrodes showed that the wave orginated in the hippocampus, in the areas known as CA3 and CA4. Microelectrode recording demonstrated that pyramidal neurons in CA3 responded to auditory stimuli and that this response was gated in a conditioning–testing paradigm (Adler, Rose, & Freedman, 1986; Bickford-Wimer et al., 1990).

Gating of the response to repeated auditory stimuli has been demonstrated in the hippocampus by other workers (Vinogradova, 1975). There are two major inputs to the hippocampal formation (Figure 7.3). One is from the entorhinal cortex, which integrates sensory information from many different areas. In the rat, the entorhinal cortex receives a major projection from the medial geniculate. In primates, there are major projections to the entorhinal cortex from the superior temporal gyrus, a cortical area that itself receives information from many sensory cortical areas, including the auditory cortex. Thus, the entorhinal cortex appears to carry specific sensory information to the hippocampus. The second major input is quite different—the cholinergic input from the medial septal nucleus. This input projects directly to CA3 and CA4, as well as to other parts of the hippocampus. Interruption of this pathway by section of the fornix, the major fiber bundle between the

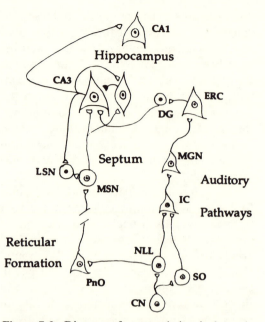

Figure 7.3. Diagram of neuronal circuits hypothesized to be involved in the gating of the P50 response. The hippocampus includes the CA1 and CA3 pyramidal areas of Ammon's horn, the dentate granule cell (GC), and the entorhinal cortex (ERC). For CA3, an inhibitory basket neuron is also shown; its synapse is colored black. The auditory pathways connect to this area through a chain of neurons, beginning with the cochlear nucleus (CN) and progressing through the superior olive (SO), inferior colliculus (IC), and medial geniculate nucleus (MGN). The nucleus of the lateral lemniscus (NLL) also sends auditory information to the reticular formation, at the level of the pontine nucleus oralis (PnO). Through unknown pathways, the reticular neurons activate the medial septal neurons (MSN) in the septum, which are also part of an excitatory feedback loop from the lateral septal nucleus (LSN). The reticular formation responds only to the conditioning stimulus. The result may be that the septal neurons excite the CA3 pyramidal neurons, so that the response to the activity coming through the ERC is enhanced. The inhibitory basket cells of CA3 are also activated, however, so that response to a subsequent stimulus is suppressed because the CA3 pyramidal cells are now inhibited. Thus, the reticuloseptal input to the hippocampus subserves the function of sensory gating.

septum and the hippocampus, causes the hippocampus to lose its gated response to repeated stimuli. The septum is thought to carry information from the brainstem to the hippocampus. The complete neuronal cir-

cuit is unknown, even in laboratory animals. Some anatomists have described direct pathways from the brainstem to the septum, whereas others favor relays through the hypothalamus or other areas. It is likely, however, that the same area of the brainstem involved in startle is also responsible for the regulation of hippocampal activity in the septum. We have found that pontine reticular formation neurons show gated response to auditory stimuli, and that stimulation in this area can suppress subsequent response to test pulses of auditory stimuli (Bickford-Wimer & Freedman, 1989).

Can the animal model be used to direct further clinical inquiries? To attempt to verify the model, we performed several clinical investigations. For example, we recorded from the hippocampal gyrus in neurosurgical patients using subdural electrodes implanted as part of their evaluation for temporal lobe epilepsy. We found that an evoked response could be recorded in this area that was much larger than the response recorded at the skull surface. Furthermore, the wave changed from positive to negative as the recording site was moved across the hippocampal gyrus. This inversion of polarity is consistent with the origin of the P50 wave in the hippocampus (Freedman, 1991).

We also have been interested in the effects of cholinergic drugs in schizophrenia, because acetylcholine is a major neurotransmitter in the pathway from the medial septal nucleus to the hippocampus. Anticholinergic drugs at high doses are known to produce psychotic phenomena, particularly hallucinations and delusions. Schizophrenics are frequently heavy smokers and have sometimes reported to us that they find nicotine the most helpful drug for their psychosis. Because nicotine acts primarily through cholinergic receptors, this effect may suggest an attempt at self-medication. Physostigmine, a drug that blocks the destruction of acetylcholine by the enzyme acetylcholinesterase, sometimes has been reported to have an antipsychotic effect in both mania and schizophrenia.

HOW CAN THE MODEL OF SCHIZOTAXIA BE VERIFIED?

Theories of human brain function based on animal models have much heuristic value, but verification of the details of their correspondence to actual pathophysiological mechanisms is inherently difficult. That difficulty is not surprising, because it is the inherent problems in working with human brains that caused the foray into animal models in the first place. The most practical methods for verification would seem to involve a genetic approach, based on the preliminary evidence that schizotaxia may be inherited.

If schizotaxia could be reliably identified, its presence could be compared to the presence of genetic markers from various chromosomal locations, taking advantage of the existence of maps of these markers, most of which are polymorphisms (i.e., regions of DNA that often differ between unrelated individuals). If schizotaxia cosegregates with one of these genetic polymorphisms in the families of schizophrenics, there is further evidence that it is indeed an inherited trait. In favorable cases, the genetic map locations can lead to the identification of the actual aberrant gene. If this gene coded for some component within the neurobiological pathway from brainstem to limbic forebrain, there would be confirmatory evidence for the neurobiological features of the hypothesis as well.

This approach is sometimes called "reverse genetics." Usually genetic approaches can be undertaken only if the phenotype of the aberrant gene is fully understood at the biochemical level (i.e., which amino acid in the protein is incorrect). Then, the aberrant nucleotide sequence is deduced and the gene is searched out. Here, the protein identity is completely unknown. If the gene is to be identified, it will be only because it is near a polymorphic marker that happens to cosegregate with it. It should be pointed out that this is not a foolproof technique, primarily because of its dependence on chance cosegregation of the marker and the phenotype. Large families are needed, so that many segregations can be observed. Even with large families, which are rare for schizophrenic people, it is necessary to pool data from many families. If schizophrenia is not a homogeneous disease, however, so that there are different genes responsible for schizotaxia in different families, data from one family, if added to data from another family, could cause confusion. There may also be chance cosegregations, in which a marker codistributes, even though there is no actual linkage. Because the technique is based on a statistical association rather than a causal linkage, such artifacts are possible. This may be the explanation for problems associated with failure to confirm the chromosome 5 location for schizophrenia (Kennedy et al., 1988; Sherrington et al., 1988).

HOW DOES SCHIZOTAXY ALTER BRAIN FUNCTION?

Although genetic confirmation for a particular form of schizotaxia may not occur in the near future, it may still be worthwhile to think about the implications of schizotaxia, as we currently understand it, for brain function. Although not as definitive a test as genetic identification, a definition of schizotaxia would seem to carry more weight if it accounted for all the known facts about schizophrenia and perhaps predicted some new ones. Our definition started with a deficit in sensory gating and moved to a putative identification of the pathway between the pontine reticular formation and the hippocampus as the site of the deficit. We give as examples several ways in which the definition can be extended to encompass other phenomena.

One way to extend the definition is to consider the purpose of sensory gating and how its disruption would alter other behaviors. The CA3 neurons of the hippocampus project to several areas, but the principal projection is to CA1. CA1 is primarily concerned with short-term or working memory. It is sometimes said that the hippocampus forms a cognitive map, so that an individual can remember where he or she is, as well as other aspects of the present context. Very small lesions in CA1 are sufficient to disrupt this memory function entirely, and, in addition, all long-term memory functions are also lost, except perhaps for the retrieval of some old memories (Butters & Miliotis, 1985). Why are sensory gating and memory connected? One possibility is that the memory capability is easily overloaded. To avoid memorizing everything, sensory gating is needed to filter out repetitive information that is less likely to be of interest. Thus, background noise such as the refrigerator or traffic or even other people's conversation does not have to enter memory.

Failure of the gating system in CA3 might disrupt both long- and short-term memories. The intrusion of new information into CA1 might disrupt its ability to keep track of the present context, perhaps leading to the distraction and disorientation noted in acutely psychotic individuals. Intrusion of new material might also lead to the formation of aberrant memories, formed on misconstrued notions of the present. These sorts of problems can also be seen in schizophrenics, who are frequently plagued by memories of past events that seem delusional. For example, one of our patients told us that a teacher had put a curse on him in a foreign tongue. He vividly remembered her mumbling something that he could not quite understand. He is now convinced that it was a curse.

Our most vivid memories are thought to be key features of our personality. If they are formed from misperceived information, they may become a nidus for future psychopathology. Psychoanalysis, for example, holds that the witnessing of a primal scene, intercourse between father and mother, which cannot be fully comprehended by the child, can be a nidus for future neurosis in the adult (Tobin, Offenkrantz, & Freedman, 1978). Studies of post-traumatic stress disorder point to a similar problem with information overload during the trauma, so that its memories can take years to comprehend and accept. Not infrequently, a trip back to the battlefield is necessary to organize all the memories. In schizophrenia, the memo-

ries often seem to arise from misunderstanding a seemingly ordinary interaction. Because schizotaxia is thought to be a genetically determined defect, the problem is more chronic than post-traumatic stress disorder and more global than the psychosexual conflict of neurosis. Thus, more aspects of the personality may be disrupted. Although schizophrenic patients may make impressive gains in psychotherapy by recalling some early memories and working through their meaning, the disease process that created them may still be active, so that new misunderstandings occur as well. It is our experience that therapeutic relationships with schizophrenics frequently end after several years with a jumble of vivid memories about the therapist, some of which may be misperceptions. Only a few patients seem to be able to learn to sort through and correct a significant portion of their aberrant and delusional memories.

What about the schizotaxic relatives who are not delusional? They apparently share the gating deficit but not the psychosis. Monozygotic twins who are discordant for schizophrenia are of special value for the assessment of the genetic determinism of psychopathology, because they share all genetic factors. Therefore, differences between them would seem to indicate nongenetic factors that influence the expression of schizotaxia as schizophrenia. One such factor is the size of the anterior hippocampus, which is smaller in the twin who has schizophrenia (Suddath, Harrison, Torrey, Casanova, & Weinberger, 1990). We have made a similar finding in sibling pairs that share the P50 gating abnormality. The sibling with schizophrenia has a smaller anterior hippocampus. These findings are consistent with Meehl's (1962) hypothesis that schizotaxia might result in schizophrenia, if there were additional problems in brain function. The monozygotic twin study suggests that the additional problem may not be genetically based. Perinatal problems, such as anoxia during delivery or in utero viral infections, have been suggested as causal factors. Such insults might usually cause variations in intelligence but not specifically cause psychosis, except in the presence of genetically determined schizotaxia.

Damage in the hippocampus has been localized to a number of sites, including Ammon's horn (CA1 through CA3), the dentate hilus (CA4), and the parahippocampal gyrus (Jeste & Lohr, 1989). The functional significance of differences between schizophrenics and their clinically unaffected siblings in these brain areas may best be considered in interaction with the deficit in sensory gating. If the hippocampus were normal, as in the unaffected siblings with gating deficits, the increased information flow might be tolerable because CA1 would be able to process it. New material might not be well screened, but it might at least be correctly identified and hence not as likely to give rise to an aberrant memory. Thus, the trait would not be disabling.

Relatives of schizophrenics, including their children, have an increased risk of schizophrenia, but they have also been anecdotally noted to include supernormal individuals as well. Creativity has been the most frequently noted trait. The presence of supernormal individuals may simply result from a selection process: a group that did not become schizophrenic would be skewed toward persons with normal or better than normal brain function. It is also possible that sensory gating may be a protective factor that prevents the hippocampus from being overwhelmed but may also keep it from occasionally obtaining some interesting information. A person without this sensory gating mechanism might be particularly good at picking up extraneous information that others would automatically filter out. Whether or not this extraneous information is the basis of creativity is not easy to determine, but one aspect of creativity is often the juxtaposition of hithertofore unrelated ideas. There is only one empirical test of the idea that sensory gating deficits are advantageous. Cromwell reported that relatives of schizophrenics with a similar sensory gating deficit (if inferred from redundancy deficit) had a significantly higher socioeconomic status than their siblings without the gating deficit (De Amicis, Wagstaff, & Cromwell, 1986).

Thus, this elaboration on the function of the sensory gating mechanisms led us to several new hypotheses: first, a hypothesis of psychosis as a disorder of memory and, second, a hypothesis of why schizotaxia becomes schizophrenia in only some of the individuals of a particular family. There are a number of other ways to elaborate on the biology of schizotaxia. We have suggested that the pathway from brainstem to hippocampus is malfunctional. The discussion above centered on the psychological consequences of that malfunction. We could also ask a series of questions about its biology. The brain does not generally reserve a specific set of genes to form one neuronal pathway. Rather, the biology is repeated all over the brain, and sometimes even outside the brain, in the peripheral nervous system. Therefore, we might also ask if we can make predictions about other biological features of schizophrenics or their relatives. The obvious problem with such an approach is that one has first to identify a particular feature and then be able to study it in a large number of schizophrenics and their relatives. The advantage of the approach is that it potentially makes use of the large body of information on the neurobiology of the brain that has been acquired by basic scientists.

For example, the ventral septohippocampal pathway has a number of unusual features. Unlike most cholinergic pathways, it is relatively poor in muscarinic receptors, particularly in humans (Zilles, 1988). Ganglionic-type cholinergic receptors are also underrepresented (Wada et al., 1989). In contrast, cholinergic receptors that bind the snake venom α-bungarotoxin are very common in this region (Clarke, Schwartz, Paul, Pert, & Pert, 1985). This type of cholinergic receptor thus shares pharmacological properties with the neuromuscular junction. A second unusual feature is that the septohippocampal pathway is dependent on nerve growth factor, even in adults. Most growth factors are primarily active during the early development of the nervous system. However, the hippocampus secretes nerve growth factor throughout adult life (Ayer-LeLeivre, Olson, Ebendahl, Seiger, & Persson, 1988). The septal neurons have receptors for nerve growth factor and, if they are not in contact with nerve growth factor, they die. Thus, after lesion of the septohippocampal pathway, the septal neurons soon disappear unless a new source of nerve growth factor is provided (either by an infusion or by implantation of cells that can make the factor). Few other neurons in the brain are similarly dependent on a constant supply of a growth factor.

These two bits of biological information might lead to further identification of the schizotaxic factor. For example, one might look at the function of other α-bungarotoxin–sensitive sites. The neuromuscular junction is one such site. Neuromuscular problems long have been described in schizophrenia research. Chemical, anatomical, and electrophysiological deficits all have been described. One particular abnormality involves an apparent decrease in the number of alpha motor neurons innervating the muscle. This abnormality is seen in the relatives of patients as well (Meltzer, 1976). A second type of neuromuscular abnormality has been demonstrated functionally. Schizophrenics have diminished ability to make smooth ocular pursuit movements as they follow a predictable slow-moving target such as a pendulum. This deficit is also shared by their relatives (Holzman et al., 1974). Although a defect in a central mechanism of visual attention is one of the postulated mechanisms for the diminished control of eye movements, a peripheral deficit in the neuromuscular junction is also possible.

Nerve growth factor also has a biology that encompasses several aspects of both the peripheral and the central nervous system. Because the gene for nerve growth factor has been identified and sequenced, there are other means available to test hypotheses about its role. For example, measurement of nerve growth factor messenger RNA levels is possible in brain tissue obtained at autopsy. The sequence of nerve growth factor can be determined, to see if there are alterations in the genetic code for this important

growth factor. DNA for sequencing this particular gene can be obtained readily from white blood cells. The intensive examination of a single gene is sometimes called the candidate gene approach, because a single gene is targeted for investigation. By comparison, the linkage mapping approach treats all areas of the genome equally. Each approach has its advantage and its pitfalls. The advantage of the candidate gene approach is that the genetic abnormalities are identified directly rather than by statistical association. Thus, large families are not needed. Furthermore, the abnormality can exist in only a small percentage of patients. Identification of a genetic abnormality that causes schizophrenia in only a small proportion of patients is difficult with linkage, but quite feasible for the candidate gene approach. The disadvantage is that one must already know a great deal about the gene in question. Generally, it must already have been isolated and its genetic code sequenced. The choice of candidate is critical. If a wrong candidate is chosen, such as a growth factor rather than its receptor, the candidate gene method would not give positive information. Even negative information might be valuable, however, given the definitive nature of gene sequencing. If one knew for certain that a particular coding sequence were normal for a protein of biological importance, such as nerve growth factor, one could move on to new directions. This level of certainty is rarely found in clinical research.

THE FUTURE OF SCHIZOTAXIA

The future is already on us, in the sense that modern tools of molecular biology such as linkage mapping and gene sequencing are already in use to try to define the neurobiological basis of the concept put forth by Meehl almost three decades ago. It is remarkable that the concept of schizotaxia should have such far-reaching consequences.

Now that the research has been set in motion, it might be useful to ask if the concept has been fully exploited or, conversely, if it has been overextended. It would seem that the intensive study of the relatives of schizophrenics, with an eye to identifying schizotaxic biological features, has been successful. What has been lacking is an attempt to integrate the findings. We have too few data on the cosegregation of the various disorders that have been noted in the relatives of schizophrenics. It will be important to note if they are all pleitrophic manifestations of the same trait or if different traits are present in the families, all or most of which must be inherited to produce schizophrenia. Some evidence favors the single-gene model, whereas other evidence favors multigenic models in which a number of abnormal genes are passed through the family. In the latter type of model, when a particular family member reaches a threshold of genetic abnormalities, schizophrenia is expressed. The multigenic model represents the most serious challenge to the concept of a single schizotaxic factor.

The concept of studying relatives, even in the absence of clinical illness, has immense appeal. They are frequently better motivated than, or at least not as negativistic, as their schizophrenic relative. There are no nonspecific effects of brain damage or medication exposure to worry about. Drug abuse is less common. There is rarely danger of precipitating an exacerbation of psychosis. Even if a number of genes are necessary to produce schizophrenia, it would still seem advantageous to be able to study one at a time in a relative. The problem is how to know which relatives carry genes for schizotaxia. The monozygotic twins discordant for schizophrenia provide one source, albeit rare. The fact that none of their genes differ from those of their schizophrenic relative limits their usefulness for some studies, particularly linkage, where genetic differences are as important as genetic similarities. The evoked potential and other tests may seem too crude to support technologically sophisticated genetic and neurobiological investigations, but there may also be a bootstrap effect, in which the phenotype is adequate to allow enough biological and genetic analysis to improve the definition of the phenotype.

The concept of schizotaxia also seems to be underexploited for prevention research. Regardless of the mode of inheritance that is eventually found for schizophrenia, it is clear that the genes are much more widespread in the families of schizophrenics than the illness itself. The prevention of brain injury in this group would seem to be an excellent way to decrease the incidence of schizophrenia. Ability to identify schizotaxia would define a population at risk, in whom studies of such interventions could be performed.

Finally, the concept of schizotaxia has an unexploited role in the design of new treatments. Our current treatments for schizophrenia are all directed at the dopamine receptor. It has become clear that these treatments are effective for acute psychoses but do little to alter the long-term progression of the illness. This clinical experience fits with the finding that alterations in dopaminergic activity correlate primarily with acute psychotic episodes. Schizotaxic features such as abnormal gating of the P50 evoked potential and abnormal smooth pursuit eye movements seem to be independent of alterations in dopamine activity. Pursuit of their neurobiology in coordinated human and animal experiments might provide an entirely new approach to the psychopharmacological treatment of schizophrenia.

REFERENCES

Adler, L. E., Gerhardt, G. A., Franks, R., Baker, N., Nagamoto, H., Drebing, C., & Freedman, R. (1990). Sensory physiology and catecholamines in schizophrenia and mania. *Psychiatry Research, 31,* 297–309.

Adler, L. E., Pachtman, E., Franks, R. D., Pecevich, M., Waldo, M. C., & Freedman, R. (1982). Neurophysiological evidence for a defect in neuronal mechanisms involved in sensory gating in schizophrenia. *Biological Psychiatry, 17,* 639–654.

Adler, L. E., Rose, G. M., & Freedman, R. (1986). Neurophysiological studies of sensory gating in rats: Effects of amphetamine, phencyclidine, and haloperidol. *Biological Psychiatry, 21,* 787–798.

Ayer-LeLeivre, C., Olson, L., Ebendahl, T., Seiger, A., & Persson, H. (1988). Expression of the beta-nerve growth factor gene in hippocampal neurons. *Science, 240,* 1339–1341.

Bickford-Wimer, P. C., Nagamoto, H., Johnson, R., Adler, L. E., Egan, M., Rose, G. M., & Freedman, R. (1990). Auditory sensory gating in hippocampal neurons: A model system in the rat. *Biological Psychiatry, 27,* 183–192.

Bickford-Wimer, P. C., & Freedman, R. (1989). Neurophysiological evidence for the gating of hippocampal auditory responses by pontine reticular formation neurons. *Neuroscience Abstracts,* 180.13.

Braff, D. L., Stone, C., Callaway, E., Geyer, M., Glick, I., & Bali, L. (1978). Prestimulus effects on human startle reflex in normals and schizophrenics. *Psychophysiology, 15,* 339–343.

Butters, N., & Miliotis, P. (1985). Amnestic disorders. In K. M. Heilman & E. Valenstein (Eds.), *Clinical neuropsychology* (pp. 403–451). New York: Oxford University Press.

Clarke, P. B. S., Schwartz, R. D., Paul, S. M., Pert, C. B., & Pert, A. (1985). Nicotinic binding in rat brain: Autoradiographic comparisons of (3-H)-acetylcholine, (3-H)-nicotine, and (125-I)-alpha-bungarotoxin. *Journal of Neuroscience, 5,* 1307–1315.

Davis, M., Gendleman, D. S., Tischler, M. D., & Gendleman, P. M. (1982). Primary acoustic startle circuit: Lesion and stimulation studies. *Journal of Neuroscience, 2,* 791–805.

De Amicis, L. A., Wagstaff, D. A., & Cromwell, R. L. (1986). Reaction time crossover as a marker of schizophrenia and of higher functioning. *Journal of Nervous and Mental Disease, 174,* 177–179.

Freedman, R. (1991). Elementary neuronal dysfunction in schizophrenia. *Schizophrenia Research, 4,* 233–243.

Holzman, P. S., Proctor, L. R., Levy, D. L., Yasillo, N. J., Meltzer, H. Y., & Hurt, S. W. (1974). Eye-tracking dysfunctions in schizophrenic patients and their relatives. *Archives of General Psychiatry, 31,* 143–151.

Jeste, D. V., & Lohr, J. B. (1989). Hippocampal pathological findings in schizophrenia. A morphometric study. *Archives of General Psychiatry, 46,* 1019–1024.

Kennedy, J. L., Giuffra, L. A., Moises, H. W., Cavalli-Sforza, L. L., Pakstis, A. A., Kidd, J. R., Castiglone, C. M., Sjogren, B., Wetterberg, L., & Kidd, K. K. (1988). Evidence against linkage of schizophrenia to markers on chromosome 5 in a northern Swedish pedigree. *Nature, 336,* 167–170.

Meehl, P. E. (1962). Schizotaxia, schizotypy, schizophrenia. *American Psychologist, 17,* 827–838.

Meltzer, H. Y. (1976). Neuromuscular dysfunction in schizophrenia. *Schizophrenia Bulletin 2,* 106–135.

Pickar, D., Labarca, R., Linnoila, M., Roy, A., Hommer, D., & Paul, S. M. (1984). Neuroleptic-induced decrease in plasma homovanillic acid and antipsychotic activity in schizophrenic patients. *Science, 225,* 954–957.

Sherrington, R., Brynjolfsson, J., Petursson, H., Potter, M., Dudelston, K., Barraclough, B., Wasmuth, J., Dobbs, M., & Gurling, H. (1988). Localization of a susceptibility locus for schizophrenia on chromosome 5. *Nature, 336,* 164–167.

Siegel, C., Waldo, M., Mizner, G., Adler, L. E., & Freedman, R. (1984). Deficits in sensory gating in schizophrenic patients and their relatives. *Archives of General Psychiatry, 41,* 607–612.

Suddath, R., Harrison, G. W., Torrey, E. F., Casanova, M. F., & Weinberger, D. R. (1990). Anatomical abnormalities in the brains of monozygotic twins discordant for schizophrenia. *New England Journal of Medicine, 322,* 1616–1619.

Swerdlow, N. R., Braff, D. L., Geyer, M. A., & Koob, G. F. (1986). Central dopamine hyperactivity in rats mimics abnormal sensory gating of the acoustic startle response in schizophrenics. *Biological Psychiatry, 21,* 23–33.

Tobin, A., Offenkrantz, W., & Freedman, R. (1978). A psychodynamic hypothesis about heroin addiction, prostitution, and suicide: An acting-out of conflicts about parenting. *International Journal of Pschoanalytic Psychotherapy, 7,* 602–608.

Venables, P. (1964). Input dysfunction in schizophrenia. In B. A. Maher (Ed.), *Progress in experimental personality research* (pp. 1–47). New York: Academic Press.

Vinogradova, O. (1975). Functional organization of the limbic system in the process of registration of information: Facts and hypotheses. In R. L. Issacson & K. H. Pribram (Eds.), *The hippocampus: Vol. 2. Neurophysiology and behavior* (pp. 1–70). New York: Plenum Press.

Wada, E., Wada, K., Boulter, J., Deneris, E., Heineman, S., Patrick, J., & Swanson, L. W. (1989). Distribution of alpha2, alpha3, alpha4 and beta2 neuronal nicotinic receptor subunit mRNAs in the central nervous system: A hybridization histochemical study in the rat. *Journal of Comparative Neurology, 284,* 314–335.

Zilles, K. (1988). Receptor autoradiography in the hippocampus of man and rat. *Advances in Anatomy, Embryology and Cell Biology, 111,* 61–80.

Part III

INFORMATION PROCESSING: BEHAVIORAL AND PSYCHOPHYSIOLOGICAL STRATEGIES

8

Schizophrenics' Reaction Time: North Star or Shooting Star?

RICHARD A. STEFFY
IRWIN WALDMAN

> . . . one research strategy . . . is to seek out those findings which have been constantly replicated. The reaction time (RT) studies are the closest thing to a north star in schizophrenia research. (Cancro, Sutton, Kerr, & Sugerman, 1971)

Several decades of research prior to 1971 led Robert Cancro and his colleagues to declare reaction time the "north star" measure of schizophrenic performance deficits. Time and again laboratory measures showed that reaction time indices discriminated schizophrenics' from nonschizophrenics' performance with remarkably little error. In this chapter we ask if Cancro and his colleague's enthusiasm about reaction time measures continues to be justified. Have alterations in procedures, use of better control groups, attempts to establish risk for the disorder, and various methodological developments in the past two decades continued to enjoy success? This update begins with a brief review of the pre-1970 work.

EARLY REACTION TIME STUDIES

Two teams laid the foundation for the enthusiastic use of reaction time measures in schizophrenia research. One started in the early 1930s at Worcester State Hospital under the direction of David Shakow, and continued after 1954, in collaboration with Ted Zahn and other colleagues at the National Institute of Mental Health (NIMH). The second group originated at the New York State Psychiatric Institute under the leadership of Joseph Zubin, with colleagues Sam Sutton, Gad Hakerem, and others. Both of these teams used varieties of a *simple* reaction time (SRT) paradigm in their probes of schizophrenic attentional difficulties. As depicted in Figure 8.1, simple reaction time—to be distinguished from choice reaction time—requires a single, unambiguous motor reaction on all trials, in most cases a finger lift from a telegraph key. As schematized in Figure 8.1, each trial is initiated with a key press after a ready signal initiates the trial. The key press begins an experimenter-controlled delay (preparatory interval) before an imperative signal commands the lift response. Reaction time is defined as the time elapsed between imperative signal onset and finger lift.

Shakow's and Zubin's teams differed in the stimulus features they manipulated during the reaction time trial series. The latter's paradigm shifted the quality and modality of the imperative signal, using an unpredictable series of low or high tones and red or green lights to signal response from trial to trial. In the New York group's work, preparatory interval variation was small (typically a 1.5- to 3.5-second delay), whereas Shakow's Worcester–NIMH group used

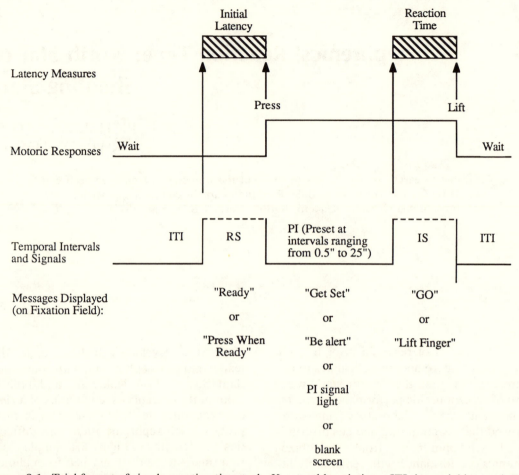

Figure 8.1. Trial format of simple reaction time task. Key to abbreviations: ITI, intertrial interval; RS, ready signal; PI, preparatory interval; IS, imperative signal. Dashed lines indicate duration is dependent on length of subject's pause before responding.

wider temporal variations (from 0.5 to 25.0 seconds) but kept the imperative signal constant.

Decades of research with both paradigms showed good discriminatory power in study after study. The modality shift procedure, for example, when featuring shifts from visual to auditory trials, yielded significant schizophrenic–normal differences in seven out of eight studies (Mannuzza, 1980). Cancro et al. (1971), using a modality shift procedure, found a strong prognostic association between reaction time indices and measures of clinical recovery.

Studies investigating temporal factors—variations in the length of preparatory interval duration and the format of pre-

paratory interval presentation (regular versus irregular)—also have been quite successful. Shakow's *set index* yielded non-overlapping distributions of scores for schizophrenics and controls in an early report by Rodnick and Shakow (1940). The set index is an aggregate measure reflecting latency and the point of crossover (as operationalized by the intersect of the regular and irregular gradients):

$$SI = \tfrac{1}{2}\left(\frac{M_{7.5\,R}}{M7.5} + \frac{M_{15\,R}}{M15}\right)MH + \left(\frac{M_{2R}}{M4R} \times M2\,R\right)$$

where M2, M4, M7.5, and 15 are the mean performance values at those preparatory interval durations, MI is the mean performance value of the irregular trials, MR is the mean performance value of the regular trials, and MH is the highest mean latency obtained. Using that index, Rosenthal, Lawlor, Zahn, and Shakow (1960) found a .89 correlation between reaction time and mental health ratings in a sample of schizophrenics. Various other measures that were built on Shakow's procedure, such as a redundancy deficit index and distraction-based reaction time procedure, also have shown good ability to discriminate schizophrenics from psychiatric controls, and process from reactive schizophrenics (Bellissimo & Steffy, 1972, 1975; Steffy & Galbraith, 1975).

The fact that simple variants of reaction time should emerge to be powerfully sensitive to schizophrenic processes may seem intuitively unlikely. In contrast to face-valid measures of deviant language or thought processes, a simple finger retraction seems a remarkably trivial, peripheral behavior to accord guiding light, "north star" status in the study of schizophrenic patients. Furthermore, as depicted in Figure 8.2, schizophrenic reaction time is a highly variable behavior offering apparently a quite noisy representation of functioning. However, the Shakow, Zubin, and other research teams

continually found highly reliable results from contrasts of schizophrenics' and other subjects' latencies (average and variance). Of particular importance, early workers saw order in the highly variable performances, particularly in response to stimulus variations they had introduced. For example, within a single-subject protocol as depicted in Figure 8.2, most of the extremely slow performance (high peak responses) resulted from conditions wherein a short-preparatory-interval-duration trial had been preceded by a long-duration trial, illustrating a phenomenon that Zahn, Rosenthal, and Shakow (1963) defined as a prepreparatory interval (or PPI) effect. Also, isotemporal sets (a series of consecutive trials with the same preparatory interval duration) marked on Figure 8.2 illustrate the rapidly increasing latencies that we have found typical of schizophrenics' performance when redundancy is introduced into reaction time trials.

From such observations, the special sensitivity of schizophrenic patients to the impact of subtle, seemingly insignificant, task variation in attention-demanding measures became a major focus of early investigations. Nonetheless, various theoreticians proposed quite different mechanisms to ac-

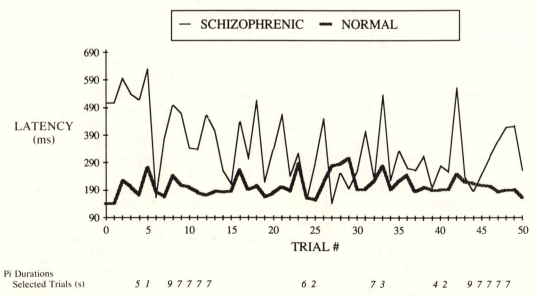

Figure 8.2. A sample reaction time series from a normal control and a schizophrenic patient.

count for the observed performance deficits. Shakow's (1962, 1963) Segmental Set Theory, for example, emphasized schizophrenics' short span of attention. In his view, these patients failed to maintain a "major set"—a sharp focus of attention—for more than a few seconds at a time. Shakow found that a variety of extraneous, task-related or self-generated stimulations quickly disrupted the performance of schizophrenics (Shakow, 1962). In support of Shakow's model, investigations of preparatory interval duration variation showed that the advantage of a series of *regular* (isotemporal) trials over an *irregular* (unpredictable) series was lost for schizophrenic subjects when trial durations exceeded 4 or 5 seconds. In contrast, normal controls profit from predictable series for much longer intervals. Figure 8.3 illustrates the difference that regular and irregular formats make across short- and long-duration trials for schizophrenic patients and for normal controls, as found in the classic Rodnick and Shakow (1940) reaction time study. The conspicuous feature of their finding—and one that was often repeated in subsequent studies—was the short-duration intersection of regular and irregular performance gradients in schizophrenic patients. This finding was taken as an indication of patients' failure to sustain sharp levels of vigilance for more than a few seconds, with estimates varying from 2 to 6 seconds across early investigations. From these findings Shakow developed the position that schizophrenics have an *excessively weak* attentional capacity.

Both Shakow and Zubin developed theories of attention dysfunctions characterizing schizophrenic disorders in general and reaction time deficits in particular, but they differed in their view of the mechanism of the deficit. In contrast to Shakow, Zubin (1975) attributed schizophrenics' performance deficits to an *abnormally strong* attentional persistence. In short, Zubin argued that schizophrenics are unable to shift their set to accommodate changes in task demands. This view was based on the finding that schizophrenics are significantly more im-

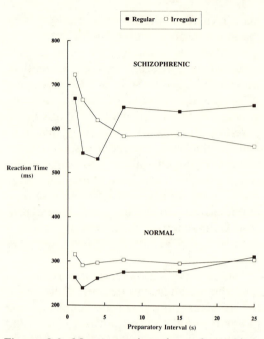

Figure 8.3. Mean reaction times for schizophrenic patients and normal control subjects plotted as a function of preparatory interval duration and regularity of presentation. (*Source:* Redrawn from Rodnick, E. H., & Shakow, D. [1940]. Set in the schizophrenic as measured by a composite reaction time index. *American Journal of Psychiatry, 97,* 214–225. Copyright 1940, the American Psychiatric Association. Reprinted by permission.)

paired than controls on reaction time trials in which a shift in the modality of the imperative signal used on a previous trial had occurred, despite the fact that the same finger lift response was required of all conditions. That is, whenever a trial with tone imperative signal is followed by a light imperative signal trial, or a light–tone order (contramodal condition), schizophrenics are found to be relatively more impaired than when a low- to high-tone or a red to green light (ipsimodal) shift occurred (e.g., Sutton & Zubin, 1965).

Other evidence for abnormal persistence in schizophrenics' laboratory task performance that supported Zubin's concept of disorder came from the already cited prepreparatory interval effects studied by the NIMH group. For example, Zahn et al. (1963) observed that the temporal features (preparatory interval) of any trial tended to have an impact on performances given on subsequent trials. If, for example, a long-preparatory-interval-duration trial preceded a short-duration trial, the latter reaction time was significantly slower than for other short-duration trials, especially those preceded by a trial of equal duration (Nideffer, Neale, Kopfstein, & Cromwell, 1971). Zahn, Rosenthal, and Shakow (1961) also showed that the arrangement of the previous block of trials has a significant impact on subsequent performances. Likewise, in our work we have reported response-produced proactive factors. That is, if the response time (independent of preparatory interval duration) of any given trial is excessively slow, it is likely to be followed by a slower-than-average performance on the next trial in schizophrenic patients (Steffy, 1978).

Shakow's reaction time paradigm yielded another impression of the strongly persistent impact of previous experiences on schizophrenics' deficits, although it was not well accommodated in his theorizing. It may be recalled that Shakow based his view that schizophrenic patients are unable to maintain a major set on the fact that regular (isotemporal) trial formats enhanced their speed of performance over random-appearing irregular trials for only short durations of a few seconds, whereas normal controls profit from regularity for much longer duration trials. However, the data in many of the early studies suggested that regularity not only failed to aid schizophrenics' performance on long trials but seemed actually to impede it. Rodnick and Shakow's classical findings, depicted in Figure 8.3, show the *strong form* of a *crossover pattern* in which short regular trial performances are faster but long regular trial performances are slower than irregular trials for the schizophrenic subjects. These findings suggest not just an absent but rather a deleterious proactive effect of the regularity.

Although the significance of the "preparatory interval duration × regularity" interaction in these early data (Rodnick & Shakow, 1940) was not analyzed, the regular–irregular trial differences (calculated separately for each preparatory interval duration) revealed a significant difference at an .05 level of confidence, even for the 25-second preparatory interval. Similar-appearing patterns in other research (e.g., Venables & O'Conner, 1959) make the strong crossover pattern credible, and Bellisimo and Steffy (1972, 1975) were inspired from these patterns to test further the impact of long-duration regular trials. Their work, with an altered paradigm, showed highly reliable crossover patterns and significant *redundancy-associated deficit* (indicating slower regular than irregular trial performances at long preparatory interval durations), as depicted in Bellissimo's findings (see Figure 8.4).

The Bellissimo–Steffy procedure used a series of four-trial miniblocks of regular (isotemporal) trials imbedded within a basically irregular series, instead of the longer separate blocks of regular and irregular trials used by Shakow, Zahn, and their co-workers. As schematized in Figure 8.5, the trial arrangements using *embedded sets* allow comparisons of irregular trials (taken from the first item of the isotemporal series) with regular trials (taken from the fourth item of the isotemporal series) that reflect the impact of regularity on performance, but are no further removed in time from each other than three trials away.[1] Subsequent research with this procedure in various labs yielded highly significant crossover patterns (tested as an interaction between preparatory interval duration and regularity) and redundancy deficit (assessed by comparisons of regular versus irregular samples taken at each long preparatory interval) in schizophrenic patients (e.g., Bohannon & Strauss, 1983; De Amicis & Cromwell, 1979; Schneider & Cauthen, 1982; Steffy & Galbraith, 1974, 1980; Strauss, Bohannon, Kaminsky, & Kharabi, 1979). Moreover, the pattern

---

1. Irregular trial estimates can be obtained from trials of a similar preparatory interval duration sampled several trials after the regular estimate to counterbalance the typical order of occurrence in embedded set designs. This refinement did not alter our results, although it appears to give increased sensitivity in recent results reported by Spohn (see Chapter 16, this volume).

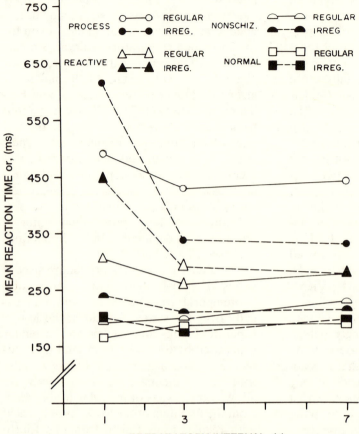

Figure 8.4. Mean reaction times for process and reactive schizophrenics, nonschizophrenic patients, and normal control subjects using "embedded sets" procedure to explore reaction time crossover. (*Source:* data published by Bellissimo and Steffy [1972]. Copyright 1972 by the American Psychological Association. Reprinted by permission.)

seems robust in response to motivational and training challenges designed to reduce deficit (Kaplan, 1974; Steffy & Galbraith, 1980).

Of special interest to the study of proactive influences on schizophrenic performance deficit, analyses of trends over the sets of four trials reliably showed decrements in the third and fourth trials relative to the first and second trials. As apparent in Figure 8.6, set position effects analyzed by Bellissimo and Steffy (1972) showed an immediate gain on trial two—thus reflecting the expected prepreparatory–preparatory interval effect (Nideffer et al., 1971; Zahn et al., 1963)—that gave way to impaired performance on the last two trials. Moreover, Bernstein's (1976) dissertation reported performance decrements far greater than the levels expected from fatigue that extended after the isotemporal set to the next four trials. From analyses of his own study and

four other previously published data sets, Bernstein observed a slowing trend of approximately 1 ms/trial across an irregular series, a 12- to 15-ms slowing per trial within an isotemporal series containing long-preparatory-interval trials, and an 8-ms/trial decrement in immediate postisotemporal set trials.

The overall impact of these findings indicates strongly impairing proactive influences at work in schizophrenic reaction time and suggests that process schizophrenics show an exceptional sensitivity to prevailing stimulus conditions. Although the findings of shift, prepreparatory interval, and regularity factors are not in a strict sense incompatible with the Segmental Set Theory, neither are they easily explained as products of excess distractibility or loss of major set. We believe such findings are better accomodated by Cromwell and Dokecki's (1968) "disattention theory," Sal-

Blocked Procedure (Shakow):

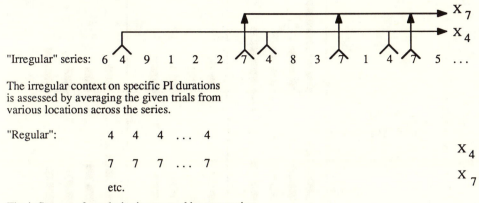

"Irregular" series: 6   4   9   1   2   2   7   4   8   3   7   1   4   7   5 ...

The irregular context on specific PI durations
is assessed by averaging the given trials from
various locations across the series.

"Regular":   4   4   4   ...   4

                    7   7   7   ...   7

              etc.

The influence of regularity is assessed by computing
the average of a block of isotemporal trials.

Embedded Set Procedure (Steffy):

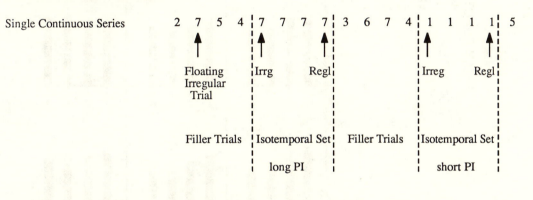

The "redundancy" effect as measured by Steffy is Trial 4 minus
Trial 1 in an isotemporal set. Cromwell measures the average of the 2nd,
3rd, and 4th trials (as reflecting regularity) minus the 1st irregular trial.

Figure 8.5. Simple reaction time trial arrangements.

zinger's (1971) "immediacy hypothesis,"
and Steffy and Galbraith's (1975) "inhibitory process deficits" models. Without be-
laboring the subtleties of the various models
here, it can be noted that recent reviews of
their strengths and weaknesses conclude
that no single theory has yet given a full explanation of the schizophrenic reaction time
performance deficit data, but each of the
various approaches from the time of Shakow forward has clarified some aspects of
schizophrenic patient dysfunctions (see,
e.g., reviews by Chapman & Chapman,
1973; Cromwell, 1975, 1984; Nuechterlein,
1977; Steffy, 1978). We have no argument

with those conclusions; our purpose in this
chapter is to update the account of reaction
time studies, reviewing what has been
learned from procedural variations, improved subject controls, and efforts to use
reaction time measures to predict clinical
outcome.

TASK FACTORS EXPLORED IN SCHIZOPHRENIC REACTION TIME STUDIES

Temporal Factors

The central feature of Shakow's simple reaction time paradigm is the preparatory in-

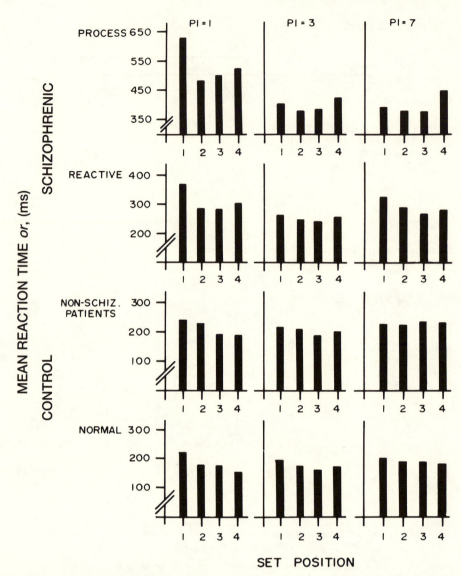

Figure 8.6. Mean reaction times for four set positions in "embedded set" depicted for three preparatory interval (PI) durations and four pathology groups. (*Source:* data published by Bellissimo and Steffy [1972]. Copyright 1972 by the American Psychological Association. Reprinted by permission.)

terval or duration. Shakow happened on its relevance in his early studies of schizophrenic slowness. As reported in his 1962 review, the Worcester State lab investigated a variety of motoric behaviors to discern the lowest level of neuromuscular complexity at which the clinical indications of slowness would be manifest. This goal proved harder than had been imagined. Huston's dissertation research found normal patellar reflex speeds indicating that spinal reflexes were intact in schizophrenics (Huston, Shakow, & Riggs, 1937). Subse-

quent research showed adequacy—at least among the most cooperative schizophrenic subjects—in tapping and pursuit rotor speed tests. Only in simple reaction time measures did vast schizophrenic–normal differences emerge. Insofar as the finger movement requirement of tapping speed and reaction time measures were roughly equivalent, Shakow reasoned that the temporal interval, and the attentional demands that the reaction time procedure added, were critical to schizophrenic slowness.

Trial duration factors. As indicated above, Shakow's comparison of response speeds under regular and irregular trial formats allowed estimates of a subject's ability to maintain a sharp degree of vigilance. The length of preparatory interval duration at which regularity of presentation no longer conferred a performance advantage over irregular trials was used to index attentional capacity. In the wooly domain of psychopathology, such precision was most welcome, and the preparatory interval duration dimension became a key feature of Shakow's theorizing. The point of intersection of regular and irregular trial data—plotted over preparatory interval duration—was found in different labs to occur at short durations for schizophrenics. Bellissimo and Steffy (1975) challenged the stability of the point of intersection by using a wide variety of preparatory interval durations, whereas Steffy and Galbraith (1974) tested the effects of variation in intertrial intervals, but these authors found no wider variation in intersects beyond the 2- to 6-second range reported in the early papers.

It may be of interest to note that reaction time studies with schizophrenic populations in the past two decades show a trend toward the use of shorter preparatory interval durations (from 1 to 10 seconds), probably because schizophrenic crossover consistently has occurred by 6 or 7 seconds and redundancy deficit (differences between regular and irregular trials) is robust at 7 seconds. Consequently, longer preparatory interval durations (11 to 25 seconds) have been less frequently investigated in recent literature. Nonetheless, Rosenbaum has argued that dropping longer trials may be shortsighted if reaction time measures are being used to study attentional impairment across conditions (within-subject comparisons) and in groups at risk for the disorder, in schizophrenia spectrum disorders, and in psychopathologies other than schizophrenia. In Rosenbaum's work, for example, schizotypic university students showed regular–irregular intersects at approximately 10 seconds, in contrast to 6 seconds for schizophrenic patients and 18 seconds for normal control subjects (Rosenbaum, Chapin & Shore, 1988).

Remote temporal factors. Because schizophrenic patients seem unable to maintain a high degree of vigilance in trials extending longer than a few seconds, it may seem surprising that their performance is found to show the effects of previous trial events, sometimes minutes later. Illustrative of these extended influences are the already mentioned effects of the previous trial's preparatory interval (the prepreparatory interval), the previous trial's response time, and the effects of earlier blocks of trials. To explore further the time course of impairments that develop during a series of reaction time trials, Steffy and Galbraith (1974) examined the effects of trial cadence on redundancy deficit. A within-subject comparison of typically used 2-second intertrial intervals with longer, 7-second intertrial intervals found magnitudes of redundancy deficit substantially reduced when longer rest periods (intertrial intervals) were used. The authors argued that their findings more strongly supported an inhibitory process dysfunction than a segmental set interpretation of redundancy deficit. The former model hypothesized that an inhibitory suppressive potential builds up from trial to trial; hence, a longer rest between trials could be expected to dissipate inhibition more thoroughly, and thereby result in lower amounts of deficit. This view derives from the tenets of Hullian theory (Hull, 1943). In contrast, if redundancy deficit reflected a weakened allocation of attention associated with length of delay, then Shakow's position implies that longer intertrial intervals would lead to increased deficit. Since Zahn (1970) had previously found no intertrial interval effect on reaction time deficit, a modified segmental set hypothesis would expect *no greater* deficit from a longer intertrial interval. It would not, however, predict a reduction in deficit resulting from a longer intertrial interval, as was obtained in our study of intertrial interval effects.

In summary, the performance decay

noted in long-preparatory-interval-duration isotemporal sets, the trial-by-trial proactive influences, the lingering impairment noted on several trials after the embedded sets, and the reduction in redundancy deficits obtained from extending the rest periods between trials collectively lead to the impression that schizophrenic performances suffer from long-persisting sources of interference. Consequently, these recent findings tend to confirm the view shared by Shakow and Zubin that schizophrenics' deficits reflect their susceptibility to interference from even the most subtle of extraneous task factors.

Extrinsic Stimulation Effects

If schizophrenics show special sensitivity to subtle, nonspecific events occurring during trial foreperiods (preparatory intervals) and to factors associated with the mere arrangement of trials, it stands to reason that specific stimuli occurring before or during reaction time trials also will have substantial impairing effects on schizophrenic performances. In fact, the data available clearly suggest that schizophrenics' performances are quite vulnerable to discrete stimuli imposed into the reaction time task. Even when such stimuli are informative and have been shown to facilitate performance levels of other subjects, task-concurrent stimuli will generally impair process schizophrenics' performances.

Zubin's group, we have already noted, appreciated the special sensitivity of schizophrenic patients to stimulus changes during reaction time performances. A crossmodal shift in the imperative signal of adjacent trials—particularly from a visual to an auditory signal—reliably yielded a significant decrement, even in trials in which the subjects were informed about the impending trial or successfully anticipated the shift in a pretrial correct guess (Spring, 1980; Waldbaum, Sutton, & Kerr, 1975). The remarkable feature of this finding is the fact that substantial impairment results even though the change from one imperative signal to another has no task relevance. The same finger lift response was required on all trials.

In dissertation research conducted in our lab, Green (1974) extended the investigation of the effects of irrelevant stimulation on process schizophrenic reaction time performance. Green studied the effect of a prestimulation procedure that simply required the subjects to listen—and not respond—to a series of 20 two-second tones with an intertone interval of approximately 3 seconds presented immediately before reaction time testing. The prestimulation procedure varied tone intensity (two levels of 50 and 95 db) and the time between the prestimulation and the test trials (immediate to 24 hours). Green found a large direct relationship in schizophrenic patients between the intensity of the prestimulation tones and the latencies obtained in a test series. The prestimulation impaired only the schizophrenic patients, not the control subjects. He also observed similar prestimulation results from bright lights preceding an auditory test series.

The prestimulation effect was observed only if the test trials were conducted immediately after the prestimulation trials (about a 10-second interval transpired between the end of the prestimulation series and the the beginning of reaction time testing). Green noticed in particular that the greatest impairment from prestimulation occurred in the first half—approximately the first 10 minutes of testing—of the 50 test trials we used. The prestimulation effect was not observed in conditions in which prestimulation and testing were separated by a half hour or more.

Green's finding of substantial reaction time performance decrement from the most intense (95-db) prestimulation is quite remarkable when one recalls that *increases* in the intensity of the imperative stimulus repeatedly have been shown to improve—to "normalize"—schizophrenic reaction time performances (one ordinarily observes a monotonic decrease in schizophrenic and normal latencies with increases in the intensity of the imperative stimulus) (Grisell & Rosenbaum, 1964; King, 1962; Rosenbaum, Mackavey, & Grisell, 1957; Venables & Tizard, 1958). In fact, Green showed the expected relationship between the intensity of the imperative signal and reaction time speed. That is, both schizophrenics and controls showed steadily faster latencies as imperative signal intensity levels were increased across five levels (ranging from 50 to 95 dB). Because the same range of stimulus intensity was used during the prestimulation as in the imperative signal amplitude manipulation, but yielded an inverse relationship between prestimulation intensity and speed, Green concluded that the *time* at which an extraneous stimuli occurs is an all-important consideration in understanding the impact of stimulation on schizophrenic performance deficits.

Green's conclusion is consistent with diverse other findings. In studies attempting to use aversive stimuli as motivational agents to "normalize" schizophrenic reaction time, the time at which the aversive stimulus is presented has proven to be important. Lang (1959) contrasted a 116-dB white noise delivered under an "escape" condition (i.e., concurrent with the imperative signal and terminated with the response), with an "avoidance" condition (allowing subjects to avoid the loud tone by producing a response faster than their predetermined average latency). Lang found that the escape condition facilitated schizophrenics' reaction time performance but the avoidance condition did not. Karras (1962) replicated the escape condition finding, and also reported that persisting background stimulation was not helpful to schizophrenic performance. Various other studies that have examined continuous white noise played as background stimulation during reaction time trials have produced a mixed picture, showing facilitation from more intense signals on some trials but not on others (Pascal & Swenson, 1952), and showing pervasive stimulation being helpful to some subjects (e.g., the more withdrawn) but not to others (the more paranoid), as reported in a study by Tizard and Venables (1957).

Studies of Temporal Course of Extraneous Stimulus Effects

A close examination of the impact of extra signals given during reaction time perform-

ances was suggested by data collected in a University of Pennsylvania dissertation by Mo (1968). Mo examined the effect of a simple informative cue, provided verbally to announce a change in preparatory interval duration on the next trial after a series of regular (5-second preparatory interval) reaction time trials. Contrasted with a no-information group, subjects in the informative cue condition simply were told that the next trial would be shorter (or longer) than the last trial. A fairly complex result emerged from this operation. In contrast to alcoholic and normal control subjects, who were scarcely influenced at all, the schizophrenic patients showed a large interaction between the information factor (information versus nothing said at all) and the direction of the shift (a shift from a 5-second to an 8-second preparatory interval, or from a 5-second to a 2-second interval). In brief, schizophrenic subjects given no information showed a better performance on the shift to the 8-second trials, but showed a much slower performance if shifted to the 2-second preparatory interval. Schizophrenic subjects given information showed the opposite pattern of results: a substantially slower performance after the shift to the 8-second and a relatively fast performance after the shift to a 2-second trial duration. In a subsequent study, Mo investigated a cued shift from preparatory intervals of 5 seconds to intervals on a subsequent trial of from 1 to 10 seconds. These results confirmed that the "preparatory interval duration × information" interactions observed in the first study, because schizophrenics' responses given information were little impaired at 2 seconds, maximally impaired at 6 to 8 seconds, and showed improvement at 9 or more seconds.[2]

The performance gradients portrayed in Mo's data gave further reason to attend to

2. Although Mo did not present an irrelevant information cue—which would have allowed him to evaluate the effect of the intrusion independently of the content or relevance of the message—it is clear that a signal prior to the trial had a substantial impact on performance, dependent on the time elapsing between the "early cue" and the signal to respond.

the temporal aspect of extraneous physical stimuli in understanding schizophrenic deficit. To investigate the time course more closely, we devised a *probed reaction time* procedure that allows the charting of variations in latency for a few seconds after unexpected extraneous stimuli.

Probed Reaction Time Results

In an initial investigation of our probed reaction time procedure, Steffy and Galbraith (1974) delivered an extraneous ("distractor") stimulus toward the end of a block of regular trials. The distractor probes were two-pronged, including a brief 25,000-foot-candle flash of light occurring instantaneously at the finger press and meaningless alteration to the fixation field—a border of Xs around a visual warning signal (the words BE ALERT) presented during the preparatory interval. To assess the impact of this probe stimulus at various intervals of time, we examined blocks of preparatory interval durations ranging from 1 to 9 seconds in which the probes were embedded. Because long-duration regular trials are a likely occasion for performance decrement in process schizophrenic patients, we reasoned that extra stimulation added to the beginning of a trial should provide an amplification of this expected decrement. In the probed reaction time procedure, variation in the preparatory interval duration provides an occasion to examine the time course of the impairment caused by multimodal extraneous stimuli.

Our expectations were supported. Relative to reactive schizophrenics, other psychiatric patient controls, and normal control subjects, two separate samples of process schizophrenic patients showed the same pattern of response decrement across time. As found in data published by Steffy and Galbraith (1975), and depicted in Figure 8.7, impairment was observed for the shortest preparatory intervals sampled (1 and 3 seconds), followed by recovery in mid-range intervals (5 seconds), and then followed by impairment again at the longest delay (9 seconds). This temporal course has features remarkably similar to those obtained by Mo,

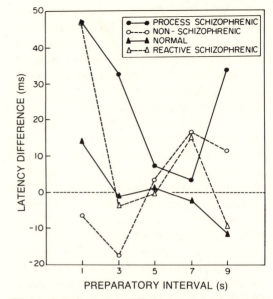

Figure 8.7. Latency difference scores obtained by four pathology groups on probed RT trials. (*Source:* data published by Steffy and Galbraith [1975]. Copyright 1972 by the American Psychological Association. Reprinted by permission.)

although displaced by approximately 2 seconds. If Mo's verbal instruction occurred approximately midway during the intertrial interval, his extraneous stimulus occurred 2 to 3 seconds earlier than when we fired our probe stimulus. Recalibrating the paradigms for this time difference makes the time of the optimal performance and the later occurring impairment nearly identical in our two labs.

Within the process group, we also observed that the pattern of recovery and subsequent impairment showed strong relations to pathology level of the process subjects as indexed by the Elgin Prognostic Scale (Wittman, 1941). These relationships confirm the relevance of the late-occurring impairment to clinical functioning.

The probed reaction time pattern described in the Steffy and Galbraith (1975) paper has been validated in subsequent studies directed toward disentangling the contribution of the two stimulus features used in the original work. As reported by Steffy (1978), variation in light intensities (comparing 25,000- and 100,000-foot-candle exposures) yielded additive levels of overall impairment but did not interact with the preparatory interval duration. The U-shaped pattern of impairment, recovery, and further decrement seems limited to the presence of the alteration in the fixation field that is displayed throughout the preparatory interval of the probe trial, and not the presence of the momentary flash of bright light. Once again, relatively subtle and irrelevant stimulus features seem to play a major role in schizophrenic performance deficits.

It is interesting in this respect to recall other examples in the schizophrenia literature wherein subtle and presumably facilitating informative stimulus conditions were seen to offer schizophrenics little advantage (Zahn, 1970), or even to exert a detrimental influence. For example, in a study by Cromwell, Rosenthal, Shakow, and Zahn (1961), schizophrenics were found to suffer a disadvantage on trials in which they not only knew the length of the preparatory interval, but in which they took responsibility for setting the dial for the length of duration themselves. Subjects in that investigation were given a dial with five levels of preparatory interval duration to test the impact of "autonomy," in contrast to the typical experimenter-controlled duration of the preparatory interval. Chronic schizophrenic patients demonstrated slower reaction time in the conditions of autonomy, and indicated that they found those trials less desirable, than in the experimenter-controlled trials. The opposite pattern was observed for the normal control subjects for both latency of response and stated desirability.

In summary, the detrimental effects of various signals imposed into the reaction time paradigm and the variation in levels of impairment that seem to occur over the preparatory interval durations give clear indication of the reaction time task's special advantage in exploring properties of schizophrenic deficits. Future research should test various models of the specific mechanisms of schizophrenia that may account for these patients' proneness to interference from extrinsic stimuli. To account for redundancy deficit and probe reaction time findings, we have favored models that

feature arousal modulation dysfunctions consistent with Pavlov's (1941) theorizing, as refined by Epstein and Coleman (1970). According to these authors, schizophrenics suffer an imbalance in excitatory and inhibitory opponent processes. Epstein has described schizophrenics' inhibitory response to have an "all or none" character. When aroused, their inefficient inhibitory functions provide either too little or too much damping of autonomic activity. As observed in many studies, schizophrenics rarely give a smoothly balanced response proportional to the stimulation received (e.g., Fenz & Velner, 1970). Consistent with that view, the impact of extraneous stimulation before or during reaction time trials shows considerable evidence of disrupted processing in the process schizophrenic samples we have studied.

Physiological Mapping of Preparatory Interval Duration

A promising, but rarely employed, investigative approach that is suggested by an arousal-modulation dysfunction model is the mapping of physiological changes associated with performance variation during behavioral tests. Reaction time measures, because of their requirement for still, attentive postures lasting several seconds, can serve as an excellent stage for physiological measurement. That is, physiological assays of most-impaired and least-impaired trials (or series of such trials) may help clarify the nature of schizophrenics' performance deficit.

Bradley's (1976) dissertation, for example, was successful in discriminating redundancy deficit patterns from redundancy-facilitated (normal) patterns with the aid of heart rate and blood volume–pressure measures. Specifically, he found robust triphasic heart rate patterns (accelerating–decelerating–accelerating) to develop across trials in regular sets that showed steady improvement (faster responses) from the first to last trial. Bradley also observed a progressive shift toward greater blood volume–pressure in sets in which redundancy was observed to facilitate performance. By contrast, the sets of trials yielding a slower trend (redundancy deficit) were characterized by a simpler biphasic heart rate pattern. These findings were viewed as consistent with established links between the autonomic nervous system and attentional functions found in physiological studies of normal subjects (Lacey, 1967; Obrist, Sutterer, Howard, Hennis, & Murrel, 1973). Their work, and that of others attempting to link physiological indices to schizophrenic-sensitive attentional measures (such as size estimation [McCormick, 1974] and the Continuous Performance Test (CPT) [Friedman, Vaughan, & Erlenmeyer-Kimling, 1978]), hold promise for expanding our knowledge of the mechanisms of deficit. For example, close examination of physiological patterning may yield fresh hypotheses about the nature of schizophrenic disorders. Tecce's (1972) study of schizophrenic's contingent negative variation patterns during reaction time trials showed sluggish recovery (return to baseline) after the motor response, a finding that suggests a neural basis for weak shifting of attention. Patterson's demonstration (personal communication) of a weak subcortical electrophysiological response to the earliest (preperceptual) processing of visually displayed information among schizophrenic patients may account for the remarkable impairments noted at the shortest preparatory intervals in our probe reaction time findings.

These physiological linkages also may help refine the measurement properties of reaction time tasks. Remarkable "north star" levels of discrimination have been observed from reaction time technology—not just between schizophrenics and normal subjects but in contrasts among various psychopathologies and within the schizophrenic spectrum as well—but they could be better. Problems of measurement error might be rectified by the study of physiological concomitants of behavioral tests in order to clarify the extent of deficit. Bradley's study, for example, noted that heart rate measures during redundancy-deficited isotemporal sets found not only a less-articulated heart rate pattern on the fourth (regular) trial, but also tended to show a significantly lower basal heart rate on all trials in the set. Should these patterns of basal and phasic heart rate be replicable, they suggest means of discriminating between "true" and "error" redundancy deficit patterns for testing the external validity of reaction time indices. Although the literature reviewed in the next section shows considerable evidence of validity, there is room for improvement when one ventures to use reaction time as a measure of individual differences. Improved validity would be particularly helpful in ascertaining schizophrenia vulnerability in relatives (De Amicis & Cromwell, 1979; De Amicis, Huntzinger, & Cromwell, 1981) and in comparing the impact of schizophrenia with the impact of epilepsy (Botwinick, Brinley, & Robbin, 1959), aging (Strauss, Wagman, & Quaid, 1983), and other psychopathologies.

DISCRIMINATING POWER OF REACTION TIME MEASURES

The nonoverlapping distributions of schizophrenic and normal "set index" scores in the Rodnick and Shakow (1940) study quickly established the reputation of reaction time measurement. Until researchers noted that the latency component accounted for most of the variation in the set index, it was widely used in a number of early major studies (e.g., Rosenthal et al., 1960; Tizard & Venables, 1956; Zahn & Rosenthal, 1965).

A purer measure of the effect of the regularity manipulation is indexed by the redundancy deficit measures of Bellissimo and Steffy (1972). This measure is composed of the latency difference between regular and irregular long-preparatory-interval-duration trials; nonetheless, it is frequently referred to as *reaction time crossover,* or RTX, to reflect the test of the interaction between preparatory interval and regularity effects. We will use the RTX label in this section of the literature review, because our convention is to test *both* the interaction as well as the simple effects of regularity at each preparatory interval. Authors vary in their preferences regarding specific tests and cut-off points. Whereas our lab has used a simple difference score of the fourth (regular) minus the first (irregular) trial in isotemporal sets of four trials, Cromwell's team uses an average of the second through fourth trial to represent regularity.

Independent of procedural variations, the various reaction time indices have proven remarkably sensitive to schizophrenic pathology and are capable of discriminating schizophrenics from other psychiatric groups, and of discriminating among different schizophrenia spectrum disorders (e.g., schizophrenia, schizotypal personality disorders). Table 8.1 summarizes our search of the schizophrenic reaction time studies pursuing the Shakow tradition since the earliest Worcester papers (e.g., Huston et al., 1937). In this table the studies are categorized according to the group comparisons analyzed, and each row gives a brief indication of the major features of the reaction time design, the groups tested, the type of reaction time index used, and the results for each index. (Because the Mannuzza [1980] review of the New York group's [Zubin et al.] research gives a thorough accounting of the crossmodal paradigm results, those studies are not included in Table 8.1.)

A cursory inspection of Table 8.1 shows that both general latency and the redundancy-sensitive measures (the set index and RTX) have substantial discriminatory power in separating schizophrenics from normal subjects as well as from other psychiatric control groups. The latency measures per se have consistently provided good separation, except for the Knehr (1954) investigation, which used a somewhat unique "knob turn"—rather than the traditional finger lift—response and a remarkably long intertrial interval. Although Bohannon and Strauss (1983) also did not show significant group discrimination on the standard latency measures, they did on the RTX index. As is readily apparent in the data displayed in Table 8.1, latency measures have been used much more often than the set and RTX indices. We note that,

whenever the latter have been used, they generally yielded a strong form of the cross-over or a significant set index.

It is comforting to recognize in the second section of Table 8.1 that these measures were as useful in differentiating schizophrenic from other psychiatric patient groups as they were in differentiating schizophrenic patients from normal subjects. Examining the third section of Table 8.1, it is also apparent that both latency and the redundancy-sensitive measures are effective in discriminating among different schizophrenic subtypes. The final section of Table 8.1 examines the sensitivity of reaction time measures to differences between normal controls and nonschizophrenic patient groups. Although there are only four studies referenced, it is apparent that some modest discriminative power exists. From these latter findings, it is clear that we need to keep an open mind regarding the particular features of psychopathology that are associated with reaction time deficits.

Relative Power of Latency and Redundancy Deficit (RTX) Measures

Examining the pattern of outcomes across the many studies listed in Table 8.1, one can see that measures of general latency, set, and RTX regularly discriminated among groups. To examine the differential sensitivity among these indices, all subjects examined in our laboratory were analyzed together to test the relative power of general latency and RTX indices.

In investigations ranging across the 1970s, we amassed samples totaling 288 process schizophrenics, 36 reactive schizophrenics, 36 nonschizophrenic patient controls, and 93 nonpatient controls. To sample the spectrum of reaction time performances, five indices were scored. Two were general latency measures, one for the shortest and one for mid-length trials. (Various ranges of preparatory interval duration were sampled in the individual investigations.) Three measures were made of RTX, one each for the shortest, mid-length, and longest preparatory interval duration trials.

Table 8.1. Discriminating Power of Simple Reaction Time Measures

Investigation	Reaction time format[a]	Group differences[b]	Latency	Set index	RTX
I: Studies Contrasting Schizophrenics with Normal Subjects					
Fedio, Mirsky, Smith, and Parry (1961)	Blocked trials with signal during PI	Sz > N	S		
Huston et al. (1937)	Blocked trials	Sz > N	S		S (weak)
Jentsch (1958)	Blocked trials	Chr Sz > N	S		NS
Knehr (1954)	Blocked trials; also: PIs = 2 and 10 s, ITI = 10 s	Sz = N	NS		
	Knob turn response	Chr Sz = N			
Rodnick and Shakow (1940)	Blocked trials, PI = 0.5–25 sec	Chr Sz > N	S	S	S (strong)
Schneider and Cauthen (1982)	Embedded set	Sz > N	S	S	
Zahn, Rosenthal, and Shakow (1961)	Blocked reg trials; ascnd-descnd series	Sz > N	S		
Zahn, Rosenthal, and Shakow (1963)	Blocked irreg trials; PPI-PI effects	Sz > N	S		
Zahn, Shakow, and Rosenthal (1961)	Blocked reg trials comb short & long PIs and ITIs	Sz > N	S		
II: Studies Contrasting Schizophrenics with Other Groups					
Bellissimo and Steffy (1972)	Embedded set	Proc Sz > Reac Sz > Nonsz > N	S		S (strong)
Bellissimo and Steffy (1975)	Embedded set	Proc Sz > Reac Sz > N	S		S
Bohannon, Strauss (1983)	Embedded set	RDC Sz = RDC manic > nonpsychotic control	NS		S (strong)
Czudner and Marshall (1967)	Blocked trials	Children: Sz > MR > N	S		S (weak)
		Children: Sz = MR = N			
De Amicis and Cromwell (1979)	Embedded set	Proc Sz > Proc Sz's relatives = N	S		
		Proc Sz > Proc Sz's relatives > N			S (strong)
Greiffenstein, Lewis, Milberg, and Rosenbaum (1981)	Blocked trial	TLE > Sz = Gen E > N	S		
		Sz = TLE > Gen E = N			S (strong)
Huston and Senf (1952)	Blocked trials	Chr Sz > Acute Sz = Depr Sz > Neurotic	S	S	NS
Rosenbaum et al. (1988)	Blocked trial	Sz > Szt = MMPI elev = N	S		
		Sz = Szt > MMPI dev = N			S
Simons, MacMillan, and Ireland (1982)	Embedded set	Szt (perc) > Szt (anhed) > N			S (strong)
Tizard and Venables (1956)	Blocked trials	Chr Sz > MR = N	S	S	S (strong)
Van Dyke and Routh (1973)	Blocked trial w/short PIs; studied effects of censure	Proc Sz = Reac Sz > N	S		
Zahn and Rosenthal (1965)	Blocked trials	Acute Sz > Nonsz	S	S	S (weak)
III: Studies Examining Schizophrenic Subgroup and Dimensional Differences					
Payne and Caird (1967)	Blocks of irreg trials w/o "ready" signal; used distracting stimuli	Para > Nonpara only on distr. trials	S		
Rosenthal et al. (1960)	Blocked trials	Correlations with mental health rating	S	S	S (weak)
Strauss et al. (1979)	Embedded set	RDC Sz = DSM-II Sz			S
Tizard and Venables (1957)	Blocked: PI 8 s only	Para & social > Nonpara & withdrawn during extraneous stim	S		

[a] Key to abbreviations: PI, preparatory interval; ITI, intertrial interval; PPI, prepreparatory interval.

[b] Key to abbreviations: Sz, schizophrenic; N, normal subject; Chr Sz, chronic schizophrenic; Proc Sz, process schizophrenic; Reac Sz, reactive schizophrenic; Nonsz, nonschizophrenic patient; RDC, Research Diagnostic Criteria diagnosis; MR, mentally retarded; TLE, temporal lobe epilepsy; Gen E, generalized epilepsy; Depr Sz, depression with schizophrenia; Szt, schizotypic; MMPI elev, Minnesota Multiphasic Personality Inventory Scores elevated; MMPI dev, Minnesota Multiphasic Personality Inventory scores deviant; Szt (perc), schizotypic perceptual aberration; Szt (anhed), schizotypic (anhedonic); Para, paranoid; DSM-II, *Diagnostic and Statistical Manual of Mental Disorders* (second edition).

[c] S, significant; NS, nonsignificant.

Using a criterion of one standard deviation below the mean for 93 normal subjects, an impairment index based on the collective number of deficit scores was computed. A collective deficit score was the number of the five measures on which a subject performed less well than the −1.00 standard deviation cutoff point. This procedure yielded a satisfactory discrimination of the groups when two or greater signs were used. That is, 75% of the process schizophrenics, 50% of the reactive schizophrenics, 25% of the nonschizophrenic patients, and only 5% of the normal controls showed reaction time impairments equal to or exceeding the standard. Noting that these indices collectively provide the same levels of efficiency reported by Holzman and his collaborators for eye tracking measures (Holzman et al., 1974), and reported in the International Pilot Study of Schizophrenia investigation using the 12 most discriminating symptoms (Carpenter, Strauss, & Bartko, 1973), we can conclude that the reaction time indices are capable of discriminating schizophrenia from other disorders and schizophrenics from normal controls, as well as among schizophrenic subtypes.

To examine reaction time efficiency in greater detail, we used MANOVAs to make several group comparisons. As presented in Table 8.2, the five indices were simultaneously analyzed to test specific differences among: (a) the normal controls versus all three patient groups, (b) the nonschizophrenic patient controls versus the two schizophrenic groups, and (c) the process versus reactive schizophrenics. The general differences among the four groups are also presented in the first row of the table. As may be seen in the left-most column, the five reaction time variables collectively were highly significant in all four of these group discriminations. The remainder of the data in Table 8.2 give the univariate results for each of the indices. Each of the general latency scores makes a significant—and in most cases a quite large—contribution to the group discriminations. The amount of redundancy deficit found in the short and mid-length preparatory intervals is naturally quite small, because the short-interval regular trials have been consistently found to yield faster speeds among all groups in this literature than the irregular trials. With respect to the long preparatory interval indices of redundancy deficit, however, significant R^2 contributions are made by these regular and irregular comparisons. In the process versus reactive schizophrenic contrast, the long-preparatory-interval RTX makes the greatest contribution among all the measures—including a difference superior to the general latency measures. Only in the nonschizophrenic versus schizophrenic contrast do long-preparatory-interval RTX trials give a relatively weak, although statistically significant, yield. In conclusion, these findings suggest that the general latency scores are indeed the best contributors, but some additional advantage is real-

Table 8.2. Diagnostic Group Differences in Reaction Time ($N = 444$)

Contrast	Multivariate results				Univariate results[a]														
	Pillai trace	Approx. F	df	p	Short PI: RT std[b]			Middle PI: RT std[b]			Short PI: RTX			Middle PI: RTX			Long PI: RTX		
					F	p	R^2	F	p	R^2	F	p	R^2	F	p	R^2	F	p	R^2
All diagnostic groups	.37	12.28	15,132	<.00	57.03	<.00	.28	36.83	<.00	.20	3.36	.02	.02	2.46	.06	.02	15.28	<.00	.09
Normal vs. patient	.24	27.32	5,438	<.00	101.192	<.00	.19	71.24	<.00	.14	0.81	.37	.00	5.83	.02	.01	20.60	<.00	.05
Nonschizophrenic vs. schizophrenic	.12	11.86	5,438	<.00	56.032	<.00	.11	24.29	<.00	.05	6.78	.01	.02	1.12	.29	.00	4.49	.04	.01
Process vs. reactive schizophrenic	.08	7.59	5,438	<.00	13.86	<.00	.03	14.96	<.00	.03	2.49	.12	.01	0.44	.51	.00	20.76	<.00	.05

[a] PI, preparatory interval; RT std, standard reaction time; RTX, reaction time crossover.
[b] The two standard reaction time variables were log transformed.

ized by adding the RTX index for long-preparatory-interval trials.

Predictive Power of Reaction Time Indices

The "north star" image of reaction time suggested by Cancro and his colleagues (1971) was derived in large part from their finding of a strong correlation between crossmodal shift effects and clinical outcome measures. The prognostic value of reaction time was not new to reaction time literature (e.g., Weaver & Brooks, 1967), but we believed the relative predictive merits of different reaction time indices needed further exploration.

Using a subset of the data examined in the MANOVA above, we were able to associate the latency and RTX indices with follow-up information of at least 1 year's duration (extending to 10 years in some cases) obtained on 104 process schizophrenic patients. In these analyses of outcome, we used as predictors several variables previously found to be effective at estimating prognosis—viz., the Ullmann–Giovanonni (1964) Process-Reactive Scale and the number of hospitalizations prior to the index hospitalization during which patients were tested—in addition to the five reaction time measures described above. In short, we were interested in examining the incremental value of reaction time indices in predicting outcome over and above clinical factors

that are (typically) predictive of subsequent adjustment. The criterion measures we used were (a) number of subsequent hospitalizations and (b) proportion of subsequent time in hospital after the time of testing.

We conducted two hierarchical multiple regression analyses (one for number of subsequent hospitalizations and one for proportion of time in hospital) in which predictor variables were entered in the following order: (1) Ullmann–Giovanonni scores, (2) prior hospitalization, (3) the two general latency measures, and 4) the three RTX measures. We found an overall multiple R of 0.45 using all of these variables to predict number of subsequent hospitalizations. The amount of unique variance in the criterion explained by each variable is described in Table 8.3. There it may be seen that the Ullmann–Giovanonni measure explained only 0.2% of the variance, whereas the number of previous hospitalizations and the proportion of time hospitalized before testing explained more than 11% of the variance. The two reaction time latency measures (entered at step 3) together explained only an extra 1.5%, whereas the three RTX measures (entered collectively in step 4) explained an additional 7%. This pattern of results indicates the merit of the redundancy deficit indices in prognosis. Insofar as our sample was composed of homogeneously chronic and process-range schizophrenic patients with extensive hospitalization ca-

Table 8.3. Case Factor and Reaction Time Variable Predictions of Number of Hospitalizations (after Testing)[a] ($N = 104$)

		Overall statistics					Step statistics				Variable statistics					1-tail
Step	Variables entered	Mult. R	R^2	F	df	p	ΔR^2	ΔF	df	p	Ry	b	S.E.	β	t	p
1	Ullmann–Giovanonni score	.046	.002	0.22	1,102	.640					.046	.012	.026	.046	0.47	.320
2	No. of hospitalizations before testing	.339	.115	4.33	3,100	.006	.113	6.38	2,100	.003	.246	.377	.115	.327	3.28	.001
	Proportion of time hospitalized before testing										.108	.566	.240	.248	2.36	.010
3	Short PI RTstd[b]	.361	.130	2.94	5,98	.016	.015	0.86	2,98	.426	.160	.395	.753	.075	0.53	.301
	Middle PI RTstd										.191	.338	.743	.066	0.46	.325
4	Short PI RTX	.448	.201	2.99	8,95	.005	.071	2.80	3,95	.044	.156	.00092	.00072	.135	1.28	.102
	Middle PI RTX										.174	.00132	.00065	.204	2.03	.023
	Long PI RTX										.207	.00081	.00094	.090	0.86	.196

[a] This variable was transformed by taking the square root of the original number and by Windsorizing extreme values.
[b] The two standard reaction time (RTstd) variables were log transformed. PI, preparatory interval.

Table 8.4. Case Factor and Reaction Time Variable Predictions of Proportion of Time Hospitalized (after Testing)[a] ($N = 104$)

		Overall statistics					Step statistics				Variable statistics					
		Mult.														1-tail
Step	Variables entered	R	R^2	F	df	p	ΔR^2	ΔF	df	p	Ry	b	S.E.	β	t	p
1	Ullmann–Giovanonni score	.202	.041	4.33	1,102	.040					−.202	−.029	.014	−.202	−2.08	.020
2	No. of hospitalizations before testing	.533	.284	13.25	3,100	<.000	.244	17.03	2,100	<.000	.321	.273	.057	.432	4.83	<.000
	Proportion of time hospitalized before testing										.330	.546	.118	.438	4.62	<.000
3	Short PI RTstd[b]	.597	.356	10.83	5,98	<.000	.071	5.44	2,98	.006	.282	−.229	.355	−.079	−0.65	.260
	Middle PI RTstd										.407	.948	.350	.337	2.71	.004
4	Short PI RTX	.606	.367	6.89	8,95	<.000	.011	0.56	3,95	.641	.105	.00017	.00035	.045	0.49	.314
	Middle PI RTX										.049	.00034	.00032	.097	1.08	.141
	Long PI RTX										.084	−.00031	.00046	−.062	−0.67	.253

[a] This variable was transformed by taking the arcsine of the square root of the original proportions.
[b] The two standard reaction time (RTstd) variables were log transformed. PI, preparatory interval.

reers, and insofar as several well-known indices of social adjustment (the Ullmann–Giovanonni and the previous hospitalization indices) were entered first into the regression equation, it is particularly impressive that reaction time measures could make independent and substantial contributions to the understanding of outcome.

These analyses were repeated (see Table 8.4) in an attempt to predict the proportion of post-testing time during which the individual was hospitalized. We obtained a multiple R of 0.61 using the same predictors as above. In contrast to the previous regression analysis, the Ullmann–Giovanonni score now explained 4% of the variance in the criterion, whereas the previous number of hospitalizations and the proportion of time hospitalized before testing explained 24% of the variance. Although reaction time measures contributed to predictions of the criterion, the contributions were different from the previous analysis. In this case, the latency measures explained 7% (when entered into the third step), whereas the redundancy deficit measures contributed only 1% (when entered at the fourth step).

The findings suggested that the different reaction time indices might be contributing in a somewhat different way to predictions of the two measures of outcome. The "proportion of time hospitalized" possibly focused on the presence of individuals with long patterns of continued stay (e.g., some patients never left the hospital after the testing), whereas the "number of hospitalizations" may have reflected "revolving door" patients who came and left the hospital with rapidity. It appears that the differential predictive yield from latency and RTX measures may reflect somewhat different patterns of patient functioning. In short, the latency measure may be more predictive of proportion of time in hospital because it is characteristic of individuals with far fewer personal resources—perhaps higher degrees of negative symptoms. We further speculate that the RTX linkage to the "number of hospitalization" criterion may result from the presence of individuals with labile or episodic qualities to their disorder, possibly reflecting a vulnerability-to-stress factor in the extreme RTX-responder patients. The value of these speculations awaits further research.

REACTION TIME INDICES AND THE DIAGNOSTIC AND STATISTICAL MANUAL OF MENTAL DISORDERS

From the literature reviewed here, it is obvious that most reaction time studies were conducted during the eras of the first and second editions of the *Diagnostic and Statistical Manual of Mental Disorders* (DSM). Our curiosity about the power of reaction time and similar measures to discriminate among disorders classified in the third edition (DSM-III; American Psychiatric Association, 1980) was served by a dissertation conducted by Connelly in 1984. In this investigation, four schizophrenia spectrum–disordered groups and two other psychiatric groups were contrasted on a variety of background factors (including hospitalization history and current functioning), as well as scores on cognitive tests and various measures of attention. Included in the investigation were four DSM-III schizophrenia spectrum diagnostic groups: Schizophrenia, Schizophreniform Disorder, Schizotypal Personality Disorder, and Schizoaffective Disorder. Bipolar Disorder and Borderline Personality Disorder were included as comparison groups.

Discriminant function analyses conducted using a set of laboratory measures and a set of background/clinical measures, and both sets together yielded remarkably clear discrimination among the six groups of 12 patients each. Using a combination of all measures, for example, discrimination accuracy was 83% or greater for any of the schizophrenic, schizophreniform, and bipolar groups. Lower accuracies for the schizotypal and schizoaffective (50%) and the borderline (25%) groups reduced the overall classification accuracy to 64%. Although far from perfect, this level of sensitivity encourages the belief that a well-constituted battery of clinically sensitive measures and laboratory attention tests can be helpful in making fairly tough differential diagnoses between schizophrenia and other DSM-III disorders, and in illuminating similarities and differences in the underlying pathology of these disorders.

Examination of "hit rates" (i.e., the percentage of true positives) per group showed a better overall yield (60% accuracy) from the laboratory tests than from the clinical measures (43% accuracy). The latter measures included indices of stress response and current functioning (from Axes IV and V), history of hospitalization, marital status, educational level, family history of disorder, and other measures of clinical adjustment. The analysis of lab measures included reaction time and other attention-demanding tests such as the Span of Apprehension, Stroop, and Digit Symbol Substitution Test. The various reaction time indices were clearly among the most efficient discriminators. For example, a short-duration (preparatory interval = 1 second) general latency measure was the best single contributor in the discriminant function analyses performed. These results indicate the continued relevance of reaction time measurement for the diagnosis of schizophrenic pathology. Moreover, these results strongly suggest continuity of diagnostic relevance from the earlier literatures to the current DSM diagnostic system.

CONCLUDING REMARKS

We continue to see substantial utility in the application of reaction time measures to the study of schizophrenia. Although other perceptual, physiological, and cognitive markers of schizophrenic pathology are now rising in popularity, reaction time has maintained its role as a major player, showing strong ability to discriminate among schizophrenic subgroups as well as between schizophrenics and other patient groups. Reaction time has an untapped potential in prognostic estimation, as the original Cancro paper argued and the Waterloo studies have strongly supported. Reflecting back on the Cancro quotation that opened this chapter, it may be said that reaction time may not qualify as the "north star," but neither is it a "shooting star." It is simply one of the "major constellations" in a laboratory technology that aids navigation toward increased understanding of the schizophrenic disorders. It is our hope that such a technology will eventually become part of an objective assessment battery used in the differential diagnosis of major mental disorders.

Clearly the study of reaction time has not yet led us to full understanding of why this index is such a reliable discriminator. That may be because it is more like a catalyst for the expression of pathological processes than it is an actual observation of the disturbed processes. It may be, for example, that the major value of reaction time rests on the simple fact that the task requires subjects to "sit quietly" for a few moments. During the reaction time task, normal and psychiatric patient groups alike tend to show physiological quieting—evidenced in heart rate deceleration, reduced respiration, baseline electroencephalogram shifts (contingent negative variation), and reduced activity in other systems. If the inhibitory controls are weak in schizophrenic pathology (Epstein & Coleman, 1970), the task requirement for damped arousal and its associated vigilance will not be sustained, and so efficiency of task performance will be impaired. From this reasoning, we suggest that the value of the reaction time task may lie less in the size of the deficit observed than in the window of opportunity it provides to examine physiological perturbations that make an appearance during the long reaction time regular trials. As work on biological substrates becomes ever more sophisticated, it may be wise for investigators to use reaction time technology as opportunities—we call them "precious moments"—for examining the concomitant central and autonomic nervous system processes that occur during the tasks. Adopting a somewhat different astronomy metaphor, reaction time and like measures may serve the same role as a high mountain top, offering a better opportunity for observation of the phenomena of interest.

In considering reaction time task utility in the clinical workplace, the Connelly (1984) study shows how differential diagnosis may be assisted by a battery of laboratory measures. Spaulding's COGLAB procedure is leading the way in developing an economical delivery system for various cognitive and perceptual–motor tests (Spaulding, Hargrove, Crineau, & Martin, 1981). Various research teams have also seen utility in "polythetic measurement strategies" (Corning, Steffy, & Chaprin, 1982). High levels of diagnostic group discriminations can be achieved with cost-effective measurement devices. The utility of reaction time measures for predicting long-term outcome is also strongly suggested by our multiple regression analyses of prognosis. We

would argue that the time is near when a standard battery of objective measures will be available to aid diagnosis. In such a vision, reaction time measures continue to enjoy an esteemed position.

REFERENCES

American Psychiatric Association. (1980). *Diagnostic and statistical manual of mental disorders* (3rd ed.). Washington, DC: American Psychiatric Press, Inc.

Bellissimo, A., & Steffy, R. (1972). Redundancy-associated deficit in schizophrenic reaction time performance. *Journal of Abnormal Psychology, 80,* 299–307.

Bellissimo, A., & Steffy R. A. (1975). Contextual influences on crossover in the reaction time performance of schizophrenics. *Journal of Abnormal Psychology, 84,* 210–220.

Bernstein, S. M. (1976). *Drift and crossover effects in the reaction time performance of schizophrenics and nonschizophrenics.* Unpublished doctoral dissertation, University of Waterloo.

Bohannon, W. E., & Strauss, M. E. (1983). Reaction time crossover in psychiatric outpatients. *Psychiatry Research, 9,* 17–22.

Botwinick, J., Brinley, J. F., & Robbin, J. S. (1959). Maintaining set in relation to motivation and age. *American Journal of Psychology, 72,* 585–588.

Bradley, I. F. (1976). *Physiological concomitants to the redundancy-associated deficit in process schizophrenia.* Unpublished doctoral dissertation, University of Waterloo.

Cancro, R., Sutton, S., Kerr, J., & Sugerman, A. (1971). Reaction time and prognosis in acute schizophrenia. *Journal of Nervous and Mental Disease, 153,* 351–359.

Carpenter, W. T., Jr., Strauss, J. S., & Bartko, J. J. (1973). Flexible system for the diagnosis of schizophrenia: Report from the WHO International Pilot Study of Schizophrenia. *Science, 182,* 1275–1278.

Chapman, L. J., & Chapman, J. P. (1973). *Disordered thought in schizophrenia.* New York: Appleton-Century-Crofts.

Connelly, W. (1984). *DSM-III Schizophrenic Disorder: Comparisons with other functional psychoses and borderline conditions.* Unpublished doctoral dissertation, University of Waterloo.

Corning, W. C., Steffy, R. A., & Chaprin, I. C. (1982). EEG slow frequency and WISC-R correlates. *Journal of Abnormal Child Psychology, 10,* 511–530.

Cromwell, R. L. (1975). Assessment of schizophrenia. *Annual Review of Psychology, 26,* 593–619.

Cromwell, R. L. (1984). Preemptive thinking and schizophrenia research. In W. Spaulding & J. Cole (Eds.), *Nebraska Symposium on Motivation, Vol. 31: Theories of schizophrenia and psychosis* (pp. 1–46). Lincoln: University of Nebraska Press.

Cromwell, R. L., & Dokecki, P. R. (1968). Schizophrenic language: A disattention interpretation. In S. Rosenberg & J. H. Koplin (Eds.), *Developments in applied psycholinguistics research* (pp. 209–261). New York: Macmillan Company.

Cromwell, R. L., Rosenthal, D., Shakow, D., & Zahn, T. P. (1961). Reaction time, locus of control, choice behavior, and descriptions of parental behavior in schizophrenic and normal subjects. *Journal of Personality, 29,* 363–379.

Czudner, G., & Marshall, M. (1967). Simple reaction time in schizophrenic, retarded, and normal children under regular and irregular preparatory interval conditions. *Canadian Journal of Psychology, 21,* 369–380.

De Amicis, L. A., & Cromwell, R. L. (1979). Reaction time crossover in process schizophrenic patients, their relatives, and control subjects. *Journal of Nervous and Mental Disease, 167,* 593–600.

De Amicis, L. A., Huntzinger, R. S., & Cromwell, R. L. (1981). Magnitude of reaction time crossover in process schizophrenic patients in relation to their first-degree relatives. *Journal of Nervous and Mental Disease, 169,* 64–65.

Epstein, S., & Coleman, M. (1970). Drive theories of schizophrenia. *Psychosomatic Medicine, 32,* 113–140.

Fedio, P., Mirsky, A. F., Smith, W. J., & Parry, D. (1961). Reaction time and EEG activation in normal and schizophrenic subjects. *Electoencephalography and Clinical Neurophysiology, 13,* 923–926.

Fenz, W. D., & Velner, J. (1970). Physiological concomitants of behavioral indexes in schizophrenia. *Journal of Abnormal Psychology, 76,* 27–35.

Friedman, D., Vaughan, H. G., & Erlenmeyer-Kimling, L. (1978). Stimulus and response related components of the later positive complex in visual discrimination tasks. *Electoencephalography and Clinical Neurophysiology, 45,* 319–330.

Green, A. A. (1974). *Effects of signal intensity, prestimulation and time controls upon simple reaction time in process schizophrenic patients.* Unpublished doctoral dissertation, University of Waterloo.

Greiffenstein, M., Lewis, R., Milberg, W., & Rosenbaum, G. (1981). Temporal lobe epilepsy and schizophrenia: Comparison of reaction time deficits. *Journal of Abnormal Psychology, 90,* 105–112.

Grisell, J. L., & Rosenbaum, G. (1964). Effects of auditory intensity on simple reaction time of schizophrenics. *Perceptual and Motor Skills, 18,* 396.

Holzman, P. S., Proctor, L. R., Levy, D. L., Yasillo, J. J., Meltzer, H. Y., & Hunt, S. W. (1974). Eye-tracking dysfunctions in schizophrenic patients and their relatives. *Archives of General Psychiatry, 31,* 143–151.

Hull, C. (1943). *Principles of behavior.* New York: Appleton-Century-Crofts, Inc.

Huston, P. E., & Senf, R. (1952). Psychopathology of schizophrenia and depression. I. Effect of amytal and amphetamine sulfate on level and maintenance of attentions. *American Journal of Psychiatry, 109,* 131–138.

Huston, P. E., Shakow, D., & Riggs, L. A. (1937). Studies of motor functioning in schizophrenia: II. Reaction time. *Journal of General Psychology, 16,* 39–82.

Jentsch, R. C. (1958). Reaction time in schizophrenia as a function of method of presentation and length of preparatory interval. *Journal of Personality, 26,* 545–555.

Kaplan, R. (1974). *The crossover phenomenon: Three studies of the effect of training and information on process schizophrenic reaction time.* Unpublished doctoral dissertation, University of Waterloo.

Karras, A. (1962). The effects of reinforcement and arousal on the psychomotor performance of chronic schizophrenics. *Journal of Abnormal and Social Psychology, 65,* 104–111.

King, H. E. (1962). Reaction-time as a function of stimulus intensity among normal subjects and psychotic subjects. *Journal of Psychology, 54,* 299–307.

Knehr, C. A. (1954). Schizophrenic reaction time responses to variable preparatory intervals. *American Journal of Psychiatry, 110,* 585–588.

Lacey, J. I. (1967). Somatic response patterning and stress: Some revisions of activation theory. In M. Appley & R. Trumbull (Eds.), *Psychological stress: Issues in research* (pp. 14–37). New York: Appleton-Century-Crofts.

Lang, P. J. (1959). The effect of aversive stimuli for reaction time in schizophrenia. *Journal of Abnormal and Social Psychology, 59,* 263–268.

Mannuzza, S. (1980). Cross-modal reaction time and schizophrenic attentional deficit: A critical review. *Schizophrenia Bulletin, 6,* 654–675.

McCormick, W. R. (1974). *Cardiac rate and size*

estimation in schizophrenic and normal subjects. Unpublished MA thesis, University of Wisconsin.

Mo, S. S. (1968). *Schizophrenic reaction time to sudden change of a fixed foreperiod.* Unpublished doctoral dissertation, University of Pennsylvania.

Nideffer, R. M., Neale, J. M., Kopfstein, J. H., & Cromwell, R. L. (1971). The effect of previous preparatory intervals upon anticipatory responses in reaction time of schizophrenic and nonschizophrenic patients. *Journal of Nervous and Mental Diseases, 153,* 360–365.

Nuechterlein, K. H. (1977). Reaction time and attention in schizophrenia: A critical evaluation of the data and theories. *Schizophrenia Bulletin, 3,* 373–428.

Obrist, P. A., Sutterer, J. R., Howard, J. L., Hennis, H. S., & Murrel, D. J. (1973). Cardiac-somatic changes during a simple reaction time task: A developmental study. *Journal of Experimental Child Psychology, 16,* 346–362.

Pascal, C., & Swensen, G. (1952). Learning in mentally ill patients under unusual motivation. *Journal of Personality, 21,* 240–249.

Pavlov, I. P. (1941). *Conditioned reflexes and psychiatry.* (W. H. Gantt, Trans.). New York: International Press.

Payne, R. W., & Caird, W. K. (1967). Reaction time, distractibility, and over-inclusive thinking in psychotics. *Journal of Abnormal Psychology, 72,* 112–121.

Rodnick, E. H., & Shakow, D. (1940). Set in the schizophrenic as measured by a composite reaction time index. *American Journal of Psychiatry, 97,* 214–225.

Rosenbaum, G., Chapin, K., & Shore, D. L. (1988). Attention deficit in schizophrenia and schizotypy: Marker versus symptom variables. *Journal of Abnormal Psychology, 97,* 41–47.

Rosenbaum, G., MacKavey, W. R., & Grisell, J. L. (1957). Effects of biological and social motivation on schizophrenic RT. *Journal of Abnormal and Social Psychology, 54,* 364–368.

Rosenthal, D., Lawlor, W. G., Zahn, T. P., & Shakow, D. (1960). The relationship of some aspects of mental set to degree of schizophrenic disorganization. *Journal of Personality, 28,* 26–38.

Salzinger, K. (1971). An hypothesis about schizophrenic behavior. *American Journal of Psychotherapy, 25,* 601–614.

Schneider, R. D., & Cauthen, N. R. (1982). Locus of reaction time change in schizophrenics and normal subject. *Journal of Nervous and Mental Disease, 170,* 231–240.

Shakow, D. (1962). Segmental set: A theory of the formal psychological deficit in schizophrenia. *Archives of General Psychiatry, 6,* 17–32.

Shakow, D. (1963). Psychological deficit in schizophrenia. *Behavioral Science, 8,* 275–305.

Simons, R. F., MacMillan, F. W., III, & Ireland, F. B. (1982). Reaction-time crossover in preselected schizotypic subjects. *Journal of Abnormal Psychology, 91,* 414–415.

Spaulding, W., Hargrove, S., Crineau, W., & Martin, T. (1981). A microcomputer-based laboratory for psychopathology research in neural settings. *Behavior Research Methods and Instrumentation, 13,* 616–623.

Spring, B. J. (1980). Shift of attention in schizophrenics, siblings of schizophrenics, and depressed patients. *Journal of Nervous and Mental Disease, 168,* 133–140.

Steffy, R. A. (1978). An early cue sometimes impairs process schizophrenic performance. In L. C. Wynne, R. L. Cromwell, & S. Matthysse (Eds.), *The nature of schizophrenia: Approaches to research and treatment* (pp. 225–232). New York: John Wiley & Sons.

Steffy, R. A., & Galbraith, K. J. (1974). A comparison of segmental set and inhibitory deficit explanations of the crossover pattern in schizophrenic patients. *Journal of Abnormal Psychology, 83,* 227–233.

Steffy, R. A., & Galbraith, K. J. (1975). The time course of a disruptive signal in the reaction time performance of process schizophrenic patients. *Journal of Abnormal Psychology, 84,* 315–324.

Steffy, R. A., & Galbraith, K. J. (1980). Relation between latency and redundancy-associated deficit in schizophrenic reaction time performance. *Journal of Abnormal Psychology, 89,* 419–427.

Strauss, M. E., Bohannon, W. E., Kaminsky, M. J., & Kharabi, F. (1979). Simple reaction time crossover occurs in schizophrenic outpatients. *Schizophrenia Bulletin, 5,* 612–615.

Strauss, M. E., Wagman, A. M. I., & Quaid, K. A. (1983). Preparatory interval influences in reaction time of elderly adults. *Journal of Gerontology, 38,* 55–57.

Sutton, S., & Zubin, J. (1965). Effect of sequence on reaction time in schizophrenia. In A. L. Welford & J. E. Birren (Eds.), *Behaviour aging, and the nervous system* (pp. 562–597). Springfield, IL, Charles C Thomas.

Tecce, J. J. (1972). Contingent negative variation (CNV) and psychological processes in man. *Psychological Bulletin, 77,* 73–108.

Tizard, J., & Venables, P. H. (1956). Reaction time responses by schizophrenics, mental defectives and normal adults. *American Journal of Psychiatry, 112,* 803–807.

Tizard, J., & Venables, P. H. (1957). The influence of extraneous stimulation on the reaction time of schizophrenics. *British Journal of Psychology, 48,* 299–305.

Ullman, L. P., & Giovannoni, J. (1964). The development of a self-report measure of the process-reactive continuum. *Journal of Nervous and Mental Disease, 138,* 38–42.

Van Dyke, W. K., & Routh, D. K. (1973). Effects of censure on schizophrenic reaction time: Critique and reformulation of the Garmezy censure-deficit model. *Journal of Abnormal Psychology, 82,* 200–206.

Venables, P. H., & O'Connor, N. (1959). Reaction times to auditory and visual stimulation in schizophrenic and normal subjects. *Quarterly Journal of Experimental Psychology, 11,* 175–179.

Venables, P. H., & Tizard, J. (1958). The effect of auditory stimulus intensity on the reaction time of schizophrenics. *Journal of Mental Science, 104,* 1160–1164.

Waldbaum, J. K., Sutton, S., & Kerr, J. (1975). Shift of sensory modality and reaction time in schizophrenia. In M. L. Kietzman, S. Sutton, & J. Zubin (Eds.), *Experimental approaches to psychopathology* (pp. 167–176). New York: Academic Press, Inc.

Weaver, L. A., & Brooks, G. W. (1967). The prediction of release from a mental hospital from psychomotor test performance. *Journal of General Psychology, 76,* 207–229.

Wittman, P. (1941). A scale for measuring prognosis in schizophrenic patients. *Elgin State Hospital Papers, 4,* 20–33.

Zahn, T. P. (1970). Effects of reductions in uncertainty on reaction time in schizophrenic and normal subjects. *Journal of Experimental Research in Personality, 4,* 135–143.

Zahn, T. P., & Rosenthal, D. (1965). Preparatory set in acute schizophrenia. *Journal of Nervous and Mental Disease, 141,* 352–358.

Zahn, T. P., Rosenthal, D., & Shakow, D. (1961). Reaction time in schizophrenic and normal subjects in relation to the sequence of a series of regular preparatory intervals. *Journal of Abnormal and Social Psychology, 61,* 161–168.

Zahn, T. P., Rosenthal, D., & Shakow, D. (1963). Effects of irregular preparatory intervals in reaction time in schizophrenia. *Journal of Abnormal and Social Psychology, 67,* 44–52.

Zahn, T. P., Shakow, D., & Rosenthal, D. (1961). Reaction time in schizophrenic and normal subjects as a function of preparatory and intertrial intervals. *Journal of Nervous and Mental Disease, 133,* 283–287.

Zubin, J. (1975). Problems of attention in schizophrenia. In M. L. Kietzman, S. Sutton, & J. Zubin (Eds.), *Experimental approaches to psychopathology* (pp. 139–166). New York, Academic Press.

9

Perception and Cognition in Schizophrenia

DAVID R. HEMSLEY

Clearly the abnormal behaviors and experiences that we characterize as schizophrenic require analysis at a number of levels—social, behavioral, cognitive, psychophysiological, and biochemical. A major task is to demonstrate how these are interrelated. An approach that views schizophrenia as a disturbance of information processing appears promising as a means of linking biological and social factors relevant to the disorder. Such research is best carried out within the framework of models of normal functioning, "by relating the concepts and objects of clinical observation to the concepts and experimental data from general psychology" (Cohen & Borst, 1987, p. 189).

Disturbances of cognition have long been viewed as among the most distinguishing features of schizophrenia. On attention, Kraepelin (1919) observed:

It is quite common for them to lose both inclination and ability on their own initiative to keep their attention fixed for any length of time . . . there is occasionally noticed a kind of irresistible attraction of the attention to casual external impressions." (pp. 6–7)

He also noted that patients "lose in a most striking way the faculty of logical ordering of their trains of thought" (p. 101). More generally, he observed that "Mental efficiency is always diminished to a considerable extent" (p. 23). Observations such as these are a necessary beginning to the understanding of schizophrenics' cognitive impairment.

Some patients are able to provide a vivid description of the way in which their perceptions and/or thinking are altered. This frequently takes a more subtle form than the report of hallucinatory experiences or delusional beliefs. Matussek (1952) described a patient who was aware of "a lack of continuity of his perceptions both in space and over time—He saw the environment only in fragments. There was no appreciation of the whole. He saw only details against a meaningless background" (p. 92). Another patient reported,

I may look at a garden, but I don't see it as I normally do. I can only concentrate on details. For instance, I can lose myself in looking at a bud on a branch, but then I don't see anything else. (p. 92).

In a similar vein, McGhie and Chapman (1961) described an extended interview study of newly admitted schizophrenics. They concentrated on changes in the patients' experiences, and presented the findings in the form of selected quotations. Typical were the following: "Everything seems to grip my attention, although I am not particularly interested in anything"; "Things are coming in too fast. I lose my grip of it and get lost. I am attending to everything at once and as a result do not attend to anything"; "My thoughts get all jumbled up. I start thinking or talking about something but I never get there." The authors argued that the primary disorder in schizophrenia is a decrease in the selective and inhibitory function of attention, and that many other cognitive, perceptual, affective, and behavioral abnormalities could be seen as resulting from this primary attentional deficit.

The most ambitious aim of psychological research in this area is to specify a single cognitive dysfunction, or pattern of dysfunction, from which the various abnormalities resulting in a diagnosis of schizophrenia might be derived: as Matussek (1952) put it, "to render understandable in psychological terms that which (in Jaspers' 1913 [1963] view) is 'not understandable' " (p. 90). To this end, there has a been a considerable research effort directed at demonstrating psychological deficits specific to schizophrenia—that is, tasks on which schizophrenics perform particularly poorly. However, the results of such research are often theoretically elaborated in two ways. Oltmanns and Neale (1978) wrote:

First the single empirical measure which has been assessed is assumed to index a more general construct. Second, it is then postulated that the construct which is implicated in the deficit is causally related to schizophrenia and can account for a variety of schizophrenic behaviours. (p. 198)

The first of these stages is dependent on an agreed-on model of normal cognitive functioning, and the use of tasks that tap a particular function. Much early research on cognitive abnormalities used tasks unrelated to such models, and findings were therefore difficult to interpret.

The information-processing approach has become dominant in research into adult cognitive processes, and therefore forms the basis for most current work on cognitive abnormalities. It aims to "make explicit the operations, stages, and processes that occur in the time between stimulation and the observed response" (Haber & Hershenson, 1973, p. 158) and "to describe the limits and characteristics of these processes" (Underwood, 1978, p. 2). It is claimed that such models specify more precisely the relationship between observed task performance and inferred function, and therefore one might more clearly identify the way in which schizophrenics are cognitively impaired.

However, this approach is not without difficulty because, although current models of human cognition share many important features, it cannot be claimed that there is an agreed-on model. A further problem is that schizophrenics tend to perform poorly on most cognitive tasks.

SELECTIVE ATTENTION

The issue of selectivity in human information processing has always been central to psychology. Underwood (1978) wrote: "attention may be used for selecting information which is to be perceived, and for selecting that which is to be responded to, as well as selecting for any number of intermediate or subordinate processes" (p. 247). It may therefore be viewed as the major control process in the passage of information through the system as a whole. Of particular interest in this context are the mechanisms relating to awareness, because many of the key symptoms of schizophrenia clearly represent alterations in conscious experience. However, there are obvious difficulties in mapping constructs that have been generated to explain task performance onto experiential phenomena. My own work derived considerably from that of Broadbent (e.g., 1971) and led to the suggestion that schizophrenics fail to establish appropriate response biases, and hence do not make use of temporal and spatial redundancy to reduce information-processing demands (Hemsley, 1990).

In a general sense, models of normal cognitive functioning accept that perception is dependent on an interaction between the presented stimulus and stored memories of regularities in previous input. The latter result in "expectancies" or "response biases" and serve to reduce information-processing demands. Norman and Bobrow (1976) made a distinction between "data driven" and "conceptually driven" processing, and it is clear that at different times, and for different individuals, either the stimulus or the expectation may exert the greater influence on perception. If schizophrenics are indeed less able to make use of the redundancy and patterning of sensory input, it should be possible to construct tasks on which it would be predicted that they would perform better than normal subjects. This would be the result of the normal subjects forming expectancies that were inappropriate to the stimulus presented. However, it is unlikely to be a straightforward endeavor because the magnitude of this effect must be great enough to counteract schizophrenics' generally lowered performance resulting from such factors as poor motivation.

One study (Brennan & Hemsley, 1984) did indicate "superior" performance by nonparanoid schizophrenics. This made use of the phenomenon of "illusory correlation," the report by an observer of a correlation between two events that in reality are not correlated. It is particularly likely to occur when the two events have a strong associative connection, and it may be viewed as a way in which prior expectations influence, and in this case mislead, subjects. It was therefore predicted that nonparanoid schizophrenics would produce weaker illusory correlations than normal subjects (i.e., their reports would more closely correspond to reality). Magaro (1980) has argued that the nature of the cognitive abnormality shown by nonparanoid is quite distinct from that of paranoid schizophrenics. The latter are seen as relying on a rigid conceptual guiding of information processing; hence Magaro would predict stronger illusory correlations in paranoid subjects. In terms of Norman and Bobrow's (1976) distinction, the nonparanoid schizophrenic might be seen as characterized by "data-driven" processing. Across the three tasks employed, the nonparanoids showed the weakest and the paranoids the strongest tendency to report illusory correlations. The normal subjects were in an intermediate position; such a pattern of results is not easily interpretable in terms of either a generalized deficit or lowered motivation.

CONTROLLED VERSUS AUTOMATIC PROCESSING

The distinction between controlled and automatic processing of information is prominent in much research on normal cognitive processes (e.g., Schneider & Shiffrin, 1977), and has recently influenced the study of schizophrenics' cognitive abnormalities. Schneider and Shiffrin's theory attempted to integrate work on the related areas of visual search, short-term memory search, and selective attention. Controlled processes are temporary sequences of operations under the control of the individual. They require attention, are often serial in nature, and involve demands on limited processing capacity. Although subject to interference by other simultaneous controlled processing, and relatively slow, they can be flexibly adapted to task requirements. In contrast, automatic processes are viewed as involving the activation of a fixed sequence of mental operations in response to a particular input configuration. They involve direct access to long-term memory (i.e., past regularities) and occur outside conscious awareness. Extensive practice results in the development of automatic processing, which, once established, is relatively inflexible and difficult to suppress.

Currently there is considerable interest in the suggestion that, in schizophrenia, conscious capacity-demanding processing is required to complete cognitive operations that are usually completed automatically. This is of particular interest because there is increased emphasis on the need to establish links between disturbances of cognition and schizophrenic symptoms. Venables (1984) pointed out that a failure of automatic processing would result in activity proceeding at the level of consciously controlled sequential processing. In the study by McGhie and Chapman (1961) of patients' reports of their experiences, one said, "I have to do everything step-by-step; nothing is automatic now. Everything has to be considered." A disturbance of automatic processing would be consistent with those studies demonstrating greater decrements in schizophrenics' performance when processing load is increased, because automatic processes serve to expand capacity by reducing the load on controlled processes. Related to this proposal is Frith's

(1979) suggestion that "the basic cognitive defect associated with schizophrenia is an awareness of automatic processes which are normally carried out below the level of consciousness" (p. 253).

There is thus some convergence of views that the dysfunction in schizophrenia is at the interface of automatic/preconscious processes and controlled/conscious processes, resulting in intrusions and discontinuities in conscious experience.

CONCLUSIONS ON PERCEPTUAL/ COGNITIVE ABNORMALITIES

It is apparent that, in considering schizophrenics' disturbances of perception and cognition, researchers have drawn on a number of theoretical models. These often differ radically in their assumptions concerning the nature of normal information processing. It is clearly hazardous to attempt to interpret studies in a different framework from those in which they were designed. Nevertheless, let us consider seven current views as to the nature of schizophrenics' cognitive impairment (Table 9.1) (Hemsley, 1987a).

Several models of normal cognition suggest that awareness of redundant information is inhibited to reduce information-processing demands on a limited-capacity system. The change from controlled to automatic processing on a task may be seen as including a gradual inhibition of awareness of redundant information (Schneider & Shiffrin, 1977). A related position has been developed by Posner and his colleagues (e.g., Posner, 1982). They distinguish automatic processes and conscious attention, the former not giving rise to awareness and the latter involving awareness and closely associated with "a general inhibitory process" (p. 173). Cognitive abnormalities in schizophrenia might then be seen as related to a weakening of inhibitory processes crucial to conscious attention. Such a disturbance would result in the intrusion into awareness of aspects of the environment not normally perceived, as reported by patients in McGhie and Chapman's (1961)

Table 9.1. Current Views on the Nature of Schizophrenics' Cognitive Impairment

1. "The basic cognitive defect . . . is an awareness of automatic processes which are normally carried out below the level of consciousness" (Frith, 1979, p. 233).
2. "There is some suggestion that there is a failure of automatic processing in schizophrenia so that activity must proceed at the level of consciously controlled sequential processing" (Venables, 1984, p. 75).
3. Schizophrenics "concentrate on detail, at the expense of theme" (Cutting, 1985, p. 300).
4. Schizophrenics show "some deficiency in perceptual schema formation in automaticity, or in the holistic stage of processing" (Knight, 1984, p. 120).
5. Schizophrenics show a "failure of attentional focusing to respond to stimulus redundancy" (Maher, 1983, p. 19).
6. "Schizophrenics are less able to make use of the redundancy and patterning of sensory input to reduce information processing demands" (Hemsley, 1987a, p. 181).
7. Schizophrenics "do not maintain a strong conceptual organization or a serial processing strategy . . . nor do they organize stimuli extensively relative to others" (Magaro, 1984, p. 202).

Reproduced with permission from Hemsley, D. R. (1987). An experimental psychological model for schizophrenia. In H. Hafner, W. F. Gattaz, & W. Janzarik (Eds.), *Search for the causes of schizophrenia* (p. 182). Heidelberg: Springer-Verlag.

study and noted by Matussek (1952). Two of the quotes in Table 9.1 (1 and 3) clearly indicate that cognitive performance is disrupted by the intrusion of material normally below awareness. The others can be related to a weakening of the influence of spatial and temporal regularities on perception.

How might these views be brought together and linked to the abnormal experiences characteristic of schizophrenia? In a very general sense the models of Broadbent, Shiffrin and Schneider, and Posner and his colleagues may be seen as illustrating the way in which the spatial and temporal regularities of past experience influence the processing, and more speculatively the awareness, of current sensory input. I have therefore argued (Hemsley, 1987a) that it is a weakening of the influence of stored memories of regularities of previous input on current perception that is basic to the schizophrenic condition. A related position recently has been put forward by Patterson (1987), who suggested that there is "a failure in the automaticity with which prior experience may be recreated in parallel with current stimulus input in schizophrenia (with concomitant failures in future orientation or contextually generated expectancy)." (p. 555) The recent evidence in support of this formulation is presented later in this paper.

INFORMATION-PROCESSING DISTURBANCES AND SYMPTOMS OF SCHIZOPHRENIA

It is clearly of some importance that "information processing deficits be shown to be related to more complex forms of psychopathology in schizophrenia, as a means for validating the deficit and demonstrating that it is not trivial" (Spohn, 1984, p. 347). In a similar vein, Anscombe (1987) has noted that "there remains a gap between the computer terminology in which attentional theories are couched, and the patient's experience of schizophrenia" (p. 291). The possible link between disordered speech and information-processing disturbance is relatively straightforward, and Harvey, Earle-Beyer, and Levinson (1988) have

demonstrated that susceptibility to distraction is an important and specific predictor of discourse failures in schizophrenia. However, for other important schizophrenic phenomena, such as hallucinatory experiences and delusional beliefs, the connection is far less straightforward. A simple attempt at such a link is presented in Figure 9.1.

It is convenient to distinguish two areas of theorizing and related experimentation. The first (e.g., Frith, 1979) seeks to account for the principal positive symptoms of schizophrenia in terms of the cognitive impairment. The second argues that certain aspects of schizophrenics' functioning may reflect the action of control mechanisms that "involve conscious and unconscious psychological processes that focus on regulating the amount of demand faced to fit the adaptive capacity available" (Strauss, 1987, p. 85).

As indicated in the previous section, Frith's (1979) model relies heavily on the distinction between preconscious and conscious processing of information. He suggested that thought disorder, hallucinations, and delusions may be seen as the results of

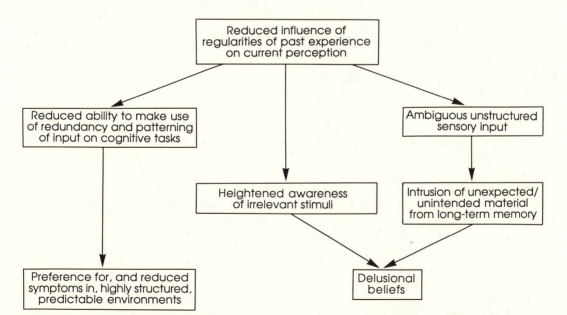

Figure 9.1. Model of cognitive abnormalities and symptoms of schizophrenia. (Reproduced with permission from Hemsley, D. R. [1987]. An experimental psychological model for schizophrenia. In H. Hafner, W. F. Gattaz, & W. Janzarik [Eds.], *Search for the causes of schizophrenia* [p. 183]. Heidelberg: Springer-Verlag.)

a defect in the mechanism that controls and limits the contents of consciousness. Delusions may be built up not only on the basis of hallucinatory experiences, but also as a result of attention being captured by incidental details of the environment. Normally, such an aspect of the situation would not reach awareness, but its registration leads to a search for reasons for its occurrence. Anscombe (1987) has extended this to suggest that certain of the patient's thoughts may be imbued with a significance that is out of proportion to their real importance, simply because they happen to capture the attentional focus. He went on to argue that both internally and externally generated perceptions *"are not placed in a context of background knowledge"* (emphasis added) and that this "results in the coming to awareness of hasty and alarming appraisals by preattentive processes" (p. 256). A patient of mine, recalling his psychotic experiences, noted that the co-occurrence of two events led immdiately to an assumption of a causal relationship between them. It was as if previous "non–co-occurrences" were completely ignored. Anscombe's position is clearly similar to the suggestion made in the previous section that the core abnormality in schizophrenia is a weakening of the influence of the regularities of past experience on current perception, and Matussek (1952) has argued that the extent to which the context is loosened crucially determines the severity of the disorder.

Matussek went on to suggest that, when the perceptual context is disturbed, the question arises as to whether other contextual relationships may be found. He quotes a patient as saying, "Out of these perceptions came the absolute awareness that my ability to see connections had been multipled many times over" (p. 96). Objects sharing certain qualities that had become prominent were seen as being linked in some significant way. Maher (1983) has also proposed that the pathology of schizophrenia "involves an inability to exclude from intrusion into consciousness material from either external stimulation or internally stored associations that would normally be excluded

on the basis of its irrelevance to the task situation in which the patient is performing" (p. 35). This he attributes to a failure to make use of the redundancies of sensory input to permit the optimum deployment of attention.

Because it has proved difficult to establish reliable behavioral concomitants of hallucinatory experiences, research in this area is of necessity largely based on self-report. Two issues must be distinguished. The first is why certain internally generated perceptions are experienced as deriving from external sources. The second concerns the determinants of occurrence of such experiences. Slade (1976) put forward a model of schizophrenic hallucinations that dealt primarily with the latter issue. This indicated three major areas of potential psychological research: (a) the investigation of factors within the individual predisposing to the development of hallucinations, (b) the role of arousal in triggering the hallucinatory phenomena, and (c) the influence of varying sensory input on the likelihood of hallucinatory experiences. All three have since proved productive. For example, Cooklin, Sturgeon, and Leff (1983) have demonstrated a significant association between the onset of hallucinatory periods and a rise in the rate of spontaneous fluctuations in skin conductance, although it was not possible to clarify the direction of cause and effect.

Relevant to the third area of potential research noted above, and of most concern to this paper, is the extensive literature on sensory/perceptual deprivation in normal subjects. It is clear that unstructured input may result in abnormal perceptual experiences, which Leff (1968) suggested "overlap considerably with those of mentally ill patients" (p. 1507). For example, in a study by Jakes and Hemsley (1986), brief exposure to unpatterned visual stimulation produced reports of complex visual sensations, the extent of which related both to the Psychoticism (P) scale of the Eysenck Personality Questionnaire and Launay and Slade's (1981) hallucination scale. It has also been possible to demonstrate the short-term manipulation of auditory hallucinations in a group of schizophrenic patients by means of alterations in auditory input (Margo, Hemsley, & Slade, 1981). The greatest reduction in hallucinatory experiences occurred when a response was required of the subject; for passive conditions the experiences were inversely related to the structure and attention-commanding properties of the input.

Such research offers no direct explanation of the occurrence of schizophrenic hallucinations, only of the extent to which they may vary under brief manipulations of input. The findings are, however, consistent with Frith's (1979) suggestion that, because auditory hallucinations represent an awareness of preconscious incorrect interpretation of auditory stimuli, they are likely to increase in conditions of ambiguous sensory input. Hartmann (1975) has speculated that "possibly something in the realm of ability to pattern sensory input, or interact with it, may be involved in the inhibitory factor [for hallucinatory experience]" (p. 73). The greater incidence of auditory as opposed to visual hallucinations in schizophrenia has been linked to the fact that "the visual background is one of patterned stimuli, the auditory background is in general less structured. Thus the latter may be considered more ambiguous, hence more open to interpretation or reconstruction in the direction of affective need" (Feinberg, 1962, p. 72).

As indicated above, it has been proposed (Hemsley, 1987a) that the schizophrenic condition is characterized by a reduction in the influence of the regularities of past experience on current perception. This, it was suggested, resulted in ambiguous, unstructured sensory input. One might therefore argue that hallucinations are related to a cognitive impairment that, even under normal conditions, results in ambiguous messages reaching awareness and hence fails to inhibit the emergence of material from long-term memory. George and Neufeld (1985) have referred to an interaction between the "spontaneous retrieval of information stored in [long-term memory] and sensory processing, the latter having an inhibitory effect on the former" (p. 268). A similar argument is put forward by Rund (1986): "Schizophrenics, possibly because of a sensory overload, . . . are more susceptible to such a direct flow between long term storage and the sensory storage level" (p. 532).

Models of this kind imply at least two dimensions on which schizophrenics may vary: first, the extent of the reduction in "perceptual organization" or structuring of input; and second, the extent to which a given level of disorganization results in the unexpected/unintended emergence of material from long-term memory. This more complex formulation appears necessary because there is only a limited relationship between disordered thinking and the occurrence of auditory hallucinations.

Hoffman (1986) has recently presented a model that emphasizes the intendedness of imagery production as an important factor influencing the experience of hallucinations. Unintended verbal imagery is experienced as externally generated. A related view is put forward by Frith (1987). Here, positive symptoms are seen as resulting from a failure to monitor willed intentions. The schizophrenic has thoughts, or performs an action, that he or she is not aware of having willed (i.e., the action is are "unintended"). In this context it is worth recalling William James' (1890) distinction between the substantive and transitive aspects of conscious experience, the latter linking the substantive parts together and giving consciousness its distinctive "stream-like" attributes. A quality of the transitive parts of consciousness emphasized by James is that they are intentional or goal directed, and he argued that personal identity is given to thought by (a) fundamental resemblance between phenomena forming part of the stream and (b) long-term continuity before the mind. Where the stream of consciousness is disrupted, psychopathology results. Hemsley (1987b) has suggested that unexpected internally generated experiences may be attributed to external events, and hence correspond to hallucinations, and went on to argue that the occurrence of such experiences might be related to an abnormality in Broadbent's (1971) pigeonholing mechanism, such that the thresholds for inappropriate intrusions into awareness are not raised by the immediately preceding contents of consciousness. The use of the term "inappropriate" of course raises the question, "inappropriate to what?", and Hoffmann's model provides the answer: "inappropriate to the intended imagery production." He also refers to "expectations" being violated and hence the verbal imagery being experienced as alien. Pigeonholing is viewed as a mechanism whereby expectancies influence perception, and a defect in this "could result in highly improbable categorizations on the basis of minimal evidence" (Collicutt & Hemsley, 1981, p. 204).

Although there are marked individual differences in the course of schizophrenic symptoms, there is a tendency for positive symptoms to decrease and negative symptoms to become more prominent (e.g., Pfohl & Winokur, 1982). Hemsley (1977) argued that the pattern of cognitive deficits shown by schizophrenics might usefully be seen as resulting in a state of "information overload," and that the strategies of processing employed by normal subjects in situations of experimenter-induced overload could be relevant to an understanding of schizophrenic behavior. In particular, it was proposed that certain of the negative symptoms of schizophrenia, such as social withdrawal, poverty of speech, and retardation, might, for certain individuals, represent adaptive strategies, learned over time, to minimize the effect of the cognitive impairment. It may also be speculated that the search for meaning in the altered experiences may diminish over time, as actions based on this search prove ineffective or counterproductive. As Anscombe (1987) put it: "less and less the subject forms his own impressions, and more and more he is impinged upon by his environment" (p. 254). In addition to chronicity, at least three factors might be expected to influence preferred strategies, and hence the form of behavioral abnormality. First are individual differences independent of the psychosis, such as personality and intelligence. For example, Frith (1979)

noted that premorbid intelligence may influence a subject's ability to construct the complex belief system necessary to explain all the irrelevant percepts of which he or she becomes aware. Second is severity of impairment: Pogue-Geile and Harrow (1988) concluded that the evidence is supportive of the view that negative symptoms "may represent a severity threshold on a continuum of liability to schizophrenia" (p. 437). Hemsley (1977) also pointed out that it may be possible to maintain a stable delusional system in the face of limited intrusions of percepts into awareness, but that beyond a certain level they may be replaced by the more transient belief systems characteristic of the nonparanoid schizophrenic. Finally, there are environmental influences: it is possible that the most acceptable methods of adaptation in many settings involve withdrawal and lowered responsiveness.

The model presented in Figure 9.1 suggests that cognitively impaired schizophrenics should function best in highly structured environments. In support of this, we have recently shown (MacCarthy, Hemsley, Schrank-Fernandiz, Kuipers, & Katz, 1986) that schizophrenics' key relatives scoring highly on "critical comments," when assessed on the Expressed Emotion rating scale (Vaughn & Leff, 1976), reported responding to problem behaviors in a more variable and unpredictable way. It was speculated that, as a result, they may provide more ambiguous information about their own feelings and the kind of behavior they expect from the patient, and that this may influence the likelihood of relapse.

RECENT RESEARCH

Our attempts to provide evidence in support of the basic formulation have drawn on both the literature on normal cognition and that of animal learning theory; the latter has become increasingly "cognitive." Thus there has been a growth of interest in the effects of amphetamine on selective attention in animals, and the possible implications for models of schizophrenia. Lubow, Weiner, and Feldon (1982) have argued that the latent inhibition paradigm is an effective way of manipulating attention in animals and that this may provide a link with the attentional disturbance prominent in schizophrenia. In the first stage of this paradigm, a stimulus is repeatedly presented to the organism; in the second stage, the preexposed stimulus is paired with reinforcement in any of the standard learning procedures, classical or instrumental. When the amount of learning is measured, relative to a group that did not receive the first stage of stimulus preexposure, it is found that the stimulus-preexposed group learn the new association much more slowly. This is interpreted as indicating a reduction in the deployment of attention to a predictable redundant stimulus.

The paradigm is illustrated in Figure 9.2. It has been shown in animals that latent inhibition is disrupted if amphetamine is administered in both the preexposure and test phases. Lubow et al. (1982) wrote: "Output is controlled, not like in the intact animal, by the integration of previous stored inputs and the prevailing situational conditions, but only by the latter" (p. 103). The distinction between "data-driven" and "conceptually driven" processing was discussed above, optimal performance being dependent on an interaction between the stimulus presented and stored memories of regularities in previous inputs that result in expectancies or response biases. Lubow et al. (1982) suggested that animals under the influence of amphetamine may be viewed as unable to utilize acquired knowledge in a newly encountered situation. They wrote: "Not having the capacity to 'use' old stimuli, all stimuli are novel. Therefore such an organism will find itself endlessly bombarded with novel stimulation, resulting perhaps in the perceptual inundation phenomena described in schizophrenia" (p.

104). There are clear similarities to the suggestion that schizophrenics fail to make use of the redundancy and patterning of sensory input to reduce information-processing demands.

Pursuing this line of research, we have recently demonstrated that latent inhibition is disrupted in acute schizophrenics showing positive symptoms (Baruch, Hemsley, & Gray, 1988), as shown in Figure 9.3, where higher scores represent more rapid learning. Clearly the acute schizophrenics tend to perform better in the preexposure condition. It was argued that these results are consistent with their being in a hyperdopaminergic state. Chronic medicated subjects performed more normally. In addition, latent inhibition for the acute group normalized following 6 to 7 weeks of antipsychotic medication, as can be seen in Figure 9.4. All except the acute preexposure group showed a simple practice effect. The performance of the acute group on the first occasion of testing was particularly interesting because, on the preexposure condition, they performed *better* than normal subjects as a result of their continued attendance to the "redundant" stimulus. Their first-test performance therefore cannot be attributed to a nonspecific loss of efficient cognitive functioning, but points rather to a specific reduction in the ability to ignore irrelevant stimuli.

We have recently investigated a second phenomenon, Kamin's (1969) blocking effect, which possesses many of the same features as latent inhibition. This paradigm (Figure 9.5) again involves a preexposure phase in which the experimental group learns an association between two stimuli $(A - X)$; control subjects learn either no association or a different one at this stage. Both groups are then presented with pairings between a compound stimulus $(A + B)$

		Test
Pre-exposure (PE) group	A-A------A-A	A-X
No pre-exposure (NPE) group	------------	A-X

Figure 9.2. Latent inhibition paradigm. In normal subjects, preexposure to stimulus A reduces the rate of learning the A-X association. This is usually interpreted as reflecting a reduction in the deployment of attention to a redundant stimulus.

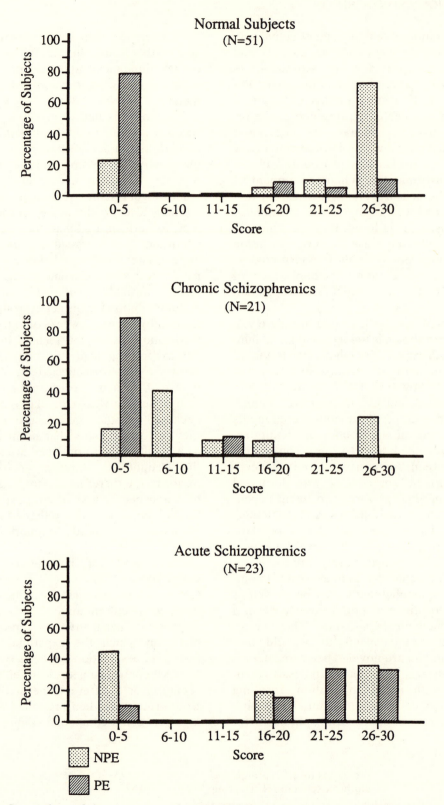

Figure 9.3. Comparison of three groups on latent inhibition task. (Reproduced with permission from Baruch, J., Hemsley, D. R., & Gray, J. A. [1988]. Differential performance of acute and chronic schizophrenics in a latent inhibition task. *Journal of Nervous and Mental Disease, 176,* 598–606.)

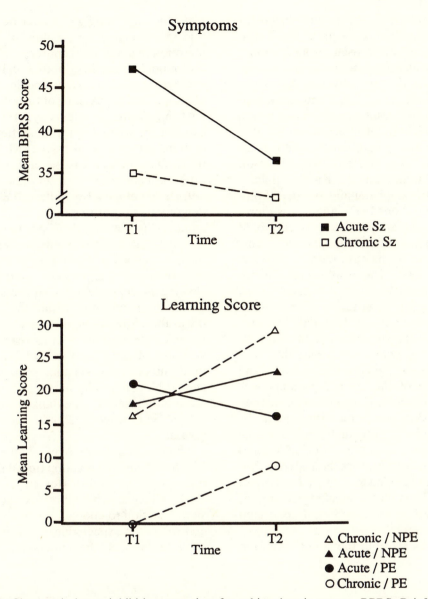

Figure 9.4. Changes in latent inhibition over time for schizophrenic groups. BPRS, Brief Psychiatric Rating Scale. Reproduced with permission from Baruch, J., Hemsley, D. R., & Gray, J. A. [1988]. Differential performance of acute and chronic schizophrenics in a latent inhibition task. *Journal of Nervous and Mental Disease, 176,* 598–606.)

	Phase 1	Phase 2	Test
Blocking group	A-X	(A + B)-X	B-X
Control group	-------	(A + B)-X	B-X

Figure 9.5. "Blocking" Paradigm. In normal subjects, the control group learns the B-X relationship faster than the blocked group. This is usually interpreted as reflecting reduction in attention to stimulus B in Phase 2 by the blocked group, because it is found to predict nothing additional to that predicted by A (i.e., it is "redundant").

and X. Finally both groups are tested for what they have learned about the B − X relationship. The preexposed group demonstrates less learning about the B − X relationship than do the controls; this is the blocking effect. There is general agreement that it arises as a result of a process in which attention to B is reduced because it is found to predict nothing additional to what is already predicted by A (Pearce & Hall, 1980). Like latent inhibition, the Kamin effect is abolished by amphetamine (Crider, Soloman, & McMahon, 1982), and it was therefore predicted that the blocking effect would be reduced in acute schizophrenics. This was found to be the case (Jones, Gray, & Hemsley, 1992). The results are summarized in Figure 9.6, which presents rank means on trial to criterion; here higher scores represent slower learning. The normal subjects showed the usual blocking effect, but the acute schizophrenics performed worse in the control condition. The performance of the chronic patients was somewhat difficult to interpret because they performed very poorly on both conditions. (We have subsequently developed a simple blocking task in an attempt to clarify this.) When mean scores were considered, the acute patients tended to perform better than normal subjects on the blocking condition, but the distribution of scores necessitated analyses by ranks.

The results for both the latent inhibition

and blocking paradigms could be conceptualized as indicating a failure of selective attention in acute schizophrenia. However, the model presented above deliberately avoided this terminology and instead emphasized the "weakening of the influence of past regularities" (Hemsley, 1987a), because there are tasks in which different predictions are generated by the two formulations. One such task is the choice reaction time procedure of Eriksen and Eriksen (1974), developed by Miller (1987). They demonstrated that reaction time to a target stimulus is increased when the context flanking that target stimulus previously has been associated with a different target stimulus requiring a competing response. This slowing is dependent on subjects making use of the regularities within the task, and it was therefore predicted that acute schizophrenics should fail to show reaction time slowing. In contrast, the "selective attention" model suggests that schizophrenics should be abnormally aware of, and hence more influenced by, the flanker stimuli; reaction time slowing should therefore be greater.

The procedure employed is illustrated in Figure 9.7, and the reaction time data in Figure 9.8 (from Jones, Hemsley, & Gray, 1991). Chronic schizophrenics showed the same reaction to cue validity as the normal controls—the expected increase in reaction time. In contrast, the acute schizophrenics

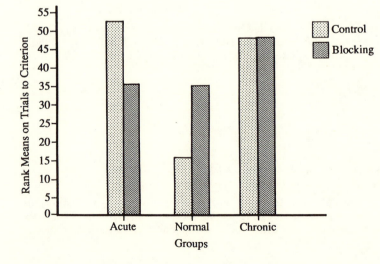

Figure 9.6. Old blocking performance of schizophrenics and normal subjects. (Reproduced with permission from Jones et al., 1992.)

Central stimulus A—press right button

Central stimulus B—press left button

88 trials in total:

$$\left.\begin{array}{ll} \text{XAX} & 40 \\ \text{YBY} & 40 \end{array}\right\} \text{'Valid' trials}$$

$$\left.\begin{array}{ll} \text{XBX} & 4 \\ \text{YAY} & 4 \end{array}\right\} \text{'Invalid' trials}$$

Figure 9.7. Modified "Eriksen" flanker task. (Reproduced with permission from Miller, J. [1987]. Priming is not necessary for selective attention failures: Semantic effects of unattended unprimed letters. *Perception* and *Psychophysics, 41,* 419–434.)

were uninfluenced by cue validity, consistent with the 1987 formulation. Subsequent analyses of error rates by hand of response have, unfortunately, somewhat complicated the picture. For right-handed responses, error rates did not differ across conditions for any group. The reaction time data are therefore interpretable as a "weakening of the effects of past regularities." For left-handed responses, however, the error rate increased markedly in the invalid condition, and this was particularly so for the acute schizophrenics. This makes the reaction time data for left-handed responses difficult to interpret. Further experiments are

obviously necessary to clarify this, but the results for the right hand are intriguing given the current interest in possible left hemisphere dysfunction in schizophrenia (see Early, Chapter 2, this volume).

In summary, since 1987, the further evidence in support of the model is as follows:

1. Acute schizophrenics show a reduction in latent inhibition.
2. Acute schizophrenics show a reduced blocking effect.
3. Acute schizophrenics are less disrupted in their performance by improbable flanker stimuli, at least when right-handed responses are considered!

It is tempting to speculate further on the possible biological bases of such disturbances of information processing. It has frequently been argued (e.g., Weinberger, Wagner, & Wyatt, 1983) that pathology of the limbic system is associated with schizophrenia. More specifically, the hippocampus and nucleus accumbens have been discussed as possible regions of the brain that might be affected, and neuropathological studies have provided some support for this view (e.g., Falkai & Bogerts, 1986). The hippocampus is an extensively researched brain structure, and there are several theo-

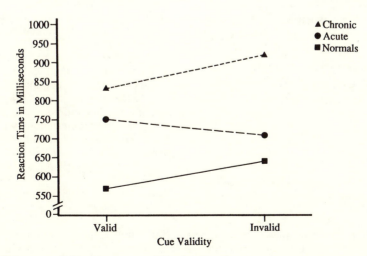

Figure 9.8. Performance of three groups on "flanker" task. (Reproduced with permission from Jones, et al. 1991.)

ries as to its function (see Schmajuk, 1984). However, Olton, Wible, and Shapiro (1986) have suggested that "The hippocampus may be the brain structure that allows each of the various components of a place and an event to be linked together and compared with other places and events" (p. 354). In a related formulation, Gray (1982) has argued for the role of the hippocampus in the comparison of actual and expected stimuli: if there is a mismatch, there is increasing attention to that input. Could a defect in this system relate to a weakening of the effect of "expectancies" on current perception? This possibility has been elaborated by Schmajuk (1987), who argued for the utility of the hippocampally lesioned animal as a model for schizophrenia. In view of the discussion in the preceding paragraph, it is of particular interest that both latent inhibition (Kaye & Pearce, 1987) and "blocking" (Soloman, 1977) are disrupted by damage to the hippocampal formation. Schmajuk (1987) argued that the "dopamine" theory is reconcilable with his model because hippocampal dysfunction might result in an increase in dopamine receptors in related brain structures such as the nucleus accumbens.

From this brief discussion it is clear that psychological and biological models of psychotic symptomatology, in particular those relating to the prominent disturbances of information processing, are converging in intriguing ways. There is an increasing emphasis on failures of integration of previous experience with current stimulus input, resulting in "inappropriate 'affective' and 'significance' assessments of the ongoing stimulation" (Patterson, 1987, p. 562).

REFERENCES

Anscombe, R. (1987). The disorder of consciousness in schizophrenia. *Schizophrenia Bulletin, 13,* 241–260.

Baruch, J., Hemsley, D. R., & Gray, J. A. (1988). Differential performance of acute and chronic schizophrenics in a latent inhibition task. *Journal of Nervous and Mental Disease, 176,* 598–606.

Brennan, J. H., & Hemsley, D. R. (1984). Illusory correlations in paranoid and non paranoid schizophrenia. *British Journal of Clinical Psychology, 23,* 225–226.

Broadbent, D. E. (1971). *Decision and stress.* London: Academic Press.

Cohen, R., & Borst, V. (1987). Psychological models of schizophrenic impairments. In H. Hafner, W. F. Gattaz, & W. Janzarik (Eds.), *Search for the causes of schizophrenia* (pp. 189–202). Heidelberg: Springer-Verlag.

Collicutt, J. R., & Hemsley, D. R. (1981). A psychophysical investigation of auditory functioning in schizophrenics. *British Journal of Clinical Psychology, 20,* 199–204.

Cooklin, R., Sturgeon, D., & Leff, J. (1983). The relationship between auditory hallucinations and spontaneous fluctuations of skin conductance in schizophrenia. *British Journal of Psychiatry, 142,* 47–52.

Crider, A., Soloman, P. R., & McMahon, M. A. (1982). Attention in the rat following chronic d-amphetamine administration: Relationship to schizophrenic attention disorder. *Biological Psychiatry, 17,* 351–361.

Cutting, J. (1985). *The psychology of schizophrenia.* London: Churchill Livingstone.

Eriksen, B. A., & Eriksen, C. W. (1974). Effects of noise letters upon the identification of a target letter in a non search task. *Perception Psychophysics, 16,* 143–144.

Falkai, P., & Bogerts, B. (1986). Cell loss in the hippocampus of schizophrenics. *European Archives of Psychiatry and Neurological Sciences, 236,* 154–161.

Feinberg, I. (1962). A comparison of the visual hallucination in schizophrenia with those induced by mescaline and LSD-25. In L. J. West (Ed.), Hallucinations. New York: Grune & Stratton.

Frith, C. D. (1979). Consciousness, information processing and schizophrenia. *British Journal of Psychiatry, 134,* 225–235.

Frith, C. D. (1987). The positive and negative symptoms of schizophrenia reflect impairments in the perception and inhibition of action. *Psychological Medicine, 17,* 631–648.

George, L., & Neufeld, R. W. J. (1985). Cognition and symptomatology in schizophrenia. *Schizophrenia Bulletin, 11,* 264–285.

Gray, J. A. (1982). *The neuropsychology of anxiety.* Oxford, England: Oxford University Press.

Haber, R. N., & Hershenson, M. (1973). *The psychology of visual perception.* New York: Holt, Rinehart and Winston.

Hartmann, E. (1975). Dreams and other hallucinations: An approach to the underlying mechanism. In R. K. Siegel & L. J. West (Eds.), *Hallucinations: Behavior, experi-*

ence and theory (pp. 71–79). New York: John Wiley.

Harvey, P. D., Earle-Beyer, E. A., & Levinson, J. C. (1988). Cognitive deficits and thought disorder: A retest study. *Schizophrenia Bulletin, 14*, 58–66.

Hemsley, D. R. (1977). What have cognitive deficits to do with schizophrenic symptoms? *British Journal of Psychiatry, 130*, 167–173.

Hemsley, D. R. (1990). *Information processing and schizophrenia*. In E. Straube, & K. Hahlweg [Eds.]. *Schizophrenia: Concepts, vulnerability and intervention*. New York: Springer-Verlag.

Hemsley, D. R. (1987a). An experimental psychological model for schizophrenia. In H. Hafner, W. F. Gattaz, & W. Janzarik (Eds.), *Search for the causes of schizophrenia* (pp. 179–188). Heidelberg: Springer-Verlag.

Hemsley, D. R. (1987b). Hallucinations: Unintended or unexpected? *Behavioral and Brain Science, 10*, 532–533.

Hoffman, R. E. (1986). Verbal hallucinations and language production processes in schizophrenia. *Behavioral and Brain Science, 9*, 503–548.

Jakes, S., & Hemsley, D. R. (1986). Individual differences in reaction to brief exposure to unpatterned visual stimulation. *Personality and Individual Differences, 7*, 121–123.

James, W. (1890). *The principles of psychology*. London: Macmillan.

Jaspers, K. (1963). *General psychopathology*. (M. W. Hamilton & J. Hoenig, Trans.). Manchester, England: Manchester University Press. (Original work published 1913).

Jones, S. H., Gray, J. A., & Hemsley, D. R. (1992). Loss of the Kamin blocking effect in acute but not chronic schizophrenics. *Biological Psychiatry, 32*, 739–755.

Jones, S., Hemsley, D. R., & Gray, J. A. (1991). Contextual effects on choice reaction time and accuracy in acute and chronic schizophrenics: Impairment in selective attention or in the influence of prior regularities. *British Journal of Psychiatry, 159*, 415–421.

Kamin, L. J. (1969). Predictability, surprise, attention and conditioning. In B. A. Campbell & R. M. Church (Eds.), *Punishment and aversive behaviour* (pp. 279–296). New York: Appleton-Century-Crofts.

Kaye, H., & Pearce, J. M. (1987). Hippocampal lesions attenuate latent inhibition and the decline of the orienting response in rats. *Quarterly Journal of Experimental Psychology. B, Comparative and Physiological Psychology, 39*, 107–125.

Knight, R. A. (1984). Converging models of cognitive deficit in schizophrenia. In W. D. Spaulding & J. K. Cole (Eds.), *Theories of*

schizophrenis and psychosis (pp. 93–156). Lincoln: University of Nebraska Press.

Kraepelin, E. (1919). *Dementia praecox and paraphrenia* (R. M. Barclay, Trans.). Edinburgh: Livingstone.

Launay, G., & Slade, P. D. (1981). The measurement of hallucinatory predisposition in male and female prisoners. *Personality and Individual Differences, 2*, 221–234.

Leff, J. P. (1968). Perceptual phenomena and personality in sensory deprivation. *British Journal of Psychiatry, 114*, 1499–1508.

Lubow, R. E., Weiner, J., & Feldon, J. (1982). An animal model of attention. In M. Y. Spiegelstein & A. Levy (Eds.), *Behavioural models and the analysis of drug action* (pp. 89–107). Amsterdam: Elsevier.

MacCarthy, B., Hemsley, D. R., Schrank-Fernandez, G., Kuipers, E., & Katz, R. (1986). Unpredictability as a correlate of expressed emotion in the relatives of schizophrenics. *British Journal of Psychiatry, 148*, 727–731.

Magaro, P. A. (1980). *Cognition in schizophrenia and paranoia*. Hillside, NJ: Lawrence Erlbaum.

Magaro, P. A. (1984). Psychosis and schizophrenia. In W. D. Spaulding & J. K. Cole (Eds.), *Theories of schizophrenia and psychosis* (pp. 157–230). Lincoln: University of Nebraska Press.

Maher, B. A. (1983). A tentative theory of schizophrenic utterance. *Progress in Experimental Personality Research, 12*, 1–52.

Margo, A., Hemsley, D. R., & Slade, P. D. (1981). The effects of varying auditory input on schizophrenic hallucinations. *British Journal of Psychiatry, 139*, 122–127.

Matussek, P. (1952). Studies in delusional perception. *Psychiat. v. Zeitschrift. Neurol., 189*, 279–318.

McGhie, A., & Chapman, J. (1961). Disorders of attention and perception in early schizophrenia. *British Journal of Medical Psychology, 34*, 103–116.

Miller, J. (1987). Priming is not necessary for selective attention failures: Semantic effects of unattended unprimed letters. *Perception Psychophysics, 41*, 419–434.

Norman, D. A., & Bobrow, D. G. (1976). On the role of active memory processes in perception and cognition. In C. N. Cofer (Ed.), *The structure of human memory* San Francisco: Freeman.

Oltmanns, J. T. F., & Neale, J. M. (1978). Abstraction and schizophrenia: Problems in psychological deficit research. *Progress in Experimental Personality Research, 8*, 197–243.

Olton, D. S., Wible, C. G., & Shapiro, M. L. (1986). Mnemonic theories of hippocampal function. *Behavioral Neuroscience, 100,* 852–855.

Patterson, T. (1987). Studies towards the subcortical pathogenesis of schizophrenia. *Schizophrenia Bulletin, 13,* 555–576.

Pearce, J. M., & Hall, G. (1980). A model for Pavlovian learning: Variations in the effectiveness of conditioned but not of unconditioned stimuli. *Psychological Review, 87,* 532–552.

Pfohl, B., & Winokur, G. (1982). The evolution of symptoms in institutionalized hebephrenic/catatonic schizophrenics. *British Journal of Psychiatry, 141,* 567–572.

Pogue-Geile, M. F., & Harrow, M. (1988). Negative symptoms in schizophrenia: Their longitudinal course and prognostic importance. *Schizophrenia Bulletin, 11,* 427–439.

Posner, M. I. (1982). Cumulative development of attentional theory. *American Psychologist, 37,* 168–179.

Rund, B. R. (1986). Verbal hallucinations and information processing. *Behavioral and Brain Science, 9,* 531–532.

Schmajuk, N. A. (1984). Psychological theories of hippocampal function. *Physiological Psychology, 12,* 166–183.

Schmajuk, N. A. (1987). Animal models for schizophrenia: The hippocampally lesioned animals. *Schizophrenia Bulletin, 13,* 317–327.

Schneider, W., & Shiffrin, R. M. (1977). Controlled and automatic human information processing. I. Detection, search and attention. *Psychological Review, 84,* 1–66.

Slade, P. D. (1976). Towards a theory of auditory hallucinations: Outline of a hypothetical 4-factor model. *British Journal of Social and Clinical Psychology, 15,* 415–423.

Soloman, P. R. (1977). Role of the hippocampus in blocking and conditioned inhibition of rabbits nictating membrane response. *Journal of Comparative and Physiolological Psychology, 91,* 407–417.

Spohn, H. (1984). Discussion. In N. D. Spaulding & J. K. Cole (Eds.), *Theories of schizophrenia and psychosis* (pp. 345–359). Lincoln: University of Nebraska Press.

Strauss, J. S. (1987). Processes of healing and chronicity in schizophrenia. In H. Hafner, W. F. Gattaz, & W. Janzarik (Eds.), *Search for the causes of schizophrenia* (pp. 75–87). Heidelberg: Springer-Verlag.

Underwood, G. (Ed.). (1978). *Strategies of information processing.* London: Academic Press.

Vaughn, C. E., & Leff, J. P. (1976). The influence of family factors on the course of psychiatric illness: a comparison of schizophrenia and depressed neurotic patients. *British Journal of Psychiatry, 129,* 125–137.

Venables, P. H. (1984). Cerebral mechanisms, autonomic responsiveness and attention in schizophrenia. In W. D. Spaulding & J. K. Cole (Eds.), *Theories of schizophrenia and psychosis.* (pp. 47–92). Lincoln: University of Nebraska Press.

Weinberger, D. R., Wagner, R. L., & Wyatt, R. J. (1983). Neuropathological studies of schizophrenia: A selective review. *Schizophrenia Bulletin, 9,* 193–212.

10

Comparing Cognitive Models of Schizophrenics' Input Dysfunction

RAYMOND A. KNIGHT

The large number of chapters in this volume that discuss the role of input or attentional dysfunctions attests to the central importance of such dysfunctions in schizophrenia. Attention–information-processing (AIP) deficits predate the onset of psychosis and constitute a consistent trait, distinguishing subgroups of schizophrenics during both the acute and remitted stages of the disorder's course (Nuechterlein & Dawson, 1984). In her integration of the research employing the high-risk strategy, Asarnow (1988) argued that AIP deficits can be found in subgroups of children at risk for schizophrenia from middle childhood. Moreover, they are especially prevalent among those risk samples who subsequently experience difficulties coping during adolescence (Erlenmeyer-Kimling & Cornblatt, 1987). Asarnow (1988) concluded that early AIP deficits may be associated specifically with a risk for schizophrenia.

Despite the mounting evidence that some form of an input or attention dysfunction is a critical deficit in schizophrenia, there is little agreement about what particular underlying cognitive–perceptual processes are responsible for schizophrenics' deficiencies on attentional tasks (e.g., Knight, 1984; Magaro, 1984; Nuechterlein & Dawson, 1984; Venables, 1984). Indeed, there is not even consensus about what research strategies are best suited to solving the methodological problems that plague investigations of schizophrenics' cognitive deficits (Chapman & Chapman, 1973, 1978; Frith, 1989; Knight, 1984, 1987, 1989; Neufeld, 1984; Widlocher & Hardy-Bayle, 1989). Ultimately, the strategy battle will be decided by the progress in deficit specification that each approach yields. The purpose of this chapter is to summarize the results of several recent AIP studies completed in my laboratory, to assess their contribution to specifying deficient perceptual–cognitive processes among schizophrenics, and to compare the explanatory power of several theories of schizophrenics' cognitive deficiencies for the data I have reviewed. A companion chapter (Knight, 1992) presents a more detailed account of the recent findings from my laboratory. The present chapter briefly summarizes that research and concentrates on the comparison among models.

THE PROCESS-ORIENTED APPROACH

In my programmatic approach to deficit specification I have followed a process-oriented strategy (Knight, 1984, 1987). This approach involves forming a network of specific, reliable, theoretically related tasks that have been explored in depth on normal samples, and using this network to assess various levels and types of information processing in schizophrenics. The strategy hinges on the ability to use theoretical models to predict what response *patterns* should occur across these tasks under conditions of adequate and inadequate process functioning. It is the pattern of performance across tasks and not the performance on any one task that is important. Experiments are constructed so that each explanatory model, even the general deficit model, predicts a distinguishable pattern of results. Thus, the tasks become analogous to consistency hurdles (Meehl, 1978) and the competing models must jump all the hurdles (i.e., accurately predict the pattern of performance) to be judged valid.

COGNITIVE RESEARCH PROGRAM

Earlier work in my laboratory using Sperling's (1960) partial report paradigm (Knight, Sherer, & Shapiro, 1977) strongly suggested that poor premorbid schizophrenics (those with inadequate social and sexual histories prior to onset of their disorder) had deficiencies in the initial stages of their information processing, either in the encoding of information in iconic storage (Neisser, 1967; Sperling, 1960) or in the transfer of information stored in this buffer to subsequent stages of processing (Dick, 1974). Iconic storage is a high-capacity, uncoded, veridical store that was hypothesized to decay rapidly (between 250 and 1,000 ms after stimulus offset). Schizophrenics' purported deficit in this earliest cognitive stage was corroborated by their performance in another paradigm, structural backward masking (Saccuzzo, Hirt, & Spencer, 1974).

Structural backward masking is a phenomenon in which a masking stimulus, presented in the same location as and a short duration after the onset of a target stimulus, interferes with the processing of this target stimulus. Typically, in normal subjects a high-intensity "pattern" mask, which is a visually structured but meaningless image, interferes with the processing of the target. This occurs when it is presented within approximately 100 ms of the onset of the target—that is, within 100 ms SOA (stimulus onset asynchrony). The SOA is the interval between the onset of the target and the onset of the mask. For schizophrenics, and most consistently for negative-symptom (Green & Walker, 1984, 1986) and poor premorbid schizophrenics (Saccuzzo & Braff, 1981), the pattern mask has been found to interfere with the processing of the target stimulus at longer ranges—up to 250 or 300 ms.

Identifying the Stages Within "Iconic Storage"

The interpretation of what processes might be deficient in schizophrenics' early processing was clarified by significant advances in the understanding of early visual processing in the mid-1970s. Data from several different paradigms indicated that iconic memory comprised two distinguishable stages (Coltheart, 1980; Kroll & Hershenson, 1980; Phillips, 1974; Potter, 1975, 1976; Potter & Levy, 1969). Figure 10.1 presents a schematic representation of these two stages, adapted for illustrative purposes from the results of Phillips' (1974) matching task for uncoded block patterns (cf. Figures 2 and 3, 8 × 8 matrix in Phillips, 1974, p. 285). The ordinate presents the percentage of correct matches, and the abscissa presents the interstimulus intervals between the block patterns. The characteristics of the two stages listed in the figure summarize the results of a number of studies (e.g., Intraub, 1984; Kroll & Hershenson, 1980; Loftus & Ginn, 1984; Loftus, Hanna, & Lester, 1988; Phillips, 1974; Potter, 1975, 1976; Potter & Levy, 1969).

The first stage, which Phillips (1974) called the sensory store, is hypothesized to be a high-capacity, rapidly decaying storage. As illustrated in Figure 10.1, it decays within 100 ms to the level of the short-term visual memory. Phillips (1974) demonstrated that information in this store is tied to spatial position and is sensitive to structural backward masking. Elements in this store are quickly identified and transferred to subsequent stages in parallel (Kroll & Hershenson, 1980; Phillips, 1974). This stage purportedly creates a preliminary perceptual representation of the stimulus that

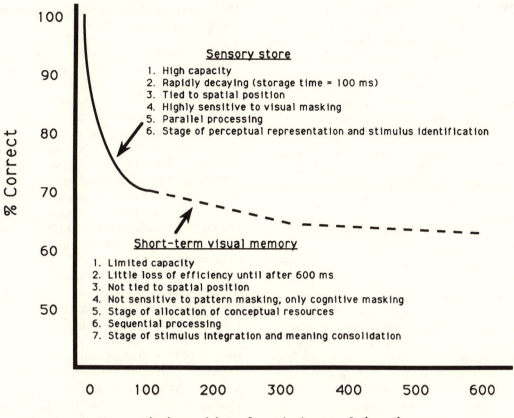

Figure 10.1. A schematic representation of the two early information-processing stages that have been the focus of several of the studies reviewed and a summary of the putative functional characteristics of each stage.

is adequate for immediate identification of the gist but is insufficient for subsequent recognition (Biederman, 1972; Loftus & Ginn, 1984; Loftus et al., 1988; Potter, 1976).

The second stage, which Phillips (1974) called short-term visual memory, is a limited-capacity storage that, as can be seen in Figure 10.1, decays more slowly than the sensory store, being efficient up to 600 ms (Phillips, 1974; Potter, 1975, 1976). It is neither tied to spatial position nor sensitive to pattern masking (Phillips, 1974). Only a cognitive mask, which requires the processing of meaningful information (Intraub, 1984; Loftus et al., 1988; Potter, 1976), disrupts this store. The interference of such a cognitive mask is directly related to its attentional demands, which are in turn determined by

the amount of new, meaningful information available in the mask (Intraub, 1984; Loftus et al., 1988). A major function of this stage is the allocation of conceptual resources to the processing of a perceptual representation, which is the product of the previous stage (Loftus et al., 1988). Elements in this store are transferred sequentially, one stimulus at a time, to subsequent stages (Kroll & Hershenson, 1980; Loftus et al., 1988; Phillips, 1974). Consequently, it involves an attentional switching from one stimulus to another (Loftus et al., 1988), and it appears to provide a brief working span in which the conceptual consolidation necessary for subsequent retention takes place (Potter, 1975, 1976).

The distinction between these stages is critical for interpreting schizophrenics' sensitivity to backward masking. If poor pre-morbids' sensory storage has a normal 100-ms duration, the pattern mask at 250 ms must be interfering with their short-term visual memory, a stage in normal subjects that is sensitive only to cognitive masking. Spaulding et al. (1980) confirmed the normalcy of schizophrenics' sensory store duration. Using a dot integration technique developed by Eriksen and Collins (1967, 1968), they demonstrated that schizophrenics' sensory store decayed at the same rate as that of nonschizophrenics and normal controls. Thus, because schizophrenics' sensory store had already decayed, the pattern mask had to be interfering with their short-term visual memory. Only a cognitive, meaningful mask and not a pattern mask interferes with the processing in this stage in normal subjects. Thus, for schizophrenics the pattern mask was apparently acting like a cognitive mask.

To test the hypothesis that both a pattern and a cognitive mask interfere with poor premorbid schizophrenics' short-term visual memory, but only a cognitive mask interferes with processing in normal subjects' short-term visual memory, we (Knight, Elliott, & Freedman, 1985) adapted Hulme and Merikle's (1976) backward masking recognition paradigm. They presented colored, naturalistic scenes as target pictures, followed at various SOAs with a pattern mask (a random array of colored shapes). To their paradigm we added a random-noise mask condition (a dense matrix randomly filled with dark or light dots), and a cognitive mask condition (photographs of real-world scenes—Potter, 1976). Consistent with our priori hypothesis, groups did not differ in their performances in the random noise condition, and sensitivity to the pattern and cognitive masks was equivalent only for the poor premorbid schizophrenics. For the poor premorbids both mask types equally disrupted processing of the target at 300 ms SOA. For normal subjects, nonschizophrenic psychotics, and good premorbid schizophrenics, only the cognitive mask interfered with processing at SOAs greater than 100 ms.

Discriminating Between Sensory Store and Short-Term Memory Deficits

Poor premorbids' equivalent sensitivity to pattern and cognitive masks in their short-term visual memory could be explained by either of two distinct processing deficits. On the one hand, the poor premorbids may not have rapidly identified the meaninglessness of the pattern mask. Consequently, they may have allocated to it processing capacity usually afforded only to a cognitive, meaningful stimulus. Such a failure to identify the gist of the mask would implicate a Stage 1, sensory store deficit (Potter, 1976). It is possible that this store might still be inferior in some aspect of its processing capability, even though it appears that it decays at the same rate for poor premorbids as for normal subjects (Spaulding et al., 1980). Alternatively, poor premorbids might be normal in their ability to identify meaninglessness (presumably a Stage 1 function), but they might have deficiencies in their short-term visual memory. Inadequacies in the functioning of this storage might make it excessively vulnerable to interference by typically ineffectual stimuli such as pattern masks.

These two alternatives make distinctly different predictions about poor premorbids' processing of meaningful and meaningless stimuli. The Stage 1 deficit hypothesis posits that poor premorbids overprocess the pattern mask because of a failure to identify its meaninglessness rapidly. Thus, it predicts that poor premorbids should be slower than controls in identifying meaningless stimuli. Such a Stage 1 deficit would also indicate that poor premorbids should have problems at all levels of meaning identification, and might only identify meaningfulness as accurately and as rapidly as controls when such meaningfulness is quite explicit.

In contrast, if the perceptual identification of meaninglessness is intact in Stage 1, but Stage 2 (short-term visual memory) is deficient, poor premorbid schizophrenics should identify meaningless stimuli as quickly as controls, but they should be less sensitive to the meaning in meaningful stimuli. This reduced meaning sensitivity could result from any of several difficulties in this stage: (a) they do not have or do not allocate ample capacity in this stage for the conceptual processing of stimuli (Loftus et al., 1988); (b) their conceptual consolidation is less complete than that of normal subjects; or (c) the long-term memories that are the product of the consolidation process in this stage (Potter, 1976) have not been sufficiently well formed to provide efficient matches to stored representations. For any of these reasons, when poor premorbids are required to make conceptual judgments about the meaningfulness of stimuli, a Stage 2 deficit would predict that they would have more difficulty recognizing the meaning in meaningful stimuli and would be slower in processing more meaningful stimuli. Not only should the pattern of their deficit in recognizing meaningfulness be different from that of a Stage 1 deficit, the level of their deficiencies also should not be as profound as a Stage 1 deficit would predict.

To test these two hypotheses we developed a reality-representation decision task with normal samples (see Knight, 1992). This task assessed the processing of perceived meaningfulness over a broad range from meaningless to meaningful stimuli. "Meaningfulness" was operationalized empirically by having undergraduates rate the representativeness of a large spectrum ($n = 319$) of art works from purely abstract to realistic. A subset ($n = 109$) of the pictures that covered both the entire range from "nonrepresentative" to "representative" and had received narrow judgment variances was selected for the reality-representation decision task. To determine the validity of this task and to assess whether our stimuli were operating in accord with the model of the first two stages, we derived and tested a series of a priori hypotheses from Kroll and Hershenson's (1980) early visual processing model. A sample of normal subjects were shown these selected pictures for short durations (100 ms and 1,000 ms) and instructed to respond as quickly as possible whether each picture represented

an object, scene, or situation in the real world ("yes" or "no"). Their answers tripped a voice-operated relay, and their reaction times were recorded from the offset of the stimulus to their response. The results of this preliminary study coincided closely with expectations and confirmed the viability of our task and our operationalization of meaningfulness.

This decision task was then presented to a new group of normal subjects, to affectively disordered psychiatric controls, and to good and poor premorbid schizophrenics. If the Stage 1 hypothesis were valid, poor premorbid schizophrenics should, relative to the controls, perceive more meaning in meaningless stimuli and respond more slowly to meaningless stimuli than to the most explicitly meaningful stimuli. If the Stage 2 hypothesis were valid, poor premorbids should perceive less meaning in meaningful stimuli and should be slower in recognizing meaningfulness, because of their purported difficulty consolidating meaning in short-term visual memory. The results were quite clear cut (see Knight, 1992). In accord with a Stage 2 deficit hypothesis, poor premorbids judged there to be the same level of meaning in nonrepresentative stimuli as other groups, but *less* meaning in the most representative stimuli. Moreover, normal subjects, those with affective disorders, and good premorbids all significantly benefited from the presence of meaning, responding relatively more quickly to meaningful than to meaningless stimuli. Poor premorbids were the only subjects who did not respond more quickly to meaningful than to meaningless stimuli. Indeed, their responses to meaningful stimuli were slightly, but not significantly, slower than their responses to meaningless stimuli. In addition, the latency of their responses to meaningless stimuli did not differ from normal subjects' reaction times to these stimuli, as the Stage 1 explanation of the backward masking deficit would require.

The results of this study directly disconfirmed the hypotheses that poor premorbids perceive more meaning in meaningless stimuli and that they are slower to perceive meaninglessness. They are therefore incompatible with the hypothesis that poor premorbids' backward masking deficit is due to a failure to recognize rapidly the meaninglessness of the pattern mask. Rather, the data suggest that poor premorbids may have some problems rapidly recognizing meaning in meaningful stimuli, a deficit that is consistent with the hypothesis that they may have difficulties in their short-term visual memory, either consolidating visual information or allocating conceptual resources efficiently.

Interfacing Short-Term Visual Memory and Perceptual Organization Deficits

These results must be integrated with the well-replicated finding that poor premorbid schizophrenics have an advantage in tasks that are facilitated by a deficit in perceptual organization. Place and Gilmore (1980) first demonstrated this superiority in a pair of numerosity tasks. They asked poor premorbid schizophrenics and drug-abusing controls to judge the number of lines presented in a display flashed for less than 20 ms. In the first task, vertical or horizontal lines appeared by themelves or with circles ("noise" condition). Schizophrenics were able to count the lines as well as controls in the no-noise condition, but they had difficulty judging numerosity when the circles were present. A clever second line-counting experiment suggested that the reason for schizophrenics' poor performance in the noise condition was not a difficulty in inhibiting the irrelevant circles but a failure to chunk the lines and circles into perceptual groups to facilitate counting. Place and Gilmore presented three categories of stimuli: (a) homogenous lines (equivalent to the no-noise condition of Experiment 1); (b) heterogeneous/adjacent lines (both vertical and horizontal lines presented in the same set with same-orientation lines grouped); and (c) heterogeneous/nonadjacent lines (with both orientation lines presented without the adjacent grouping of similar lines). Controls' performance declined from condition (a) to condition (c); schizophrenics found the three tasks equally easy, and over all three conditions were significantly better than controls. These results suggest that, before counting, controls automatically organized the lines in conditions (b) and (c), and that this organization interfered with their counting. Because schizophrenics apparently did no such automatic chunking, their perception of numerosity proceeded unabated. These results have been replicated in two other laboratories (Orlowski, Keitzman, Dornbush, & Winnick, 1985; Wells & Leventhal, 1984).

Previously, I had argued that the now disconfirmed Stage 1 deficit hypothesis provided a possible link between poor premorbids' backward masking and perceptual organization difficulties (Knight, 1984; Knight et al., 1985). Their purported inability to perceive quickly the lack of meaningful organization in the mask was hypothesized to lead to excessive processing of the pattern mask, analogous to normal subjects' processing of a cognitive mask. Our reality decision task data indicate the adequacy of poor premorbids' sensory store, and suggest by implication that some deficiency in short-term visual memory, rather than in the perceptual processing of the sensory store, may be responsible for poor premorbids' difficulty on the perceptual organization tasks.

The well-established phenomenon of automaticity, by which subjects learn with repeated exposure to respond to a group of features rapidly with limited use of attentional resources (Logan, 1990), could provide the explanatory bridge between schizophrenics' masking and perceptual organization deficits. Even though there is some controversy about the basic processes underlying the development of automaticity (e.g., Hasher & Zacks, 1979; Logan, 1988, 1990; Newell & Rosenbloom, 1981; Schneider, 1985; Shiffin & Dumais, 1981; Shiffrin & Schneider, 1977), an adequately functioning short-term visual memory is critical to all models of automaticity (see Knight, 1992). An allocation (Loftus et al., 1988) or consolidation (Potter, 1975, 1976) deficiency in short-term visual memory could limit either the experiential base or the integrative capacity necessary for the development of automatic processing, and in so doing reduce schizophrenics' ability to learn to respond rapidly and efficiently to groups of features. Such inefficiencies also could make short-term visual memory more vulnerable to interference by stimuli such as pattern masks that would otherwise not affect processing in this stage. Thus, poor premorbids' perceptual organization and backward masking deficits both can be explained by the same short-term visual memory deficit hypothesis.

Studying Strong Forms of Perceptual Organization and Symmetry

There is a wide variance both in the developmental prepotency of perceptual structures (Bornstein, Ferdinandsen, & Gross, 1981; Bornstein, Gross, & Wolf, 1978; Yonas & Granrud, 1985) and in the speed with which automatic responding to various stimuli is learned by adults (Logan, 1988, 1990). If some deficiency in short-term visual memory underlies poor premorbids' aberrant performance on certain perceptual organization tasks, an assessment of their capabilities in processing stimuli that vary in the age at which they are perceived as structural wholes and in the ease of their automization could shed light on the nature of poor premorbids' short-term visual memory processing. Therefore, in our next two studies we attempted to specify further the nature and extent of poor premorbids' difficulty learning to consolidate visual stimuli into perceptual wholes. In an effort to delimit the broad boundaries of their organizational deficiencies, we tested poor premorbids' competence on two radically different kinds of perceptual organization.

In the first study we (Knight, Elliott, & Hershenson, 1993) tested the strongest form of the perceptual organization deficit hypothesis. We focused on symmetry, because of its role as a prepotent, early-developing organizational principle (Bornstein et al., 1978, 1981). If poor premorbids were deficient in their processing of symmetrical

patterns, this would suggest a severe, pervasive problem in figural integrative abilities, and would once again question the competence of their Stage 1 sensory store. In contrast, if their sensory store were intact but their short-term visual memory were deficient, as the reality decision task has indicated, one would predict more adequate processing of symmetrical patterns. The early development of the recognition of symmetrical patterns suggests that they have structural prepotence and do not require extensive experience to be perceived automatically as wholes. A deficit in short-term visual memory is likely only to produce performance deficiencies for configurations that either demand a larger number of repeated exposures or a longer history of attentional allocation for rapid, automatic responding to develop.

The paradigm we employed (see Knight, 1992, for details and examples of stimuli) was a direct adaptation of two matching studies (Hershenson & Ryder, 1982a, 1982b). It made use of the finding that, when stimuli form a perceptual gestalt, a physical match of its internal features is inhibited but a name match is facilitated. This is especially true when the presence of overall organization is a diagnostic, which indicates that the names are the same (e.g., Fox, 1975; Mermelstein, Banks, & Prinzmetal, 1979). In both physical match and name match paradigms we used two-letter combinations that could be either symmetrical or asymmetrical and four types of symmetry (translational, horizontal-axis-bilateral, vertical-axis-bilateral, and rotational; see Weyl, 1952). We hypothesized that, if poor premorbid schizophrenics have a deficiency in their rapid perception of symmetrical configurations, symmetry should neither interfere with their physical match performance nor facilitate their name match performance. If their processing of symmetry were intact, their response patterns should parallel those of the other groups.

The results of this study were eminently clear. Symmetry interfered with the physical match for all groups equally. In the name match task, the only difference among the groups was that the poor premorbids did not learn to use the vertical-axis-bilateral symmetry as a diagnostic for a "SAME" response, as did the other groups. This does not suggest any deficit in their ability to rapidly perceive symmetrical organization, but rather suggests a failure to learn to use such organization as an efficient indicator of sameness.

The results of this study disconfirmed the hypothesis that poor premorbids' input deficiency should be characterized as a general deficiency in all forms of perceptual organization. When integrated with the results of the numerosity tasks, they suggest that poor premorbids process the elements of a stimulus as integrated wholes (i.e., organize them automatically) only when they are overwhelmed by an imposing, prepotent, or overlearned structure, like that provided by symmetry. Consistent with my interpretation of the reality decision task, poor premorbids' competence in processing symmetrical patterns supports the hypothesis that perceptual processing in their sensory store is adequate, and deficits in perceptual organization may be limited to configurations that require for their rapid, automatic processing the repeated attentional allocation and the depth of conceptual processing afforded in short-term visual memory. Indeed, this explanation is consistent with the performance differences evidenced by the poor premorbids in the vertical-axis-bilateral condition of the name match task. Here, they were clearly affected by the symmetrical organization but did not learn to use such structural information to determine quickly and efficiently that the letters in the configuration had the same name.

Manipulating Stimulus Configurations to Elucidate Processing Deficits

To elucidate further poor premorbids' Stage 1 and 2 processing, in our next study (see Knight, 1992) we investigated more directly the strategies that they implement in their early visual encoding in these stages. We chose a paradigm (Rosen & Hershenson, 1983) that allowed us to assess schizophren-

ics' wholistic and sequential processing of stimuli that had a less imposing structure. We used a visual matching task in which the arrangement of the stimuli had been found to facilitate either wholistic processing (i.e., automatically organized perceptually) or sequential processing. Four of eight unfamiliar, but simple, geometric figures were arranged in either a square (wholistic) or linear (sequential) configuration. For each configuration type there were three response conditions—same (all geometric figures the same), easy-different (all figures different), and hard-different (only one figure different). Square configurations facilitated wholistic processing because they encourage comparison of the two entire square configurations. The linear configurations encouraged element-by-element sequential comparison of the geometric figures, rather than wholistic comparison of the entire string.

Normal subjects, those with affective disorders, good premorbids, and poor premorbids were flashed same, easy-different, or hard-different versions of the square or linear configurations at either 100 or 1,000 ms. They were required to say whether the configurations they viewed were the same or different. Their responses tripped a voice-operated relay, and their reaction times were measured from the onset of the stimulus to their response. Complex patterns of responding to these conditions indicated the processing strategies that each group of subjects were employing (see Knight, 1992). Normal subjects, those with affective disorders, and good premorbid schizophrenics showed evidence of wholistic patterns of responding to square configurations and sequential, analytical patterns of responding to linear stimuli. In contrast, poor premorbids showed an unchanging response pattern to both square and linear configurations, which suggested that their initial processing of stimuli was partial and diffuse rather than wholistic and integrated, and that this preliminary pass was not followed by a sequential analysis of component parts. Additional processing time yielded improved accuracy but did not change their processing strategy.

Integrating Results: A Short-Term Visual Memory Deficit Model

The integration of these results with our symmetry matching tasks, our reality-representation decision task, and our backward masking picture task yields a consistent description of poor premorbid schizophrenics' early visual encoding. The undeviating pattern of their responding in both the square and linear conditions of the geometric shape matching task indicates that their processing of these stimuli was limited to an initial, diffuse preliminary pass. This diffuse initial processing of stimuli does not appear to have been followed by a more detailed scanning of individual elements. Either poor premorbids did not allocate adequate conceptual processing resources in their short-term visual memory to the perceptual output of their sensory store, or they allocated sufficient capacity but experienced some difficulty in the initial conceptual processing of the perceptual information. Clearly, such limited and superficial conceptual processing of the stimuli in short-term visual memory could negatively affect the quality of the memory representations that are the product of this stage, and could thereby have impact on poor premorbids' ability to automatize perceptual constructs. Such a deficiency would be consistent with their failure in Place and Gilmore's numerosity task to group similarly oriented lines automatically. In contrast, when poor premorbids encountered prepotent structures such as the symmetrical stimuli in our physical and name matching tasks, which either require minimal experience to gain an automatized, perceptually integrated status, or for which the perceptual system may be more specifically attuned, their diffuse processing was capable of rapidly encoding the structure.

Short-term visual memory hypothetically marks the beginning of conceptual processing, which operates on the output of perceptual processing (Loftus et al., 1988). In normal subjects, only a meaningful pattern mask, and not a meaningless pattern mask, disrupts the conceptual processing of a target during this stage. The fact that schizophrenics' sensory store decays within 100 ms as does that of normal subjects (Spaulding et al., 1980) indicates that the well-replicated interference of a structural backward mask at 250 to 300 ms SOA must be occurring during the operation of short-term visual memory. Conceptual masking in our picture masking paradigm purportedly occurs because the subject switches processing from one picture (the target) to the subsequently presented picture (the mask), thereby terminating the processing of the target before it is sufficiently consolidated for subsequent recognition (Loftus et al., 1988; Potter, 1976). The degree of masking in this stage is directly related to the cognitive attentional demands of the mask (Intraub, 1984; Loftus et al., 1988). Consistent with their performance on the square and linear matching tasks, poor premorbids' conceptual engagement of the target in short-term visual memory could be sufficiently weak that it is vulnerable to interference from meaningless structured information, even though they can rapidly identify such patterns as meaningless, or they may have inefficient allocation capabilities or limited attentional resources in their short-term visual memory.

Poor premorbids' allocation or consolidation difficulties in short-term visual memory, and concomitant limited perceptual automatization, also could account for the reduced perception of meaningful structures in visual stimuli that they evidenced in the reality decision task. The results of this task also disconfirm the alternative sensory store explanation for such interference. That is, it appears that poor premorbids were able to recognize as quickly as controls the meaninglessness of the pattern mask. Therefore, it is not likely that they allocated to it more conceptual resources than necessary. Rather, the alternative explanation, that some processing weakness in short-term visual memory makes this stage vulnerable to interference, appears to account better for the data. Finally, a short-term visual memory deficit accounts for their poorer picture recognition memory (see Knight, Sims-Knight, & Petchers-Cassall, 1977). Thus, the results of the series of studies that I have reviewed converge on deficiencies in short-term visual memory as a likely candidate to explain and integrate all of the results presented, and indicate that it is a reasonable heuristic construct to guide future research.

ASSESSMENT OF MODELS OF AIP IN SCHIZOPHRENIA

The series of studies presented in the previous section illustrates how our process-oriented research program has attempted to specify cognitive deficiencies in schizophrenics. In accord with the process-oriented strategy, we have used the theoretical models and the diverse paradigms developed to study early visual information processing to measure schizophrenics' perceptual and cognitive processes from multiple perspectives. We have chosen paradigms that minimize the methodological confounds produced by schizophrenics' general performance deficiencies (see Knight, 1992), and we have attempted to limit the range of processes that can account for poor premorbid schizophrenics' cognitive deficiencies. In this series of studies we pitted specific models of cognitive deficiencies against each other and allowed the contrasting patterns of responding across tasks to determine the better model. Although we did not directly contrast our models with a number of models that have been proposed by other investigators, the explanatory power of these other models can be assessed in light of the results I have discussed. Many hypothetical constructs have been proposed to account for schizophrenics' cognitive deficiencies. I focus on four that are most relevant to early visual processing.

Slowness of Processing

Saccuzzo and Braff (1981) have speculated that schizophrenics, especially poor pre-

morbids, might be deficient on tasks like backward masking, because they are slower in processing stimuli from iconic storage to their short-term memory. Short-term memory refers here not to the short-term visual memory that reaches its peak between 100 and 600 ms (Loftus et al., 1988; Phillips, 1974; Potter, 1976), but to a subsequent store that serves as an active, working memory, enduring for 3 to 20 seconds and processing information from both iconic storage and long-term memory by conscious memory routines, such as rehearsal (Atkinson & Shiffrin, 1968). As Schuck and Lee (1989) have indicated, this hypothesis is more descriptive of the observed outcome of schizophrenics' processing difficulties (less information processed) than it is a model of what is specifically aberrant in their information input. Indeed, such a speed explanation does not provide adequate mechanisms to account for schizophrenics' superiority on the numerosity tasks (e.g., Place & Gilmore, 1980).

In our backward masking picture task (Knight et al., 1985), the slowness hypothesis would predict neither the equivalence of poor premorbids' masking functions in the pattern and cognitive mask conditions nor their adequacy in the random noise mask condition. Rather, a generic slowness in processing at these early stages should simply make schizophrenics take longer than control subjects to process stimuli in all three conditions. Thus, it would seem more consistent with this hypothesis to predict that the masking potency of all three mask types would be enhanced equally relative to controls. Poor premorbid schizophrenics should not, therefore, show masking functions that are equivalent to controls in the random noise and cognitive mask conditions, but inferior in the pattern mask condition, as we found.

This disconfirmation of the global slowness hypothesis, of course, highlights Schuck and Lee's (1989) criticism of this hypothesis—its lack of specificity. It does not stipulate whether the hypothesized slowness is in the visual, sensory processing; in the generation of a perceptual representation, which is sufficient in normal subjects at 100 ms to allow the gist of a picture to be identified (Biederman, 1972; Loftus & Mackworth, 1978; Potter, 1975, 1976); in the conceptual processing that begins at 100 ms (Loftus et al., 1988); or in all these transformations in these early stages. Even if one amended the slowness theory to conform to the two-stage (sensory store and short-term visual memory) model, and argued that schizophrenics were slow in their perceptual processing of the stimulus (Loftus et al., 1988), several problems would remain. It would still not be clear why a pattern mask, which apparently only masks visual processing in the sensory store (Phillips, 1974), should interfere with the development of a perceptual representation at 200 to 300 ms, when the sensory store is no longer present (Spaulding et al., 1980). Moreover, the beginning of the cognitive processing of the stimulus is dependent on the adequacy of the perceptual representation (Loftus et al., 1988). Thus, if the time necessary for the formation of the perceptual representation is lengthened, the beginning of conceptual processing should be delayed. Would not the effects of conceptual masking be enhanced in this case?

The lack of specificity in the generic slowness model also does not provide sufficient explanatory power to account for the results of studies in which poor premorbids manifest different patterns of processing various kinds of stimuli. For example, to account for the relative differences in performance patterns that poor premorbids showed in rating and responding to meaningful relative to meaningless stimuli and in matching square and linear configurations, the hypothesis must provide greater specification about how the purported speed deficit should differentially affect the processing of various stimulus dimensions during these early stages (e.g., meaningful versus meaningless, simple versus complex). If the problem of generic slowness is not differentially related to any stimulus dimensions or kinds of information transformation, should not all schizophrenics' patterns of performance

in processing remain the same, but simply be delayed or their accuracy reduced?

Momentary Capacity Limitation

Nuechterlein and Dawson (1984), in their comprehensive review of the perceptual–cognitive results of studies on high-risk samples, argued that subsamples of those at risk for schizophrenia showed evidence for dysfunctions that affected a variety of elementary processes rather than for a more focal deficit on a single, specific process. They inferred from the studies they reviewed that deficits were most prevalent in tasks that imposed a high momentary processing load and were not found in those tasks with low processing demands. This led them to speculate that the cognitive deficiencies found both in schizophrenics and in those at risk for schizophrenia may be due to "a reduced amount of processing capacity available for task-relevant cognitive operations" (p. 193). This explanation accounts well for the Continuous Performance Test results and for the Span of Apprehension results (e.g., Asarnow & MacCrimmon, 1978, 1981; Wohlberg & Kornetsky, 1973).

The limited capacity model does considerably less well, however, explaining schizophrenics' performance on other cognitive tasks. Like the slowness model, it also suffers from a lack of specificity. It delimits neither the locus nor the cause of the capacity limitations. This results in explanatory flexibility but predictive frailty and restricted falsifiability. Indeed, before judging whether this hypothesis is compatible with the findings I have presented, one must first determine which operationalization of capacity is being assessed, as Neufeld, Vollick, and Highgate-Maynard have done (Chapter 11, this volume). In their stochastic modeling analyses of a memory search paradigm, Neufeld et al. assessed one particular operationalization of capacity, the rate at which information is transmitted. They concluded that schizophrenics do not show capacity reduction in their memory search capabilities. Because of the vagueness of the momentary limited capacity model, many operationalizations of capacity must be assessed to determine the viability of the model. Moreover, even if one operationalization shows consistent performance across various tasks, it would be necessary to determine whether the deficit was primary or secondary to some more elemental processing deficiency. Given its definitional adjustableness, one can create post hoc explanations that would account for many of the results presented, but it is unlikely that the patterns could be predicted a priori from a single definitional model.

Like the slowness of processing hypothesis, the limited capacity hypothesis would not predict the superiority of schizophrenics' performance on the numerosity tasks. A limited capacity model alone cannot explain why schizophrenics fail to chunk similarly oriented lines. In contrast, if, as Place and Gilmore (1980) suggested, schizophrenics have some deficiency in their perceptual chunking, so that features that should be processed in parallel as perceptual wholes are processed as individual features, capacity resources would be strained because of the increased processing load such a deficit would incur (Schneider & Shriffrin, 1985; Shriffrin & Schneider, 1977, 1984). Thus, a problem with either chunking or automatizing, as I have suggested, could account for apparent capacity limitations, but it is not evident how capacity limitations could account for deficiencies in chunking. If one attempted to integrate the limited capacity hypothesis with the results of the numerosity tasks by positing that poor premorbid schizophrenics either have not learned, do not implement as a processing strategy, or are not capable of processing such stimuli in parallel automatically, thereby reducing available capacity by requiring the use of conscious, capacity-demanding processing (Nuecterlein & Dawson, 1984), one would in essence be relegating the limited capacity hypothesis to the role of a secondary consequence of a more primary automatization or perceptual organization deficit (see Knight, 1984).

Poor premorbids' equivalent performance in the pattern and cognitive mask conditions in our backward masking picture study also creates some difficulties for a model that relies exclusively on limited capacity. Nuechterlein and Dawson (1984) speculated that the greater masking range of a pattern mask for schizophrenics in backward masking paradigms might be interpreted in light of the integration explanation of structural backward masking (Felsten & Wasserman, 1980; Schultz & Eriksen, 1977). In this model, when the mask is superimposed on the target, a degraded, integrated montage of mask and target is purportedly formed. Nuechterlein and Dawson suggested that schizophrenics may have more difficulty than controls processing this fused stimulus configuration, either because of a deficiency in perceptual sensitivity or because of the increased processing demand required to recognize degraded stimuli. As Schuck and Lee (1989) have pointed out, this explanation is not parsimonious, because schizophrenics and hypothetically schizotypal college students are also deficient in metacontrast backward masking paradigms, wherein the mask is adjacent to, but not superimposed on, the target (Lee, 1985; Merritt, Balogh, & Leventhal, 1986). Here no montage should be formed, and schizophrenics' backward masking deficit could not be attributed to a difficulty processing an integrated montage. Moreover, at the SOAs at which the pattern mask was still disrupting target picture processing in our picture masking paradigm (300 ms), a pattern mask should not be exerting the perceptual masking effects necessary for target–mask integration (Loftus & Ginn, 1984). Rather, it should only have conceptual masking effects (Loftus & Ginn, 1984). Thus, the masking integration model does not appear to provide an adequate bridging mechanism to allow the limited capacity hypothesis to explain schizophrenics' backward masking deficits.

An alternative bridge between the limited capacity model and schizophrenics' backward masking deficiencies could be constructed using variations of an attentional allocation hypothesis. It could be argued that schizophrenics either allocate an inappropriately large proportion of their limited available resources to processing the pattern mask or that their capacity is so limited that allocating even a small amount of attention to the pattern mask disrupts their processing of the target.

The first explanation, excessive allocation, like our original Stage 1, perceptual organization hypothesis (Knight, 1984; Knight et al., 1985), conflicts with the results of our reality decision task, discussed earlier. In that study poor premorbid schizophrenics, in contrast with all other groups, responded relatively more quickly to meaningless than to meaningful stimuli and were not significantly different from normal subjects in their rapid recognition of meaningless configurations (see Knight, 1992). Therefore, there was no evidence that poor premorbid schizophrenics allocated more processing time, and by inference capacity, to meaningless stimulus configurations (i.e., to stimuli analogous to the pattern masks). Moreover, it has been argued that conceptual processing, which is the exclusive processing mode at 300 ms after stimulus offset (Loftus & Ginn, 1984), operates on only a single picture at a time (Loftus et al., 1988). Conceptual masking is thought to constitute a target–mask attentional switch, the probability of which varies as a function of the attentional demands of the mask (i.e., the amount of perceptual data in each mask and the conceptual processing demands of each mask) (see Intraub, 1984; Loftus et al., 1988). Our pattern and cognitive masks differed on both of these dimensions, and especially on the latter. If schizophrenics' early deficit is simply a capacity limitation, why would a pattern mask, which is lower in processing demands, affect their processing more than it does that of controls, but a cognitive mask equally affect the performance of both schizophrenics and controls?

The second explanation, severe capacity limitations, also encounters inconsistencies. If the problem were that schizophrenics had such limited capacity that any attention to another stimulus was sufficient to overload their processing and exceed capacity, why did they respond appropriately to the random noise and cognitive masks, whose masking functions bracketed the pattern mask function (Knight et al., 1985)? If one argued that the pattern mask, although limited in its attentional demands, clearly had more perceptual complexity than the random noise mask and was sufficient to surpass schizophrenics' severely limited capacity, the same criticism presented above for the excessive allocation hypothesis would be apropos. How does this explanation account for the adequacy of poor premorbids' performance in the cognitive masking condition? Consequently, neither the deficient allocation nor the severely limited capacity explanation is adequate to save the limited capacity model. Neither can explain the greater masking effects of the pattern mask, and both would predict a cognitive masking deficit as well as a pattern masking deficit. Thus, the limited capacity hypothesis in its present form does not account for the results of the backward masking picture study.

Although the results of the square and linear configuration matching task experiment do not disconfirm a limited capacity explanation, the model, as currently delineated, does not provide the specificity necessary to predict the results found. Indeed, this experiment once again highlights the theory's major weakness—its lack of predictive specificity. For this model to be heuristic, the extant research relevant to capacity limitations must be integrated and an operationalization of capacity must be generated that consistently accounts for the available data. Then, this more circumscribed model must be tested in a series of studies that put it at severe risk for disconfirmation. Until it survives such a test, it will remain only a facile, post hoc explanation.

Aberrant Transients

Schuck and Lee (1989), using Breitmeyer's (1984) sustained–transient channel model of visual processing, have proposed an aberrant transient channel hypothesis to explain schizophrenics' difficulties with backward masking. Breitmeyer and Ganz's (1976; Breitmeyer, 1984) model divides the visual system into two parallel and semi-independent, but complementary, channels. One channel system, the transient system, serves to orient the organism and to direct its attention to locations in visual space that might contain novel and important information. Cells in this system are characterized by high temporal resolution (Kulikowski & Tolhurst, 1973), short latency (Breitmeyer, 1975; Cleland, Levick, & Sanderson, 1973), and relatively low spatial resolution (Kulikowski & Tolhurst, 1973; Meyer & Maguire, 1977). Thus, events of change in the visual field are quickly apprehended, and global characteristics are rapidly processed. The other channel system, the sustained system, purportedly processes structural or figural information and is essential for high-acuity tasks such as high-resolution stereoacuity and pattern perception. Accordingly, cells in this system are characterized by high spatial resolution (Kulikowski & Tolhurst, 1973; Meyer & Maguire, 1977), long latency (Breitmeyer, 1975; Jones & Keck, 1978), and both long duration and long integration time (Breitmeyer & Ganz, 1976; Meyer & Maguire, 1977), all of which are necessary for high-acuity, sustained processing tasks. The two systems work to complement each other in facilitating the processing of information. Whereas the sustained system's long integration time permits proactive inhibition of successive visual fixations, the transient system's inhibiting action serves the important function of terminating the integration within the sustained channels, thereby freeing these channels from information that might otherwise persist into the next fixation period.

As I indicated earlier, in structured backward masking a meaningless patterned mask follows the target and appears in the same location as the target. In metacontrast (backward) masking, the mask follows the target but juxtaposes rather than being superimposed on the target locus. Schizophrenics show excessive vulnerability to both kinds of backward masking (e.g., Lee,

1985; Saccuzzo & Braff, 1981). In contrast, in a paracontrast (forward) masking task, in which the mask precedes and is not superimposed on the target locus, schizophrenics have not been found deficient (Lee, 1985). Schuck and Lee (1989) have argued that the processing differences between these two kinds of masking provide critical information about schizophrenics' early input difficulties. Breitmeyer and Ganz (1976; Breitmeyer, 1984) explain these two types of masking by different neural interactions within or between sustained and transient channels. Whereas paracontrast (forward) masking is explained by intrachannel masking in the sustained channels (i.e., it is mediated by lateral inhibition of the center of receptive fields of sustained cells by their own antagonistic surrounds), backward masking (both metacontrast and structural) is attributed to interchannel inhibition of the sustained responses by transient channel activity. Because transient activity purportedly plays an important role in backward but not in forward masking, schizophrenics' differential deficit on these masking tasks implicates deviant transient channels as candidates to explain the pattern of their masking deficit (Schuck & Lee, 1989). Aberrant transient activity, whether abnormally high in amplitude, overly persistent, or lower in threshold, could account for this performance pattern (Schuck & Lee, 1989).

There are certain results in the backward masking picture study (Knight et al., 1985) that raise some questions about the aberrant transients explanation. First, poor premorbid schizophrenics showed the same responses to random noise masks as did controls (a significant masking effect at 50 ms SOA, but at SOAs of 150 ms and greater their random-noise mask conditions did not differ from the no-mask baseline condition). Consistent with other masking studies (see Breitmeyer, 1984), the transient activity elicited by these random noise dot patterns interrupted target picture processing at short SOA durations. If aberrant transient activity is responsible for poor premorbid schizophrenics' masking deficit, why did poor premorbid schizophrenics show deviant masking functions only to pattern masks and not to random noise masks? One might hypothesize that it was the difference in the spatial frequency of the masks. Whereas the small dots of the random noise mask have the appearance of a high-spatial-frequency configuration, the pattern mask had a comparatively lower spatial frequency, which could have enhanced transient activity. If this were the discriminating factor in these two conditions for poor premorbids, it would suggest a limitation of the aberrant transient deficit to particular stimulus conditions, which in turn would further restrict the explanatory power of the model.

Second, the perceptual aspects of early processing are apparently complete by 300 ms after stimulus offset (Loftus & Ginn, 1984; Loftus et al., 1988). Because a pattern mask still affected target picture processing for poor premorbid schizophrenics up to 400 ms SOA, it must have been interfering with the conceptual and *not* the perceptual processing of the target. In normal subjects interference at this stage is limited to cognitive, information-laden masks (Intraub, 1984; Potter, 1976) and appears to be determined primarily by the conceptual, attentional demands of the masking stimulus relative to the target (Intraub, 1984; Loftus et al., 1988). Whereas it is reasonable to hypothesize that excessive transient activity might enhance perceptual masking, it does not seem likely that higher amplitude transient activity, produced by a pattern mask with low attentional demands and no meaningful, conceptual information, would disrupt conceptual processing at 300 ms SOA.

Because of the alerting function that transients serve, aberrant transient activity could also contribute to the selective attention (e.g., Hemsley & Richardson, 1980; Wishner & Wahl, 1974) and sustained attention (e.g., Walker, 1981; Wohlberg & Kornetsky, 1973) deficits so frequently found in schizophrenics (Schuck & Lee, 1989). This model apparently offered a possible explanation of the discrepant findings between masking and stimulus integration studies. For example, in our perceptual integration task (Knight, Sherer, Putchat, & Carter,

1978) we minimized transient activity because we employed successive dark fields. We found no difference between the performance of schizophrenics and controls. In contrast, the various backward masking studies that have maximized transient activity have found schizophrenics deficient (see Balogh & Merritt, 1987). This explanation is not without its problems, however. Spaulding et al.'s (1980) iconic integration task did not minimize transient activity. They used light fields with black dots in their integration task and still found that schizophrenics' integration decay function did not differ from that of controls. Their results suggest that the minimization of transient activity was not the factor differentiating our original integration results from the typical masking results.

The aberrant transient activity hypothesis also has difficulty explaining schizophrenics' differential performance patterns across tasks that should be equal in their elicitation of transient activity. Poor premorbid schizophrenics' performance patterns in both the reality decision task and the square versus linear configuration matching tasks (discussed earlier) could not be accounted for by differential transient elicitation patterns in the tasks, because the tasks in each experiment were equated in their stimulus onset/offset characteristics. One would have to hypothesize that random transient discharges (B. D. Schwartz & Winstead, 1982) pulled schizophrenics' attention away from target processing, resulting in less depth of processing on certain trials. For the reality decision task, one would have to argue in addition that such activity differentially affected the processing of more meaningful stimuli, thereby making poor premorbid schizophrenics see less meaning in meaningful pictures and also not respond relatively more quickly to meaningful than to meaningless stimuli. The problem with this explanation is that controls did not require more time, and by inference more depth of processing, to recognize the greater meaning in meaningful stimuli. They responded significantly more quickly to meaningful than to meaningless stimuli.

Why, then, would aberrantly discharging transients differentially affect poor premorbids' response to meaningfulness rather than to meaninglessness? In the square–linear matching study, poor premorbid schizophrenics' failure to change their processing strategy across stimulus durations or configuration types (see Knight, 1992) could conceivably be a processing strategy resulting from undependable stimulus availability due to random transient interruption.

Schizophrenics' superiority on tasks in which automatic perceptual organization inhibits task-relevant responding constitutes one of the most serious challenges to the aberrant transient hypothesis. As currently formulated, it does not provide a mechanism to explain their perceptual chunking deficits. Some evidence (Williams, 1980; Williams & Weisstein, 1980) suggests a possible tentative link between transient channels and perceptual organization. Although a complete understanding of the relation of global analysis to neural channels has not been determined, one speculation derived from these data (Breitmeyer, 1984) is that, for brief presentations and SOAs not exceeding 50 ms, a low spatial frequency processing of global form might be carried out by transient channels. If the automatic chunking of similarly oriented lines is a transient channel perception, the aberrant transients hypothesis could provide a bridge between the backward masking and the perceptual organization task results. This linkage between transient activity and perceptual organization suggests the possibility, however, that the deficit in schizophrenics' transient functioning may exceed simple deviance in their amplitude, persistence, or threshold, and may involve some deficiency in their basic processing capability. I must conclude at this point that, although the deficient transients hypothesis provides some enticing, paradigm-specific integrations, there remain some significant problems in the precision of its characterization of the nature of schizophrenics' processing deficiencies and with the universality of its explanation. The model certainly warrants further investigation.

Inhibitory Failures

In an attempt to integrate schizophrenics' information-processing dysfunctions with critical symptoms, Frith (1979) has argued that the major symptoms of the disorder (hallucinations, delusions, and thought disorder) could be explained by positing a breakdown in the filtering mechanisms that monitor the selection of preconscious material for passage into conscious awareness. He hypothesized that schizophrenics' "nerve net" selective system does not have the capacity to generate sufficient inhibition, and consequently too many neurons become activated simultaneously. A disruption in inhibitory processes at an early stage of cognition purportedly results in the awareness at higher cognitive levels of multiple irrelevant stimuli. Consequently, schizophrenics are hypothesized to become aware of the functioning of various preconscious automatic processes and to find it difficult to select and follow out appropriate courses of action.

Because this model was generated as an explanatory construct for symptoms (Frith, 1989), rather than specifically as an integration of schizophrenics' performance on the kinds of perceptual–cognitive tasks that I have been considering, it is somewhat lacking in specificity at the more elemental level of analysis. Consequently, it is difficult in certain paradigms to generate what a priori predictions this model would make. Post hoc explanations are notoriously easy to generate but never ultimately convincing. The problems with filter deficit models in general have been discussed elsewhere (S. Schwartz, 1982). I limit my discussion to the explanatory power of this specific model for the visual input studies that have been the focus of this chapter.

There are, of course, some commonalities between this hypothesis and the short-term visual memory hypothesis that I have proposed. For instance, the latter attributes poor premorbid schizophrenics' excessive vulnerability to the presence of a backward mask to a deficiency in the functioning of short-term visual memory that makes this stage overly susceptible to interference. The major difference between the two hypotheses is that in my hypothesis (a) the consolidation of information, (b) the allocation of conceptual resources in short-term visual memory, or (c) the depth of processing of the stimulus in short-term visual memory, necessary for developing perceptual automaticity, is posited to be the primary deficit. Vulnerability to interference (in this instance failure to disregard or inhibit irrelevant stimulation) is hypothesized to be a secondary consequence. In Frith's theory, inhibition failure is primary. Although schizophrenics are hypothesized to become abnormally aware of automatic processes, no specific deficit in automaticity per se is predicted.

Because no deficit in the automatic chunking of stimuli is directly predicted by Frith's model, it is difficult to determine how the model would account for schizophrenics' failure to group similarly oriented lines in the numerosity studies. If the deficit in selective capacity or the purported consciousness of automatic processes also implies a deficit in automatic perceptual organization, how does this differ from a deficit in automaticity per se? What is the nature and extent of this deficit? How would the inhibition model account for the differential adequacy with some types of perceptual organization (i.e., the perception of symmetry) but not others (e.g., grouping similarly oriented lines)?

Frith's (1979) hypothesis also is not obviously congruent with the backward masking results. If it is simply the case that all preconscious stimuli enter schizophrenics' awareness, why should a patterned mask that occurs after a target stimulus has been perceptually encoded and is apparently being conceptually processed (Loftus & Ginn, 1984) disrupt the processing of the target? The inhibition of the mask is not a prerequisite for processing the target. Normal subjects do not inhibit the mask and can remember its content (Loftus et al., 1988). Some deficit other than inhibitory failure must be invoked.

In attempting to explain how failures of inhibition lead to auditory hallucinations, Frith (1979) proposed that the awareness of uninhibited, incorrect, early interpretations of stimuli produces hallucinations. Moreover, he argued that hallucinations should be more likely as the ambiguity of sounds increases. According to the model, the more the meaning of the stimulus is clear, the less interpretative confusion should be generated by schizophrenics' inhibition deficit. This line of reasoning might lead a proponent of this model to argue that the prepotency of certain structures, such as symmetry, creates such clear stimulus situations that the inhibition deficit is ameliorated. However, the organization pattern of the lines in the numerosity tasks is sufficiently ambiguous that the schizophrenic processes each line separately. It would seem to follow from such an argument that Frith's model would predict that, as the stimulus became clearer or as the meaningfulness of the structures increased, schizophrenics' processing deficiencies should decrease. We found, however, exactly the opposite in our reality-representation decision task. Because Frith's model focuses not on the consolidation of information per se but rather on the inability to inhibit irrelevant stimulation, the model has significant difficulty explaining why, in contrast to all other groups, poor premorbid schizophrenics were not faster to recognize meaningful than meaningless paintings and why they perceived less meaning when meaning was most clear.

Although ultimately we should be able to tie together AIP deficits with other symptoms in schizophrenia, reasoning from symptoms to early information-processing deficits, as Frith (1979) has done, is fraught with hazards, not the least of which is symptom–process equivocality. That is, the possibility exists that the same manifest symptom in psychotics may be produced by different underlying processes (see Knight, 1987, for an elaboration of this problem). Although I agree with the importance of relating AIP deficits to manifest symptoms (George & Neufeld, 1985; Knight, Elliott, Roff, & Watson, 1986; Neale, Oltmanns, &

Harvey, 1985), I would argue that greater progress will be achieved if we move from process specification to process–symptom linkage, rather than in the opposite direction (Knight, 1987).

Short-Term Visual Memory Deficit—Strengths and Limitations

Table 10.1 presents a comparative summary of how well each deficit hypothesis, as currently formulated, did in accounting for the data of the five critical studies reviewed. This table basically summarizes the preceding discussion by giving a rating on a 6-point scale to each hypothesis for each of the five studies. The table clearly illustrates the judged predictive and explanatory superiority of the short-term visual memory hypothesis. It is consistent with the results of all five studies, and it predicted the results of three out of five of these studies. In contrast, all the alternative hypotheses, including the perceptual organization hypothesis that I proposed earlier (Knight, 1984; Knight et al., 1985), are rated as inconsistent with at least two studies, and each has

at least one study that was judged to present a strong challenge to its validity.

Thus, the studies in our program have converged on short-term visual memory as a critical processing stage for explaining poor premorbid schizophrenics' inferior performance on a multitude of cognitive tasks from a variety of experimental paradigms. It has shown considerable explanatory, integrative, and predictive power for the body of studies I have reviewed. Because this hypothesis was generated within the framework of the cognitive theories that explain the performance of normal subjects on these tasks, and because it was modified in accord with the results of succeeding experiments, its predictions for these particular tasks have been quite specific. Thus, it has an advantage over the competing hypotheses that were created either (a) within only one of the paradigms reviewed (e.g., the slowness and aberrant transients hypotheses); (b) primarily within the context of paradigms not reviewed in this chapter (e.g., the momentary capacity limitation hypothesis); or (c) within the context of explaining manifest symptoms (the inhibitory

Table 10.1. Evaluative Summary of the Validity of Six AIP Hypotheses on the Five Critical Studies Reviewed

Deficit hypotheses	Studies				
	Numerosity	Picture backward masking	Reality representation decision	Symmetry matching	Square/linear configuration matching
Stage I perceptual organization	+ +	+ +	– – –	– –	–
Stage II short-term visual memory	+	+ +	+ +	+ +	+
Slow processing	– – –	– –	–	0	–
Momentary capacity limitation	– – –	– –	+	0	+
Aberrant transients	– –	–	– –	0	–
Inhibitory failure	– – –	– – –	– – –	+	– –

– – –   The data constitute a strong challenge to the hypothesis as currently formulated.
– –   The data are inconsistent with the current version of the hypothesis, but *significant* modifications in the specifications of the hypothesis could accommodate these results.
–   The data are inconsistent with the current version of the hypothesis, but *moderate* modifications in the specifications of the hypothesis could accommodate these results.
0   The data are neither consistent nor inconsistent with the hypothesis.
+   The data can be interpreted post hoc as consistent with the hypothesis, but the results could not be predicted a priori.
+ +   The results would be predicted by the hypothesis as currently formulated.

failure hypothesis). Nonetheless, the series of studies presented does pose a challenge to these alternative hypotheses. To maintain the viability of these alternative hypotheses, their proponents must increase the specificity of their theories and provide testable bridges to the data reviewed. They must generate experimental paradigms in which their models predict a priori the performance patterns found, and a short-term visual memory deficit hypothesis fails to predict these patterns.

Despite the demonstrated explanatory power and heuristic potential of the short-term visual memory hypothesis, it still has substantial limitations in its current state of development. From the vantage of the process-oriented research strategy that has guided its generation and testing, the body of results that support it has some weaknesses. Several critical propositions that buttress the logical structure of the model (e.g., the normal duration of poor premorbids' sensory store, the equivalence of their pattern and cognitive masking functions, and the normal speed of their processing of meaningless stimuli) have been supported by only a single study, rather than by the convergence of multiple studies using different paradigms. This is a basic requirement of the process-oriented strategy (see Knight, 1984). In addition, the speculations about the functioning of short-term visual memory (e.g., its putative role in learning to automatize particular perceptual organizations), although reasonable, require further empirical support.

Although this series of studies converge on short-term visual memory as a likely locus of poor premorbid schizophrenics' encoding difficulties, the exact nature of their processing inadequacies in this stage have not been specified. Indeed, clarification of the role of this stage in normal subjects' cognitive processing is only beginning, and extant data point to multiple, complex operations transpiring. One major function of this stage is the allocation of conceptual resources to processing the perceptual representation that is purportedly the product of the previous stage (Loftus et al., 1988). The

result of appropriate allocation is the conceptual processing of the stimulus and the consolidation of information for later recognition (Potter, 1976). Consequently, poor premorbids' deficit in this stage could involve a problem in attentional allocation or in consolidation or in both. Whereas an attentional allocation deficiency interfaces more easily both with evidence implicating the anterior attention system (Posner, Early, Reiman, Prado, & Dhawan, 1988; Posner & Nakagawa, 1989) and with the findings of deficits in vigilance and sustained attention tasks (Nuechterlein & Dawson, 1984), consolidation notions are more congruent with perceptual organization formulations of schizophrenics' encoding deficiencies.

Although no definitive discrimination between these two components is possible, particular findings give some basis for speculation. If the Loftus et al. (1988) model of short-term visual memory is accurate, wherein only a single picture is cognitively processed in short-term visual memory at a time, an allocation explanation would focus on whether or not the stimulus was cognitively engaged, and on the switching of such engagement. If allocation were faulty, and processing had been disrupted either by a pattern or by a cognitive mask, the consequences to target processing should be the same because the switching of attention is hypothetically an all-or-none phenomenon. This is precisely what we found in our backward masking picture study (Knight et al., 1985). Moreover, consistent with the results of this study, the allocation deficit explanation would predict a normal masking range for poor premorbids in the cognitive mask condition, because SOAs beyond 200 to 300 ms should be critical not to the initial cognitive engagement of the target, but only to the consolidation of target information. Thus, once the target was allocated appropriate resources, consolidation should proceed normally. In contrast, although it would be consistent with the consolidation deficit hypothesis that the pattern and cognitive masks would have equivalent effects up to 300 ms, greater disruptions of target processing at longer intervals in the cognitive mask condition would also be expected if poor premorbids' consolidation processes were less efficient, and especially if they were slower than those of controls.

The comparability of poor premorbids' cognitive masking range to that of controls (Knight et al., 1985) suggests that the duration of consolidation in their short-term visual memory is equivalent to that of normal subjects and that their cognitive consolidation of the target is sufficiently efficient that an adequate trace for subsequent memory has been generated by 400 ms, when the cognitive mask ceases its interference. Thus, these results present some problems for the consolidation explanation. They do not, however, allow unequivocal conclusions about the efficiency of poor premorbids' consolidation processing, which could still be deficient under these conditions. Although the allocation deficit hypothesis has an apparently slightly better fit with these results, further studies of the duration and efficiency of consolidation in poor premorbids' short-term visual memory are clearly necessary before firm conclusions can be reached.

Advances in the study of the neuropathology and electrophysiology of schizophrenia (e.g., Early, Reiman, Raichle, & Spitznagel, 1987; Freedman et al., 1987; Oke & Adams, 1987; Patterson, 1987) are providing an increasingly rich source of speculations about the physiological underpinnings of cognitive deficits in schizophrenia, and they are documenting abnormalities in the earliest components of schizophrenics' responses to stimuli. As I indicated earlier, my strategy has been to use cognitive models to guide our attempt to specify the processes underlying schizophrenics' cognitive deficiencies. I have reasoned that, when these processes were adequately isolated and understood, they would provide a solid base that could be integrated with the neuropathological and electrophysiological data, to the benefit of each domain. Other investigators (e.g., Posner & Nakagawa, 1989) have implemented an alternative strategy of using explicit anatomical models

of attentional deficits to guide their search for the processes underlying schizophrenics' cognitive deficiencies.

Ultimately, both my approach and theirs, if properly implemented, should converge on the same psychological and physiological processes. Because the linkages between a putative short-term visual memory deficit and the extant neuropathological and electrophysiological findings would constitute an important avenue of construct validation, my failure to date to make these connections constitutes another current weakness of the model that must be addressed in future research. The process orientation would demand, of course, that such linkages be made with the same model-driven, a priori specificity that is the hallmark of this strategy and that has been the key to what success it has achieved in the psychological domain. Speculative forays lacking such predictive power are likely to yield negligible spoils.

Another limitation of the short-term visual memory deficit hypothesis is the extensiveness of its application in schizophrenia. Evidence for the proposed deficit has been found only in poor premorbid schizophrenics. When schizophrenics have been dichotomized on the basis of their social competence, good premorbids, those schizophrenics with adequate social and sexual histories prior to the onset of their disorder, have shown performance patterns comparable to those of nonschizophrenic controls on almost all the cognitive tasks that I have reviewed. Yet, the good premorbids manifest the hallucinations and delusions that are characteristic of schizophrenia. Good premorbids' consistent information-processing competency and superiority to poor premorbids cannot be attributed to differences in age, amount of hospitalization, medication levels, education, or intelligence. They were not different from poor premorbids on these variables, and none of these variables correlated significantly with performance on the information-processing tasks administered.

One component on which these social competence subgroups have shown consistent differences in our samples has been negative symptoms. Whereas poor premorbids typically have negative symptoms, especially affective flattening, these symptoms have been rare in our good premorbid schizophrenics (e.g., Levin, Hall, Knight, & Alpert, 1985). Thus, our results are consistent with studies that have found that AIP deficits covary with negative, but not positive symptoms (e.g., Bilder, Mukherjee, Rieder, & Pandurangi, 1985; Braff, 1989; Green & Walker, 1984; Nuechterlein, Edell, Norris, & Dawson, 1986). Although no specific etiological model has emerged to integrate and explain the apparent heterogeneity among schizophrenics (Walker, 1987), and there is, indeed, not even a consensus about which variables are most critical for identifying homogeneous subgroups (see Knight, 1987; Knight et al., 1986), the data reviewed here suggest that early input dysfunctions certainly should be factored into any proposed explanatory models.

The subgroup differences we have found underscore two methodological lessons important for future research. First, they illustrate the importance of analyzing subgroups differences in cognitive research in schizophrenia. The unique patterns of poor premorbids' performances on various tasks would have been lost if they had been grouped with good premorbids. Thus, taxonomic as well as theoretical, a priori process specificity is critical for solving the mysteries of schizophrenics' cognitive deficiencies. Second, the subgroup differences suggest that there may be a complex relation between manifest symptoms and the processes that underlie them. It is unclear whether positive symptoms are produced by different processes than those that produce negative symptoms. Likewise, it is unclear whether symptoms are multiply determined, and whether similar behavioral manifestations covary with different underlying processes in different groups of patients. The possibility of such complex interactions between processes and overt behaviors requires us to rethink our research strategies for relating processes to symptoms, and to create designs that take into account the possible equivocality of the relations among symptoms and processes (see Knight, 1987).

CONCLUSION

The studies I have reviewed have disconfirmed some hypotheses about schizophrenics' cognitive deficiencies and have posed substantial hurdles for other hypotheses, thereby helping to reduce the number of contending models. Their cumulative evidence converges on short-term visual memory as a promising focus of future research on poor premorbids' AIP deficits. Although this research raises many new questions, it does so within the context of a process orientation whose viability has been demonstrated by its continued progress in deficit specification. Its products continue to support the validity of its solutions to the serious methodological difficulties we face (Knight, 1984, 1987).

ACKNOWLEDGMENTS

The research reported in this article was supported by Research Grant MH39640 from the National Institute of Mental Health, United States Public Health Service, and by a grant from the Scottish Rite Schizophrenia Research Program, Northern Masonic Jurisdiction, United States.

I wish to express deep appreciation to the staff and especially to the patients of Edith Nourse Rogers Memorial Veterans Hospital for their cooperation with our research program. Special thanks are due to Gregory Binus for his continued support of this research. I thank my collaborators, who have coauthored the research papers cited, and also Arthur Falk, Dara Monoach, and Edith Rosenberg, who were instrumental in gathering and analyzing the data for these studies. Finally, I thank Judith Sims-Knight, Maurice Hershenson, and Steven Kramer for helpful criticisms of an earlier draft.

REFERENCES

Asarnow, J. R. (1988). Children at risk for schizophrenia: Converging lines of evidence. *Schizophrenia Bulletin, 14,* 613–631.

Asarnow, R. F., & MacCrimmon, D. J. (1978). Residual performance deficit in clinically remitted schizophrenics: A marker of schizophrenia? *Journal of Abnormal Psychology, 87,* 597–608.

Asarnow, R. F., & MacCrimmon, D. J. (1981). Span of apprehension deficits during postpsychotic stages of schizophrenia. *Archives of General Psychiatry, 38,* 1006–1011.

Atkinson, R. C., & Shiffrin, R. M. (1968). Human memory: A proposed system and its control processes. In K. W. Spence & J. T. Spence (Eds.), *The psychology of learning and motivation: Advances in research and theory* (Vol. 2, pp. 89–195). New York: Academic Press.

Balogh, D. W., & Merritt, R. D. (1987). Visual masking and the schizophrenia spectrum: Interfacing clinical and experimental methods. *Schizophrenia Bulletin, 13,* 679–698.

Biederman, I. (1972). Perceiving real-world scenes. *Science, 177,* 77–80.

Bilder, R. M., Mukherjee, S., Rieder, R. O., & Pandurangi, A. K. (1985). Symptomatic and neuropsychological components of defect states. *Schizophrenia Bulletin, 11,* 409–419.

Bornstein, M. H., Ferdinandsen, K., & Gross, C. G. (1981). Perception of symmetry in infancy. *Developmental Psychology, 17,* 82–86.

Bornstein, M. H., Gross, C. G., & Wolf, J. Z. (1978). Perceptual similarity of mirror images in infancy. *Cognition, 6,* 89–116.

Braff, D. L. (1989). Sensory input deficits and negative symptoms in schizophrenia. *American Journal of Psychiatry, 146,* 1006–1011.

Breitmeyer, B. (1975). Simple reaction time as a measure of the temporal response properties of transient and sustained channels. *Vision Research, 15,* 1411–1412.

Breitmeyer, B. (1984). *Visual masking: An integrative approach.* New York: Oxford University Press.

Breitmeyer, B., & Ganz, L. (1976). Implications of sustained and transient channels for theories of visual pattern masking. *Psychological Review, 83,* 1–36.

Chapman, L. J., & Chapman, J. P. (1973). *Disordered thought in schizophrenia.* New York: Appleton-Century-Crofts.

Chapman, L. J., & Chapman, J. P. (1978). The measurement of differential deficit. *Journal of Psychiatric Research, 14,* 303–311.

Cleland, B. G., Levick, W. R., & Sanderson, K. J. (1973). Properties of sustained and transient ganglion cells in the cat retina. *Journal of Physiology (London), 228,* 649–680.

Coltheart, M. (1980). Iconic memory and visible persistence. *Perception and Psychophysics, 27,* 183–228.

Dick, A. O. (1974). Iconic memory and its relation to perceptual processing and other memory mechanisms. *Perception and Psychophysics, 16,* 575–596.

Early, T. S., Reiman, E. L., Raichle, M. E., & Spitznagel, E. L. (1987). Left globus pallidus abnormality in never-medicated patients with schizophrenia. *Proceedings of the National Academy of Sciences, U.S.A., 84,* 561–563.

Eriksen, C. W., & Collins, J. F. (1967). Some temporal characteristics of visual pattern perception. *Journal of Experimental Psychology, 74,* 476–484.

Eriksen, C. W., & Collins, J. F. (1968). Sensory traces versus the psychological moment in the temporal organization of form. *Journal of Experimental Psychology, 77,* 376–382.

Erlenmeyer-Kimling, N., & Cornblatt, B. (1987). The New York High-Risk Project: A followup report. *Schizophrenia Bulletin, 13,* 451–461.

Felsten, G., & Wasserman, G. S. (1980). Visual masking: Mechanisms and theories. *Psychological Bulletin, 88,* 329–353.

Fox, J. (1975). The use of structural diagnostics in recognition. *Journal of Experimental Psychology: Human Perception and Performance, 1,* 57–67.

Freedman, R., Adler, L. E., Gerhardt, G. A., Waldo, M., Baker, N., Rose, G. M., Drebing, C., Nagamoto, H., Bickford-Wimer, P., & Franks, R. (1987). Neurobiological studies of sensory gating in schizophrenia. *Schizophrenia Bulletin, 13,* 669–678.

Frith, C. D. (1979). Consciousness, information processing and schizophrenia. *British Journal of Psychiatry, 134,* 225–235.

Frith, C. D. (1989). Specific cognitive deficits in schizophrenia. *Cahiers de Psychologie Cognitive [European Bulletin of Cognitive Psychology], 9,* 623–626.

George, L., & Neufeld, R. W. J. (1985). Cognition and symptomology in schizophrenia. *Psychological Bulletin, 93,* 57–72.

Green, M., & Walker, E. (1984). Susceptibility to backward masking in schizophrenics with positive and negative symptoms. *American Journal of Psychiatry, 141,* 1273–1275.

Green, M., & Walker, E. (1986). Symptom correlates of vulnerability to backward masking in schizophrenia. *American Journal of Psychiatry, 143,* 181–186.

Hasher, L., & Zacks, R. T. (1979). Automatic and effortful processes in memory. *Journal of Experimental Psychology: General, 108,* 356–388.

Hemsley, D. R., & Richardson, P. H. (1980). Shadowing by context in schizophrenia. *Journal of Nervous and Mental Disease, 168,* 141–145.

Hershenson, M., & Ryder, J. (1982a). Perceived

symmetry and name matching. *Bulletin of the Psychonomic Society, 19,* 19–22.

Hershenson, M., & Ryder, J. (1982b). Perceived symmetry and visual matching. *American Journal of Psychology, 95,* 669–680.

Hulme, M. R., & Merikle, P. M. (1976). Processing time and memory for pictures. *Canadian Journal of Psychology, 30,* 31–38.

Intraub, H. (1984). Conceptual masking: The effects of subsequent visual events on memory for pictures. *Journal of Experimental Psychology: Learning, Memory, and Cognition, 10,* 115–125.

Jones, R., & Keck, M. J. (1978). Visual evoked response as a function of grating spatial frequency. *Investigative Ophthalmology and Visual Science, 17,* 652–659.

Knight, R. A. (1984). Converging models of cognitive deficit in schizophrenia. In W. D. Spaulding & J. K. Cole (Eds.), *Nebraska symposium on motivation, Vol. 31: Theories of schizophrenia and psychosis* (pp. 93–156). Lincoln: University of Nebraska Press.

Knight, R. A. (1987). Relating cognitive processes to symptoms: A strategy to counter methodological difficulties. In P. D. Harvey & E. F. Walker (Eds.), *Positive and negative symptoms of psychosis: Description, research, and future directions* (pp. 1–29). Hillsdale, NJ: Lawrence Erlbaum Associates.

Knight, R. A. (1989). Cognitive deficiencies in schizophrenics: Abandoning cognitive models generated for normals confuses rather than clarifies. *Cahiers de Psychologie Cognitive [European Bulletin of Cognitive Psychology], 9,* 642–649.

Knight, R. A. (1992). Specifying cognitive deficiencies in poor premorbid schizophrenics (pp. 252–289). In E. Walker, R. Dworkin, & B. Cornblatt (Eds.), *Progress in Experimental Personality and Psychopathology Research, Vol. 15.* New York: Springer Publishing Company.

Knight, R. A., Elliott, D. S., & Freedman, E. G. (1985). Short-term visual memory in schizophrenics. *Journal of Abnormal Psychology, 94,* 427–442.

Knight, R. A., Elliott, D. S., & Hershenson, M. (1993). *Perceptual organization in schizophrenics: The processing of symmetrical patterns.* Manuscript submitted for publication.

Knight, R. A., Elliott, D. S., Roff, J. D., & Watson, C. G. (1986). Concurrent and predictive validity of components of disordered thinking in schizophrenia. *Schizophrenia Bulletin, 12,* 427–446.

Knight, R. A., Sherer, M., Putchat, C., & Carter, G. (1978). A picture integration task for measuring iconic memory in schizophrenics. *Journal of Abnormal Psychology, 87,* 314–321.

Knight, R. A., Sherer, M., & Shapiro, J. (1977). Iconic imagery in overinclusive and nonoverinclusive schizophrenics. *Journal of Abnormal Psychology, 86,* 242–255.

Knight, R. A., Sims-Knight, J. E., & Petchers-Cassell, M. (1977). Overinclusion, broad scanning, and picture recognition in schizophrenics. *Journal of Clinical Psychology, 33,* 635–642.

Kroll, J. F., & Hershenson, M. (1980). Two stages in visual matching. *Canadian Journal of Psychology, 34,* 49–61.

Kulikowski, J. J., & Tolhurst, D. J. (1973). Psychophysical evidence for sustained and transient detectors in human vision. *Journal of Physiology (London), 232,* 149–162.

Lee, R. G. (1985). *A comparison of forward and backward masking in schizophrenics and controls.* Unpublished master's thesis, Bowling Green State University, Bowling Green, OH.

Levin, S., Hall, J. A., Knight, R. A., & Alpert, M. (1985). Verbal and nonverbal expression of affect in speech of schizophrenic and depressed patients. *Journal of Abnormal Psychology, 94,* 487–497.

Loftus, G. R., & Ginn, M. (1984). Perceptual and conceptual processing of pictures. *Journal of Experimental Psychology: Learning, Memory, and Cognition, 10,* 435–441.

Loftus, G. R., Hanna, A. M., & Lester, L. (1988). Conceptual masking: How one picture captures attention from another picture. *Cognitive Psychology, 20,* 237–282.

Loftus, G. R., & Mackworth, N. H. (1978). Cognitive determinants of fixation location during picture viewing. *Journal of Experimental Psychology: Human Perception and Performance, 4,* 565–572.

Logan, G. D. (1988). Toward an instance theory of automatization. *Psychological Review, 95,* 492–527.

Logan, G. D. (1990). Repetition priming and automaticity: Common underlying mechanisms? *Cognitive Psychology, 22,* 1–35.

Magaro, P. A. (1984). Psychosis and schizophrenia. In W. D. Spaulding & J. K. Cole (Ed.), *Nebraska symposium on motivation, Vol. 31: Theories of schizophrenia and psychosis* (pp. 157–229). Lincoln: University of Nebraska Press.

Meehl, P. E. (1978). Theoretical risks and tabular asterisks: Sir Karl, Sir Ronald, and the slow progress of soft psychology. *Journal of Consulting and Clinical Psychology, 46,* 806–834.

Mermelstein, R., Banks, W., & Prinzmetal, W. (1979). Figural goodness effects in perception and memory. *Perception and Psychophysics, 26,* 472–480.

Merritt, R. D., Balogh, D. W., & Leventhal, D. B. (1986). Use of metacontrast and a paracontrast procedure to assess the visual information processing of hypothetically schizotypic college students. *Journal of Abnormal Psychology, 95,* 74–80.

Meyer, G. E., & Maguire, W. M. (1977). Spatial frequency and the mediation of short-term visual storage. *Science, 198,* 524–525.

Neale, J. M., Oltmanns, T. F., & Harvey, P. D. (1985). The need to relate cognitive deficits to specific behavioral referents of schizophrenia. *Schizophrenia Bulletin, 11,* 286–291.

Neisser, U. (1967). *Cognitive psychology.* New York: Appleton-Century-Crofts.

Neufeld, R. W. J. (1984). Re: The incorrect application of traditional test discriminating power formulations to diagnostic-group studies. *Journal of Nervous and Mental Disease, 172,* 373–374.

Newell, A., & Rosenbloom, P. S. (1981). Mechanisms of skill acquisition and the law of practice. In J. R. Anderson (Ed.), *Cognitive skills and their acquisition* (pp. 1–55). Hillsdale, NJ: Lawrence Erlbaum Associates.

Nuechterlein, K. H., & Dawson, M. E. (1984). Information processing and attentional functioning in the developmental course of schizophrenic disorders. *Schizophrenia Bulletin, 10,* 160–203.

Nuechterlein, K. H., Edell, W., Norris, M., & Dawson, M. E. (1986). Attentional vulnerability indicators, thought disorder, and negative symptoms. *Schizophrenia Bulletin, 12,* 408–426.

Oke, A. F., & Adams, R. N. (1987). Elevated thalamic dopamine: Possible link to sensory dysfunctions in schizophrenia. *Schizophrenia Bulletin, 13,* 589–604.

Orlowski, B. K., Kietzman, M. L., Dornbush, R. L. & Winnick, W. W. (1985, August). *Perceptual disorganization in schizophrenia.* Paper presented at the meeting of the American Psychological Association, Los Angeles, CA.

Patterson, T. (1987). Studies toward the subcortical pathogenesis of schizophrenia. *Schizophrenia Bulletin, 13,* 555–576.

Phillips, W. A. (1974). On the distinction between sensory storage and short-term visual memory. *Perception and Psychophysics, 16,* 283–290.

Place, E. J. S., & Gilmore, G. C. (1980). Perceptual organization in schizophrenia. *Journal of Abnormal Psychology, 89,* 409–418.

Posner, M. I., Early, T. S., Reiman, E. M., Pardo, P. J., & Dhawan, M. (1988). Asymmetries in hemispheric control of attention in schizophrenia. *Archives of General Psychiatry, 45,* 814–821.

Posner, M. I., & Nakagawa, A. (1989). A cognitive neuroscience perspective to control deficits in schizophrenia. *Cahiers de Psychologie Cognitive [European Bulletin of Cognitive Psychology], 9,* 667–670.

Potter, M. C. (1975). Meaning in visual search. *Science, 187,* 965–966.

Potter, M. C. (1976). Short-term conceptual memory for pictures. *Journal of Experimental Psychology: Human Learning and Memory, 2,* 509–522.

Potter, M. C., & Levy, E. I. (1969). Recognition memory for a rapid sequence of pictures. *Journal of Experimental Psychology, 81,* 10–15.

Rosen, K. S., & Hershenson, M. (1983). Tests of a two-stage model of visual matching. *Perceptual and Motor Skills, 56,* 343–354.

Saccuzzo, D. P., & Braff, D. L. (1981). Early information processing deficit in schizophrenia: New findings using schizophrenic sub-groups and manic control subjects. *Archives of General Psychiatry, 38,* 175–179.

Saccuzzo, D. P., Hirt, M., & Spencer, T. J. (1974). Backward masking as a measure of attention in schizophrenia. *Journal of Abnormal Psychology, 83,* 512–522.

Schneider, W. (1985). Toward a model of attention and the development of automatic processing. In M. I. Posner & O. S. Marin (Eds.), *Attention and performance XI* (pp. 475–492). Hillsdale, NJ: Lawrence Erlbaum Associates.

Schneider, W., & Shiffrin, R. (1985). Categorization (restructuring) and automatization: Two separable factors. *Psychological Review, 92,* 424–428.

Schuck, J. R., & Lee, R. G. (1989). Backward masking, information processing, and schizophrenia. *Schizophrenia Bulletin, 15,* 491–500.

Schultz, D. W., & Eriksen, C. W. (1977). Do noise masks terminate target processing? *Memory & Cognition, 5,* 90–96.

Schwartz, B. D., & Winstead, D. K. (1982). Icon formation in chronic schizophrenics. *Biological Psychiatry, 20,* 1015–1018.

Schwartz, S. (1982). Is there a schizophrenic language? *The Behavioral and Brain Sciences, 5,* 579–626.

Shiffrin, R. M., & Dumais, S. T. (1981). The development of automatism. In J. R. Anderson (Ed.), *Cognitive skills and their acquisition* (pp. 111–140). Hillsdale, NJ: Lawrence Erlbaum Associates.

Shiffrin, R. M., & Schneider, W. (1977). Controlled and automatic human information processing: II. Perceptual learning, automatic attending, and a general theory. *Psychological Review, 84,* 127–190.

Shiffrin, R. M., & Schneider, W. (1984). Automatic and controlled processing revisited. *Psychological Review, 91,* 269–276.

Spaulding, W., Rosenzweig, L., Huntzinger, R., Cromwell, R. L., Briggs, D., & Hayes, T. (1980). Visual pattern integration in psychiatric patients. *Journal of Abnormal Psychology, 89,* 635–643.

Sperling, G. (1960). The information available in brief visual presentations. *Psychological Monographs, 74*(11, Whole No. 498).

Venables, P. H. (1984). Cerebral mechanisms, autonomic responsiveness, and attention in schizophrenia. In W. D. Spaulding & J. K. Cole (Ed.), *Nebraska symposium on motivation, Vol. 31: Theories of schizophrenia and psychosis* (pp. 47–91). Lincoln: University of Nebraska Press.

Walker, E. (1981). Attentional and neuromotor functions of schizophrenics, schizoaffectives, and patients with other affective disorders. *Archives of General Psychiatry, 38,* 1355–1358.

Walker, E. (1987). Validating and conceptualizing positive and negative symptoms. In P. D. Harvey & E. F. Walker (Eds.), *Positive and negative symptoms of psychosis: Description, research, and future directions* (pp. 30–49). Hillsdale, NJ: Lawrence Erlbaum Associates.

Wells, D. S., & Leventhal, D. (1984). Perceptual grouping in schizophrenia: Replication of Place and Gilmore. *Journal of Abnormal Psychology, 93,* 231–234.

Weyl, H. (1952). *Symmetry*. Princeton, NJ: Princeton University Press.

Widlocher, D., & Hardy-Bayle, M.-C. (1989). Cognition and control of action in psychopathology. *Cahiers de Psychologie Cognitive [European Bulletin of Cognitive Psychology], 9,* 583–615.

Williams, M. C. (1980). *Fast and slow responses to configurational factors in 'object-superiority' stimuli*. Unpublished doctoral thesis, State University of New York at Buffalo.

Williams, M. C., & Weisstein, N. (1980, May). *Apparent depth and connectedness produce spatial frequency specific effects on metacontrast*. Paper presented at the annual meeting of the Association for Research in Vision and Ophthalmology, Orlando, FL.

Wishner, J., & Wahl, O. (1974). Dichotic listening in schizophrenia. *Journal of Consulting and Clinical Psychology, 42,* 538–546.

Wohlberg, G. W., & Kornetsky, C. (1973). Sustained attention in remitted schizophrenics. *Archives of General Psychiatry, 28,* 533–537.

Yonas, A., & Granrud, C. E. (1985). Development of visual space perception in young infants. In J. Mehler & R. Fox (Eds.), *Neonate cognition: Beyond the blooming buzzing confusion* (pp. 45–67). Hillsdale, NJ: Lawrence Erlbaum Associates.

11

Stochastic Modeling of Stimulus Encoding and Memory Search in Paranoid Schizophrenia: Clinical and Theoretical Implications

RICHARD W. J. NEUFELD
DAVID VOLLICK
SHARA HIGHGATE

CONTEXT OF INVESTIGATION

Investigation of cognitive–behavioral aspects of schizophrenia has reaped a relatively rich harvest of data from the application of paradigms adopted from the experimental psychology of memory and cognition (for reviews, see Broga & Neufeld, 1981a; Neufeld, 1991; Spaulding & Cole, 1983). Such studies largely have been addressed to a level of analysis referred to in an influential commentary on cognitive science by Marr (1982) as "computational." A model is constructed comprising with varying degrees of formality the computations underlying observed task performance. Such computations are not constrained at this point to conform in specified ways to plausible neurological-level transactions. For example, a computational model of memory for categorical stimulus properties, such as win–loss records of sports teams, may be constructed employing concepts such as "stimulus-trace repertoire" and "trace strength," but with little formal regard for physiological mechanisms of implementation (e.g., Estes, 1976). The psychopathologist of schizophrenia is interested in how such models must be perturbed in order to accommodate performance deviations and/or deficits. Selected findings from this level of analysis form the subject matter of the present chapter.

The computational level is put into broader perspective by considering its relation to complementing levels of analysis (Figure 11.1). At the algorithmic level, efforts are made to model cognitive events according to "brain" or "computer" metaphors (see Pylyshyn, 1984; Rummelhart & McClelland, 1986). Models at this level of analysis are designed to convey more strongly actual goings on at the implementational (physiological) level, including patterns of excitation within neuronal networks. For instance, the memorial representation of categorical item properties may be modeled employing various operations of matrix algebra, with the elements of certain matrices representing actual units (neurons) of the processing system (see McClelland & Rummelhart, 1986). Considerably less work has been done on psychopathology at the algorithmic level of analysis than at the computational level of analysis, although it is far from absent from the scene. Some modeling of reduced sensitivity among schizophrenic patients to contextual stimuli governing speech, for example, has been underway

LEVEL OF ANALYSIS	METHODS OF STUDY	MOST RELEVANT LEVELS OF PSYCHOPATHOLOGY
COMPUTATIONAL	INFORMATION-PROCESSING PARADIGMS FROM THE EXPERIMENTAL PSYCHOLOGY OF COGNITION	CLINICAL SYMPTOMATOLOGY (E.G., THOUGHT-FORM DISORDER; THOUGHT-CONTENT DISORDER)
ALGORITHMIC	ASSESSMENT OF CONNECTIONISTIC MODELS OF NEURONAL ACTIVATION/INHIBITION SEQUENCES, LARGELY THROUGH COMPUTER SIMULATION (PARALLEL-DISTRIBUTED-PROCESSING MODELS), CONSTRUCTION OF "COMPUTER-METAPHORS" FOR COGNITIVE OPERATIONS	
IMPLEMENTATIONAL	NEUROPHYSIOLOGY/ NEUROCHEMISTRY; ELECTROPHYSIOLOGY	GENETICALLY-ENDOWED, AND OTHER PHYSIOLOGICAL SUBSTRATES OF PSYCHOPATHOLOGY

Figure 11.1. Levels of analysis of information processing. (*Source:* Adapted from Marr, 1982.)

(Cohen & Servan-Schreiber, 1992; see also Hoffman & Dobscha, 1989, elaborated on later in this chapter).

At the implementational level, the investigator is concerned with how cognitive transactions might be realized physically. The implementational level of analysis is composed of neurophysiological/neurochemical and electrophysiological investigations. The pursuit of clinically significant abnormalities obviously constitutes a flourishing line of study, as is evidenced strongly in the present volume.

The importance of each level of analysis to a comprehensive account of informational events mediating "behavioral output" has been stated by Marr (1982), as well as by others, working at the algorithmic level of analysis (e.g., Rummelhart & McClelland, 1986; for a less favorable view of computational and algorithmic analyses, see Edelman, 1986). A similar statement may be made here—that each level of analysis is vital to a comprehensive account of deviation in informational events mediating *abnormal* behavioral output.

Of the three levels of analysis, the computational level might be considered as having the most direct link to symptomatology; both symptom taxonomies and computa-

tional-level models are concerned with cognitive–behavioral variables. As already implied, however, the value of computational-level studies does not consist solely in their symptomatological implications. Among other contributions, this level may inform—and be informed by—the algorithmic and implementational levels.

We turn now to a set of closely related paradigms from the experimental psychology of normal memory and cognition, one of which has enjoyed fairly extensive application to the study of information processing in schizophrenia.

MEMORY AND VISUAL SEARCH PARADIGMS: LATE AND EARLY TARGET PRESENTATIONS

In a typical memory search paradigm, a subject indicates as quickly and accurately as possible whether or not a visually presented item (target item; e.g., a letter of the alphabet) is a member of a previously memorized item list *(memory set)*. Figure 11.2 illustrates the progression of events for a representative "positive trial"—one in which the target item is present in the memory set (Sternberg, 1975). In this example, after visually focusing on a fixation "X", an array

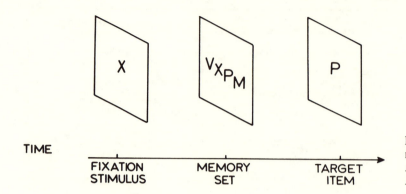

TIME

FIXATION   MEMORY   TARGET
STIMULUS   SET   ITEM

Figure 11.2. Representative memory search trial. (*Source:* Adapted from Townsend & Ashby, 1983.)

of four items is shown; the target item follows and the response is registered subsequently.

A visual search trial would proceed in a similar fashion, except the temporal locations of the target item and the item array are interchanged. Now the subject searches the visual array for the earlier memorized target, rather than searching the memory-held array for the subsequent visual target. Size of the memory set, or visual array, varies across trials, normally from one through to some subspan value. Performance as a rule is measured as reaction time associated with the respective memory set/visual array sizes. Error rates typically are low and seldom are of primary interest (however, see Link & Heath, 1975; Pachella, 1974; Schweikert, 1985).

Memory and visual search paradigms can be mixed such that, instead of one target item, several items are presented. The subject then indicates whether one of the targets is present in the memory set or, similarly, whether one of the memorized targets is present in the visual array. The composite paradigm, however, rarely has been used in studies of schizophrenia.

The emphasis in this chapter squarely is on results from memory search experiments, with reference periodically being made to visual search. Thus, we turn to a description of dimensions of memory search tasks, and to processes thought to be involved in task completion; our description ushers in findings from studies of schizophrenia.

Dimensions of Memory Search Tasks and Processes in Performance

Dimensions of variation in memory search tasks, and types of cognitive operations thought to be involved in correct responding, are sketched out here. More extensive discussions are available elsewhere (e.g., Townsend, 1974). Two dimensions have been referred to already. One of these comprises the presence versus absence on a given trial of the target item in the memory set (*positive* versus *negative* trial). Associated with this dimension is the processing division, "self-terminating versus exhaustive search." *Self-terminating* search implies that, for positive trials, examination of the memory set ceases and the response takes place once the target is encountered. *Exhaustive* search implies that all members of the memory set are examined; accordingly, exhaustive search tends to occur for negative trials. A consequence of the liaison between self-terminating–exhaustive search and positive–negative trials is that the slope of the function relating reaction time to memory set size tends to be steeper for negative trials (illustrated in Figure 11.5, below).

Serial versus *parallel* search is one of the most prominent distinctions concerning the nature of task performance. In serial search, items are considered to be examined successively (Figure 11.3a). In parallel search, examination begins on all items simultaneously (Figure 11.3b); however, examination is not completed on all items simultane-

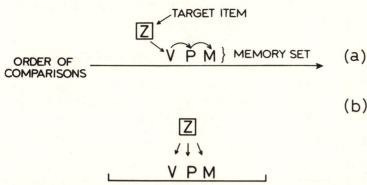

(b)

Figure 11.3. Schematic portrayal of serial *(a)* and parallel *(b)* memory search (memory set size = 3, negative trial).

ously. Rather, item completions are distributed stochastically over time.

The concept of *capacity* also is pertinent to what is to follow. Capacity is identified with the "rate" or speed of processing. It may be thought of in terms of the number of items completed in a given unit of time, or the amount of time required for completion of a single item. In the case of parallel memory search, if the rate of examining the individual items is affected by the size of the memory set—as "items are added in parallel"—the capacity of the system is *limited*. Conversely, if the individual-item rate is not affected by additional items, *unlimited* capacity is in effect. In the case of limited capacity, the additional item(s) are said to have had "direct nonselective effects on the other item-examination processes."

The final division concerning processes is that of *stochastic dependence–independence*. Suffice it to say that stochastic independence implies that the rate of processing applied to an uncompleted item is unchanged with successive completions of earlier-examined items. Stochastic dependence implies the opposite. To illustrate, in the case of limited capacity, above, the rate of processing an individual item decreases as the memory set increases. However, as items successively are completed, the "freed-up" processing resources now may be allocated to the uncompleted items, thus increasing the rate of examination applied to them (Townsend, 1974). Such stochastic dependence is a case in point of "indirect nonselective effects" among the item examination processes.

The preceding task dimensions and process descriptors have been discussed with reference to memory scanning. Other processes considered to be involved in task performance include (a) encoding, which is the translation of the raw target stimulus into a format supposedly facilitating comparison to members of the memory-held set; and (b) selection and registration of the response appropriate to the outcome of the memory search process.

Encoding putatively entails varying degrees of "elaboration" of the presenting target, depending on what exactly is being compared with respect to the memory-held items. At the simplest level, template matching requires simply the extraction of the salient physical features of the target. Encoding of names is required where name matching might be involved (e.g., accessing the same name to "A", "a", or a calligraphical "A"; Posner & Mitchell, 1967). In a task entailing memory scanning to verify simple statements, critical statement linguistic properties may be encoded into an "abstract propositional format" (Carpenter & Just, 1975). A task may require the subject to indicate if the "real-life size" of the target resembles that of a memory set item. In this instance, the target would be encoded with respect to its size properties. If the target were presented in a pictorial format (with no size cues other than pictorial content), encoding would be facilitated presumably because of a more direct activation of the "imagery system"; presenting the name of the target instead should increase the encoding load by requiring that the initial verbal representation in turn be referred to the imagery system to access size properties (Paivio, 1975).

When considering the above processes together, certain descriptors discussed above with reference to the processing of individual items in memory search once more are applicable. Processes may proceed serially or in parallel (e.g., encoding preceding versus commencing with memory scanning). In addition, one process may affect the speed of another in direct or indirect nonselective ways. Where more than one process is being considered, and several operations constitute a given process, as when several comparisons between target and memory set items must be completed, such operations may be referred to as subprocesses or stages.

In general, the slope of the choice reaction time function relating reaction time to memory set size is the focus of attention when considering the memory-scanning process; the 0 intercept of the function, in contrast, is the focus with respect to encoding and response processes (see Figure 11.4). This practice seems to retain a degree of formal legitimacy amid the undermining by developments in stochastic modeling of a number of other practices routinely in-

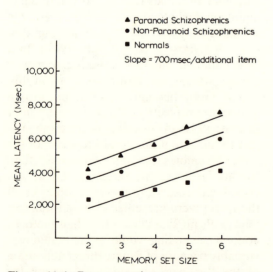

Figure 11.4. Representative memory search reaction time functions ("exhaustive-search" trials). (*Source:* Adapted from Neufeld, 1977.)

voked to interpret memory scanning and related task performance.

FINDINGS FOR SCHIZOPHRENIA

A representative pattern of results from studies of memory search choice reaction time among paranoid and nonparanoid schizophrenics and controls is presented in Figure 11.4. Detailed reviews of these studies have been presented elsewhere (Broga & Neufeld, 1981a; Neufeld, 1991). Slopes of the reaction time function are similar across groups, but intercepts for paranoid—and to a lesser extent for nonparanoid—schizophrenics are elevated. Thus, memory scanning appears to be intact but encoding and/or response processes are not. In general, the groups have had similar error rates, and so interpretations are not complicated by differential "speed–accuracy tradeoffs."

Convergent evidence indicates that the source of schizophrenic intercept elevation is slower completion of the encoding process, as follows. First, when encoding time by and large has been eliminated from intercept values through paradigmatic innovations, schizophrenic–control differences have disappeared (Neufeld, 1978). Second, estimated milliseconds required for response organization and execution processes of the variety employed in these tasks (e.g., Biederman & Kaplan, 1970) are well below the range of observed intercept values. Third, patients with unipolar affective disorders, whom one might suspect of being at least as susceptible as paranoid schizophrenics to retardation in response processes, have intercept values that are significantly lower than those of schizophrenic samples (Highgate-Maynard & Neufeld, 1986). Finally, response times have tended not to increase differentially with increased response complexity, encoding load remaining constant (Dobson & Neufeld, 1982).

The inferences to be drawn from the observations to date, then, are that paranoid (and nonparanoid) schizophrenics retain strengths in memory search but show weaknesses (nonparanoids less so) in encoding raw stimulation into a search-facilitative format. Our aim now is to examine these strengths and weaknesses from the perspective of stochastic modeling, and to draw out possible theoretical and clinical implications of the results.

Some Representative Results

A study whose results in the main are representative of those examining schizophrenic choice reaction time (CRT) memory search is that of Highgate-Maynard and Neufeld (1986). Results are representative in terms of the apparent integrity of memory search amid deficient stimulus encoding. These results are taken, then, as a case in point on which to focus our stochastic modeling considerations.

Briefly, groups of paranoid and nonparanoid schizophrenics, patients with unipolar affective disorder (nonschizophrenic psychiatric controls), and nonpatients ($n = 20$) completed a relatively demanding CRT memory search task. They were asked to indicate whether the target item (either an animal or an object) resembled a memory set item with respect to its "real-life size" ("overall magnitude"; see Paivio, 1975). Memory set sizes ranged from one through four. One half of the subjects in each group were presented with drawings of the target items, whereas the other half were presented with names of the items. Thus, encoding requirements presumably were greater in the latter case, inasmuch as the initial verbal representation of the target item would require referral to the imagery system to access the necessary size properties (see also George & Neufeld, 1984). In each condition, encoding demands exceeded considerably the mere extraction of presenting physical features, as might be sufficient in simple template matching.

Memory scanning also was considered to be relatively demanding. It required comparison between the size properties of the target item and the respective memory set items, and, additionally, the setting of these contrasts against subjective criteria of similarity in size (see Hockley & Murdock,

1987; Wright, 1977). Responses were identified as correct or incorrect according to target–memory set item proximities, defined a priori on the basis of Thurstonian discriminal-difference distributions of previous normative size ratings (detailed in Highgate-Maynard & Neufeld, 1986). Subjects were acquainted with task requirements and the nature of correct responding with the aid of practice trials; a similar number of such trials was required for each group.

Furthermore, it was ascertained that the normative ratings of item sizes (Paivio, 1975) were similarly applicable to all groups. Other precautions involve comparability of speed–accuracy tradeoffs and provision for extraneous demographic and clinical variables (e.g., age, education, IQ, hospitalization, medication).

STOCHASTIC MODELING

Stochastic modeling roughly entails specifying formally the "processing systems" possibly underlying performance of memory search, visual search, and related tasks. Emphasis here is on response latencies; however, models of relative accuracy also are available. The term "stochastic" implies that provision is made in these models for an inevitable degree of unpredictability of response times.

Candidate models of schizophrenic performance are identified as follows. The mathematically posed structures of selected models are set against observed similarities and differences in performance between schizophrenics and controls. Models whose structures can accommodate the observed data patterns are retained as tenable candidates. Of particular interest are the model parameters within those structures whose variation provides for schizophrenic performance deviations. Although emphasis is on mean response latencies, mention is made of a second performance measure that can assist in narrowing down candidate models. This measure is the *variance* in response latencies within subjects, over trials. For example, in the representative study discussed above, each subject received nine negative and nine positive trials under each memory set size. Variance in response times across each such set of nine trials potentially is informative regarding candidate models. A comprehensive account of stochastic modeling is available in a volume by Townsend and Ashby (1983).

Derivations of the formulas applied here are well beyond the mandate of this chapter, but are available elsewhere (e.g., Townsend, 1974, 1984; Townsend & Ashby, 1983). Certain extensions and elaborations are necessary for the current developments (see Appendices A and B).

One final word: it is assumed that the structure of the system operative in a given task is the same for both schizophrenics and controls (see Neufeld, 1982; Neufeld & Broga, 1981). Within selected constraints, this assumption can be relaxed in the case of encoding, the conclusions invoking the assumption remaining intact (Neufeld, 1990a). It can be shown that, at least for the data to be discussed in relation to memory search, a switch in systems as we move from schizophrenics to controls is highly unlikely.

Memory Search

The results from the representative study discussed above included a highly significant Memory Set Size × Positive–Negative Trial interaction ($p<.001$). This effect was stable across groups, levels of encoding, and combinations of those factors (p values $>.20$). Figure 11.5 presents the differences in positive–negative trial slopes corresponding to the significant interaction. Each data point is based on a total of 720 trials. This level of aggregation is ideal where the aim is to minimize sources of variance competing with the parameters of a common model structure (Neufeld & Gardner, 1990). In the present instance, then, the schizophrenics and controls performed in a similar fashion. The goal now becomes one of identifying the nature of the system evidently remaining intact despite the occurrence of schizophrenia. A model accommodating the observed pattern of means across positive and negative trials is required.

Note that the ratio of the negative to positive slopes is strikingly close to 3:1, rather than 2:1, as would be necessary, for example, for the standard serial search model. A model whose predicted mean response times are closest to this feature of the data is the "moderately limited capacity" (MLC) parallel model with stochastic independence (Townsend & Ashby, 1983).

In this model, the rate of processing applied to an individual item is determined by the number of items in the memory set (k). This rate then remains constant throughout the trial. Its value, $v(k)$, is equal to

$$(v/k)(\Sigma_i^k 1/i),$$

where v = the individual-item rate when k = 1 (i.e., no division of capacity among multiple items). A glimpse into the workings of this model is afforded by considering a set size of 2, both items being compared to the target (Figure 11.6). The rate applied to each item is $3v/4$. Following completion of one of the items (Stage 1), the uncompleted item continues to be processed at the same rate (Stage 2).

Because the two items are processed at the same rate, they have an equal chance of being completed first. The time from the beginning of the trial to the completion of the first item is known as the first intercompletion time, and that between the first and second completions is referred to as the second intercompletion time. In this model, the *expected* values of these intercompletion times—correponding to the means that would be obtained over a large number of trials—are unequal. The expected value of the first intercompletion time is $2/(3v)$, whereas that for the second is $4/(3v)$ (see Appendix A). Summing of these values, however, results in a total expected completion time for the trial [$E(T)$] of $2/v$. In general, for exhaustive processing [$E(T)_{Ex}$] of a memory set size of k, $E(T)_{Ex} = k/v$. A point to be returned to later is that models with unequal intercompletion times and those with equal intercompletion times will

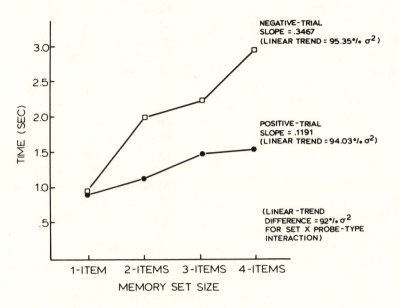

NEGATIVE-TRIAL
SLOPE = .3467
(LINEAR TREND = 95.35% σ2)
POSITIVE-TRIAL
SLOPE = .1191
(LINEAR TREND = 94.03% σ2)
(LINEAR-TREND
DIFFERENCE = 92% σ2
FOR SET X PROBE-TYPE
INTERACTION)
TIME (SEC)
3.0
2.5
2.0
1.5
1.0
.5
1-ITEM
2-ITEMS
3-ITEMS
4-ITEMS
MEMORY SET SIZE

Figure 11.5. Positive and negative trial reaction time slopes (correct responses). (*Source:* Adapted from Highgate-Maynard, 1984.) Times for memory set size = 1 are arbitrarily equated (see Townsend & Ashby, 1983).

predict variances of total completion times that are unequal, even if they predict identical mean total completion times.

Turning to self-terminating (ST) processing, we observe that

$$E(T)_{\mathrm{ST}} = k/(v\Sigma_i^k 1/i)$$

(see Appendix A). For $k = 2$, this value becomes $1.33/v$. Whereas $E(T)_{\mathrm{Ex}}$ has increased by $1/v$ from $k = 1$ to $k = 2$, $E(T)_{\mathrm{ST}}$ has increased by $0.33/v$.

As implied by the label, the item-level processing rate of the MLC model decreases as k increases, but not as drastically

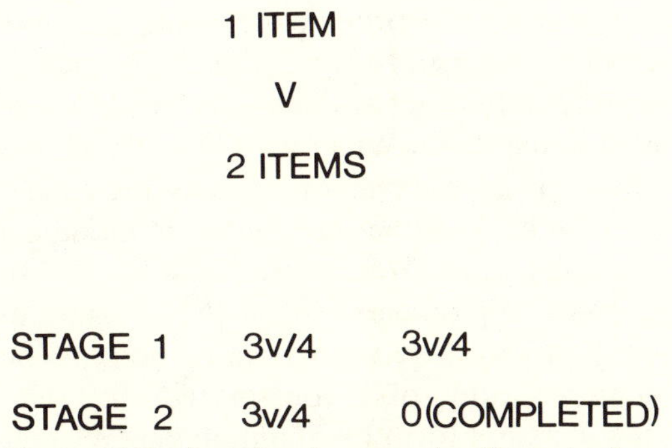

1 ITEM
V
2 ITEMS
STAGE 1 3v/4 3v/4
STAGE 2 3v/4 0(COMPLETED)

Figure 11.6. Item-level processing for a stochastically independent parallel model with moderately limited capacity and $k = 2$. (*Source:* Adapted from Townsend & Ashby, 1983.)

as it would if capacity were strictly fixed. For the fixed-capacity stochastically independent model, the item level processing rate = v/k, where v once again is the item-level rate when $k = 1$.

The fixed-capacity independent parallel model also produces an exhaustive to self-terminating net slope ratio of approximately 3:1. However, the exhaustive mean response times are curvilinear, positively accelerating with increasing k. The relative inefficiency of the fixed-capacity independent parallel model might be noted in passing. Increments in expected completion times with increasing values of k are considerably higher than are those of the MLC independent parallel model, and, for that matter, the dubiously efficient standard serial model. The latter's exhaustive processing slope is the same as that of the MLC independent parallel model. However, as mentioned, the self-terminating slope is less by a factor of two rather than approximately three.

How well do the expected completion times generated by the MLC independent parallel model fit the observed means? To throw into relief memory scanning, over and against other processes involved in performance, increments in mean completion times accompanying successive increments in memory set sizes were examined. Thus, three mean differences were available from the negative trials and three from the positive trials. The theoretical increments in completion times, as established from the model, were derived; these derived increments then represented the model's predictions, to be tested against the observed increments.

First, the rate parameter, v, was estimated using a minimum χ^2 criterion, and found to be 1.23 (items/s). With this value inserted into the model, and a corresponding loss of 1 df, an excellent fit between the model's predictions and observed values was obtained ($\chi^2_{(5)} = .108$, $p > .50$). (Recall that as fit is improved, χ^2 decreases.) (Although the result indicates a close fit, especially as combined with the relative values of the slopes, the test statistic should not be taken too literally as χ^2 [see Townsend & Ashby, 1983, p. 432].) Similar tests applied separately to each of the four groups of subjects indicated an excellent fit in every instance.

Confidence in the model fit might be enhanced by incorporating the average completion time variance for each memory set size, as well as the grand completion time means for each set size, into the calculations (see Appendix B). The benefits accruing to this added complication would include the doubling of data points for the closed solution for v, and correspondingly more pairs of observed and predicted values for the evaluation of fit (Neufeld, 1989). The inclusion of variances may be useful in eliminating certain models from among those with identical predictions of mean total completion times.

Overall, then, results are accordant with the operation of a fairly sophisticated memory search system—one that undergoes a set amount of capacity depletion with increasing k. We might imagine, for example, that an increase in k has "incentive properties" moderating somewhat a potentially more drastic depletion of the item-level rate, as would be seen with a fixed-capacity independent system. In any event, the factors responsible for the operation of the sup-

ported model evidently are not lost with the occurrence of schizophrenia.

The MLC independent parallel system may be operative in other memory search tasks resembling the present one. There are hints of its operation also in certain types of visual search tasks (e.g., the "triangle-mismatching condition" of Triesman & Paterson, 1984). The point is that the system appears to be available to schizophrenics and controls alike when it is called on by task requirements. Moreover, its operation may bestow tangible advantages over the operation, say, of the familiar standard serial processing model.

One of these advantages involves "survival value," as follows. Even a split-second gain in verifying that an external stimulus is a member of a set of memory-held stimuli signifying danger, or is a member of a set signifying positive reinforcement, potentially can spell the difference between survival success and failure in an environment that demands a quick reaction (see Edelman, 1986).

Second, certain more molar memory operations involved in day-to-day functioning stand to benefit. These are operations that putatively lean somewhat heavily on the ascertainment from memory of the presence of significant stimulus properties. The effects of positive identification that takes two thirds as long as that prescribed by the standard serial model can be compounded into substantially greater efficiency of larger scale operations in which these processes participate.

A word is in order concerning the now familiar construct of attentional or processing capacity (e.g., Kahneman, 1973; Navon & Gopher, 1980; Wickens, 1984). By far the most formal treatment of processing capacity is to be found in the stochastic modeling literature (e.g., Townsend & Ashby, 1978). It has been referred to as the amount of work the system is capable of doing. The quantification of "transmitted information," as put forth by Shannon and Weaver (1949), provides a relevant angle on this construct. With respect to the processing systems being dealt with in this chapter, capacity is identified most closely with the rate parameter, v. Concerning the system involved in memory scanning, then, the verdict on hypothetical capacity reduction in schizophrenia from this analysis is negative.

Encoding

We turn now to the encoding process, in which the group of paranoid schizophrenics especially were slower than were the other groups. Plotted in Figure 11.7 are means of negative trials for the paranoids and nonpatients across encoding loads. These results are representative of the broader set of data, in that the relevant lower and higher order interactions (all four diagnostic groups included) were nonsignificant throughout ($p > .20$). Negative-trial means are plotted because the encoding load manipulation was enhanced under this condition, for reasons not entirely clear at this point ($p < .05$). Of importance for the present purposes was the marked additivity of the group differences across levels of encoding load (p for interaction $> .80$), and the maintenance of this additivity over types of trials ($p > .24$). The mandate thus becomes one of short-listing from available models those producing additive effects of encoding load and diagnostic status.

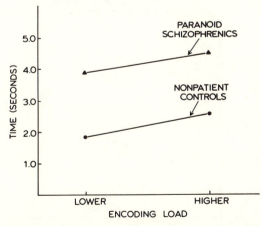

Figure 11.7. Response latency for negative trials as a function of encoding load and paranoid schizophrenia. Lower encoding load = pictorial target format; higher encoding load = verbal target format. (*Source:* Data from Highgate-Maynard, 1984.)

Our search is narrowed by knowing that our likelihood of success is greater among parallel models with limited capacity and possibly stochastic dependence, and among serial models with stochastic independence (Townsend, 1984). (Capacity limitation is not that relevant in the case of serial models because only one item is processed at a time.) With these properties in mind, two parallel models and one serial model were identified. Their candidacy is defended mathematically in Appendix B. When considering these models, it should be kept in mind that, unlike the case of memory scanning, in which there were k items in the memory set, the k subprocesses now are more "covert" in nature, in that they do not correspond to observable stimuli. Furthermore, when it comes to encoding, the self-terminating–exhaustive division is not involved because the systematic presence/absence of a target in the memory set presumably does not infiltrate this level of processing. In any case, the representative data on which we have converged for now are negative-trial specific.

One of the parallel models retained as a candidate, the MLC independent parallel model, already has been discussed. The second parallel model is one with limited capacity and displays stochastic dependence. The fixed-capacity parallel model with reallocation is sensitive to the number of subprocesses k, with its item-level rate being set at v/k. However, the completion of an item is said to "release" the associated processing capacity for application to the uncompleted items. Thus, after the first item is completed, the item-level capacity becomes $v/(k - 1)$, and so on for the remaining items, whereby the last item to be completed is processed at rate v.

Figure 11.8 presents a schematic layout of this model for $k = 2$. In this special case, $E(T) = [2(1/2\ v)]^{-1} + v^{-1} = 2/v$. In the general case, $E(T) = \Sigma_i^k\ (i\ 1/i\ v)^{-1} = \Sigma_i^k\ v^{-1} = k/v$. The standard serial model is presented schematically in Figure 11.9. Here, $E(T) = \Sigma_i^k\ 1/v = k/v$ once again.

Observe that certain models do not accommodate mean latency additivity, re-

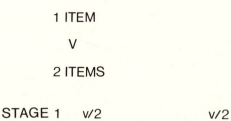

STAGE 1   v/2   v/2

STAGE 2   0(COMPLETED)   v

Figure 11.8. Schematic layout of the fixed-capacity parallel model, with reallocation, for $k =$ 2. (*Source:* Based on Townsend & Ashby, 1983.)

gardless of parameter perturbation. A representative of such a "class of models," the independent parallel model with unlimited capacity, is examined in Appendix B. What sort of parameter perturbation is required by those models that do accommodate additivity?

One possibility is alteration downward of the rate parameter, v. However, a hypothetical decline of v with paranoid schizophrenia prevents additivity of latencies in these models. Instead, an increase in the number of subprocesses required to accomplish the encoding process, denoted $g>0$, must be hypothesized (see Appendix B). Accordingly, the diagnostic status of paranoid schizophrenia in the present sample is associated not with a reduced rate of processing but with an inefficient application of an apparent intact rate of processing. Inefficiency, here, comprises extra operations required to complete the encoding process.

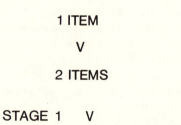

STAGE 1   V   0

STAGE 2   0(COMPLETED)   V

Figure 11.9. Schematic layout of the standard serial model, with stochastic independence, for $k = 2$. (*Source:* Based on Townsend & Ashby, 1983.)

TOWARD A COMPREHENSIVE STOCHASTIC MODEL OF PARANOID SCHIZOPHRENICS' MEMORY SCANNING TASK PERFORMANCE

The representation of paranoid schizophrenics' memory scanning performance tendered here is designed to convey strengths in memory search and deficits in encoding. Strengths in "response processes" easily could be included, but are omitted because they are not essential to the main points. As before, our formal development is simplified somewhat by extracting from the results of our representative study a subset of data making for two 2-level factors.

The mean response latencies for the paranoid schizophrenics and nonpatient controls for memory set sizes 2 and 4 (negative trials) are presented in Figure 11.10. This smaller set of means is "informationally sufficient," in that they capture key characteristics of the data: intact memory scanning, delayed completion of encoding, and additivity of effects on response latencies of the factor influencing the encoding process (diagnostic group status) and that influencing the memory process (memory set size). Regarding additivity, for the interaction spe-

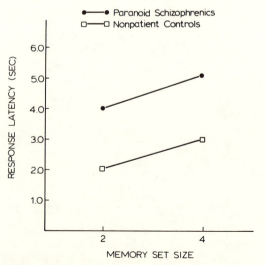

Figure 11.10. Response latency for negative trials as a function of memory set size (2 versus 4) and paranoid schizophrenia. (*Source:* Data from Highgate-Maynard, 1984.)

cific to the data presented in Figure 11.10, the value of F is .0016.

What observations must a tendered model take into account? We may enumerate the findings that at this point must be incorporated:

1. Memory search comparable to that of controls
2. Delayed completion of stimulus encoding
3. Additivity of effects on mean response latencies of factors influencing encoding and memory search
4. Operation of an MLC independent parallel model, in the case of the memory search process
5. Operation of a model yielding values for $E(T)_{Ex},k,v = k/v$, in the case of the encoding process

These observations are represented as follows. The encoding process precedes the memory search process, as seen in Figure 11.11. The processes (a) proceed serially, (b) with each being affected selectively by its associated factor and (c) with each being stochastically independent of the other. The representation has the advantage over competing representations of being parsimonious with respect to the extent findings. For example, additivity of factor effects on response latencies may be accommodated by having the processes carried out in parallel, but not without a rather complex interplay in terms of nonselective factor effects and stochastic dependence.

The upper portion of Figure 11.11 describes the transactions among the controls, whereas the lower portion describes those among the paranoid schizophrenics. In each case, the upper pair of processes depict encoding followed by memory search, where the memory set size, k, is equal to 2. The lengthened right-hand process for the lower pair in each case represents $k = 4$. Throughout, the process on the left represents encoding. In keeping with Figure 11.10, the latencies are treated as though they are averaged over encoding loads. Therefore,

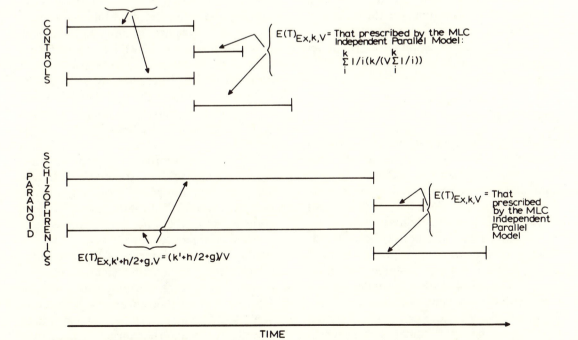

Figure 11.11. Representations of stimulus encoding and memory search for paranoid schizophrenics *(bottom)* and controls *(top)*.

under no impairment, the number of sub-processes is presented as $k' + (0 + h)/2 = k' + h/2$. The distinguishing feature of the representation for the paranoid schizophrenics is the addition of $g>0$ sub-processes to the encoding process.

The specific model best describing the encoding process may be difficult to identify. We reiterate that the requisite structure of $E(T)_{Ex}$ (item 5 above) is not unique to a specific model. There is some hope, however, of reducing the number of candidates by considering their predicted response latency variances (cf., mathematical Appendix A of Neufeld & Williamson, in press). The variances predicted by the standard serial model and the fixed-capacity parallel model with reallocation are equal to each other, but different from those predicted by the MLC independent parallel model (detailed in Appendix B). Thus, the first pair of models or the third model may be eliminated, depending on which set of predicted variances best fits with the observed variances. Whether values of the variances predicted by the first pair of models and those predicted by the MLC independent parallel model are sufficiently discrepant to permit the necessary discrimination through conventional tests of comparative goodness-of-fit, is an empirical question currently under examination.

CLINICAL AND THEORETICAL IMPLICATIONS

In educing potential clinical and theoretical implications from the foregoing developments, we address first the domain of symptomatology, most notably delusions in paranoid schizophrenia. As is the case with most correlational psychopathology, clinical inferences must take on a conservative tenor, being prefaced with appropriate caveats. Accordingly, it must be restated that, *inter alia*, the proposed stochastic model is identified with results from a certain laboratory paradigm. Furthermore, the main direction of influence between domains of observables always is contestable when one domain comprises deficits identified from labora-

tory task performance and the other comprises clinical symptomatology. A number of other issues raised when attempting to draw clinical inferences from cognitive–behavioral laboratory studies must be kept in mind; these have been discussed at some length elsewhere (e.g., George & Neufeld, 1985). Given the due cautions and qualifications, it is suggested that the formulated model may provide an informative angle on some aspects of delusions in paranoid schizophrenia.

Consider, first, memory search as represented in the tentative stochastic model. This process was identical for the paranoid schizophrenics and controls. The portrayal represents a given instance of a fairly well-documented finding: nonchronic paranoid schizophrenics draw inferences from information residing in short-term/working memory with normal speed and accuracy. This observation is consistent with clinical symptomatology comprising systematized, fairly well-integrated thought content (e.g., as noted in the *Diagnostic and Statistical Manual of Mental Disorders,* third edition, revised [DSM-III-R; American Psychiatric Association, 1987, pp. 188, 197]). Descriptions of the integrity of certain features of paranoid schizophrenic thinking have been noted in historical as well as more recent clinical observations (e.g., Cromwell, 1975; Kraeplin, 1919; Nicholson & Neufeld, in press). Findings presented here indicate that a relatively complex memory search system withstands the presence of this disorder.

Encoding, as represented in the stochastic model, presents a somewhat different story. Completion of this process is delayed because of additional component operations entering into the encoding process. Although the apparatus for extracting information and drawing inferences from stimulus material residing in memory may be entirely functional, certain material necessary for drawing correct inferences may be incomplete. Recall that in a typical memory search paradigm, an external target is presented and remains in view pending the response. Consistently responding in the keyed direction demands that the information carried by the target (e.g., relative size properties) adequately be summoned. Were the target to disappear before the encoding process had been completed, relevant information would stand to be lost. Responding may still proceed, but without the constraints imposed by the information carried by the external stimulus.

By extension, an individual for whom encoding routinely is delayed may bear an ongoing risk of missing information held by surrounding stimuli. Included may be information critical to "objectively accurate" inferences about encountered events and objects. Thus, the stochastic model suggests ways in which the processes it contains may contribute to the occurrence of false beliefs. (Contribution to other behaviors characterizing paranoid schizophrenics, including certain features of eye-movement dysfunction, have been presented elsewhere; Mather, Neufeld, Merskey, & Russell, 1991; Neufeld, Mather, Merskey, & Russell, in press; Neufeld & Williamson, in press.)

Of course, many individuals who in all likelihood have similar difficulties with stimulus encoding, including those with certain perceptual handicaps, are not inordinately prone to delusions. A clue regarding this propensity in paranoid schizophrenia may lie in a particular "response style" observed among these patients under certain laboratory conditions (Broga & Neufeld, 1981b; McCormick & Broekema, 1978; Price & Eriksen, 1966). These subjects have been especially liberal in expressing confidence in their judgments about presented stimulation. This style of responding is contrasted in some clinical groups by a degree of reticence to state the judged status of stimuli, despite *less* processing deficiency. Such a combination has characterized, for example, nonparanoid schizophrenics (Broga & Neufeld, 1981b).

Why might the product of cognitive transactions involving incomplete or fractional input commonly comprise negative content (e.g., persecutory or jealous ideation)? Moreover, why might the product most often have considerable personal, emotional significance? Such content may have a certain protective function, vis-à-vis positive, detached content. Specifically, in the company of incomplete or fractional information, erroneously assuming ill intent on the part of others may carry considerably less risk of harm than erroneously assuming benevolent intentions. That is to say, an overall defensive stance may have "survival value" in this way.

We turn now from clinical symptomatology to one of several areas of day-to-day functioning on which the current formulations might impinge. This area involves the negotiation of environmental stressors. Reduction of stress often demands personal control over environmental threats (see, e.g., Averill, 1973; Thompson, 1981). In numerous instances, effective controlling activity proceeds on the basis of threat-related information that has been encoded from environmental stimuli (Morrison, Neufeld, & Lefebvre, 1988; Neufeld, 1990b). Reduced efficiency of such processes, which are involved in stress resolution, obviously makes for increased vulnerability (see Nicholson & Neufeld, 1989; 1992; Neufeld & Nicholson, 1991). Interventions designed to minimize incidents that tax deficient processes, or that facilitate adjustment (e.g., "buying time" to compensate for retarded completion of selected processes), may be of some aid to the enterprise of "stress management" among these patients (see Wallace & Boone, 1983).

The issue of depleted attentional capacity (e.g., Kahneman, 1973) among schizophrenics has been referred to in previous sections. As noted, the model parameter that distinguishes especially paranoids' performance is one that indicates additional component steps for process completion. The data-fitting model does not include a shift with schizophrenia in values of parameters expressing processing capacity.

Finally, the current results are seen to have implications at the algorithmic level of analysis (Figure 11.1), specifically a currently well-known version called Parallel Distributed Processing (PDP; McClelland &

Rummelhart, 1986). PDP models are "connectionistic models" of neuronal functioning (Hebb, 1949), set forth to account for certain phenomena of learning and perception. The models depict patterns of activation within networks of "units" (neurons) designed to accommodate the target performance. They are implemented mathematically through a series of straightforward matrix operations. Roughly, the values of the matrix elements represent settings of neuronal units, and change iteratively and reiteratively to mimic patterns of stimulus input, or, in the case of learning, to encapsulate response requirements.

How might our computational account of encoding deficit be represented at the PDP algorithmic level of analysis? Suppose the system "responsible for encoding" was best described by one of the candidate parallel models. Suppose further that there is a degree of correspondence between the component operations at the computational level (subprocesses) and given constructs of PDP. An increase in the number of encoding subprocesses associated with paranoid schizophrenia at the computational level may imply a parallel increase in the number of PDP modules of units, or simply units, transacting the process. The expanded unit network thus embodies the PDP substrates of the computational level's increased subprocesses. In this way, reduced efficiency of process execution identified at the computational level may have correlates at the algorithmic level of analysis.

To the degree that the standard serial model is tenable at the computational level, events from a PDP perspective may take the form of additional iterations of unit-setting adjustments to converge on the target settings. One could easily imagine the starting unit settings among paranoid schizophrenics as being more distant from the target settings. Increased distance, in turn, may stem from greater attenuation of more target-compatible settings with the progression of time.

A word is in order concerning recent analyses of selected symptoms of schizophrenia carried out at the algorithmic level of analysis by Hoffman and Dobscha (1989). A relatively close match between their computer simulations and computational-level findings discussed in this chapter involves their combination of (a) relatively "unambiguous informational input" (e.g., presentation of a clearly recognizable, simple visual stimulus); and (b) several "memorized stimuli" to which the presented stimulus must be compared. The counterpart at the computational level is a memory search task entailing simple template matching (especially in light of the results of Hoffman, 1987) and positive trials (see section entitled "Dimensions of Memory Search Tasks and Processes in Performance"). Hoffman and Dobscha's results are restricted to the memory search process, and to accuracy vis-à-vis latency of the search process output. Under the conditions outlined above, normal accuracy rates would be observed among schizophrenic patients. Accordingly, empirical false-negative rates have been similar among schizophrenic patients and controls, as stated earlier.

Within the algorithmic architecture described by Hoffman and Dobscha (1989), the encoding process would correspond to translation of the presented stimulus (target) into an array of "$+1$" and "-1" values. Such an array comprises the digital format of the target required for the algorithmic version of the subsequent comparisons. The speed of this translative process, although the focal subject of this chapter, unfortunately is not directly implicated by Hoffman and Dobscha's simulation studies.

However, the above suggestions regarding possible algorithmic substrata of our candidate computational models can be accommodated within the structure of the algorithmic system used by those investigators. Specifically, the expanded network of units suggested by the tenability of our parallel models easily can be accommodated through an expanded array of target–stimulus unit settings. We simply need to specify that the temporal aspects of constructing the requisite array of $k + g$ or $k + h + g$ (to use the present notation) settings represent a "parallel Poisson process," as described here (one with ''positive stochastic dependency'' in the case of the fixed-capacity reallocation model).

Suggested algorithmic substrata of the standard serial candidate also can be accommodated. Rather than an expanded network of units, this suggestion specifies additional operations of unit-setting adjustments to achieve the relevant pattern of neuronal stimulation. With respect to the system used by Hoffman and Dobscha, this is the equivalent of saying that additional steps in the digitization process would be necessary to convert the presented target into its unit-setting array. On balance, then, although recent algorithmic-level analyses and the current computational-level analysis are not mutually confirmatory, they certainly are not incompatible.

CONCLUDING COMMENTS

In this chapter, we have journeyed from preliminary considerations surrounding the context of computational accounts of cognitive–behavioral deficit, through the construction of a stochastic model of memory scanning performance in paranoid schizophrenia to the model's clinical and theoretical implications. As with any formal approach, it has been necessary to spell out quantitatively the structure of the hypothetical models considered. Although a formal approach to the interpretation of data may lend itself to increased precision, the progression of ideas undoubtedly appears spartan at times. The proposed model, for example, addresses delusional symptomatology in a relatively mechanistic, reductionistic fashion. As a result, the approach may be indicted for not doing justice to the clinical richness of the phenomenon. Indeed, ''motivational factors'' may be necessary supplements to provide for such properties as the tenacity of delusions (see Winters & Neale, 1986). Nevertheless, on balance, the merits of formal approaches are likely to triumph over any disadvantages in vindicating their usage. Attempts to improve on eloquent apologetics presented elsewhere would be otiose (e.g., Staddon, 1984).

ACKNOWLEDGMENTS

Studies from the authors' laboratory referred to in this paper, and preparation of the manuscript, were supported by an operating grant from the Medical Research Council of Canada and a Tonnenbaum Scientist Award to the first author, and a scholarship from the Ontario Ministry of Health to the second author.

Expected Exhaustive and Self-Terminating Response Latencies for the Independent Parallel Model with Moderately Limited Capacity

The rate of processing applied to the individual item for a memory set size k, denoted $v(k)$, is equal to

$$v/k \; \Sigma_i^k \; 1/i$$

The expected exhaustive processing time, $E(T)_{Ex}$

$$= \Sigma_i^k \; 1/[iv(k)]$$

$$= \Sigma_i^k \; 1/(iv/k \; \Sigma_i^k \; 1/i)$$

$$= k/v$$

$E(T)_{ST}$, in turn,

$$= 1/v(k) = (k/v)(1/\Sigma_i^k \; 1/i)$$

where $v = $ the individual-item rate when $k = 1$, and where the target match has an equal chance for each ordinal position of completion.

This can be seen more clearly by considering the following array of expectancy values.

Because the expected time for completing one of several items (e.g., $k - 1$ of them) being processed in parallel, each at rate $v(k)$, is $1/[(k - 1)v(k)]$,

$$E(T)_{ST} = 1/k \; \Sigma_i^k \; [k/(kv(k)] + (k - 1)/[(k - 1) \; v(k)]$$
$$+ (k - 2)/[(k - 2)v(k)] + \cdots 1/v(k)$$
$$= 1/v(k) = (k/v)(1/\Sigma_i^k \; 1/i)$$

Serial position	$E(T)_{ST} \mid$ serial position $j(j = 1, 2, \ldots , k)$
1	
2	$1/[k \; v(k)]$
3	$1/[k \; v(k)] + 1/[(k - 1) \; v(k)]$
.	$1/[k \; v(k)] + 1/[(k - 1) \; v(k)] + 1/[(k - 2) \; v(k)]$
.	. . . .
.	. . . ...
k	
	$1/[k \; v(k)] + 1/[(k - 1) \; v(k)] + 1/[(k - 2) \; v(k)] + \ldots + 1/v(k)$

Identification of Models Generating Additive Effects of Encoding Load and Diagnostic Status on Response Latencies

Additive effects on response latencies of encoding load, and diagnostic status of paranoid schizophrenic–not paranoid schizophrenic, implies that the mixed second-order difference in the expected total completion times is equal to 0 (Townsend, 1984):

$$E(T; x_{a(1)}, x_{b(2)}) - E(T; x_{a(1)}, x_{b(1)})$$
$$- [E(T; x_{a(2)}, x_{b(2)}) - E(T; x_{a(2)}, x_{b(1)})] = 0$$

Here, $x_{a(1)}$ and $x_{a(2)}$ denote the lower and higher values of the encoding load factor, and $x_{b(1)}$ and $x_{b(2)}$ denote the absence and presence of paranoid schizophrenia.

We let k stand for the number of subprocesses involved in transacting the encoding process. The rate of processing (number of subprocesses completed per unit time) is denoted v. Increased encoding load is represented by an increase in k. Impairment associated with paranoid schizophrenia can be represented by (a) a further increase in k or (b) a decrease in v.

Convenient indexes of additive effects on expected response latency, $E(T)$, include the following: for case (a), the second-order difference equation with respect to k for the model-generated $E(T) = 0$. The first-order difference equation is

$$E(T)_{k+1} - E(T)_k = \Delta E(T)_k / \Delta_k = \Delta E(T)_k$$

The second-order difference equation is

$$\Delta^2 E(T)_k = \Delta E(T)_{k+1} - \Delta E(T)_k$$
$$= E(T)_{k+2} - E(T)_{k+1}$$
$$- [E(T)_{k+1} - E(T)_k]$$

For case (b), the partial derivative with respect to v of the first-order difference equation with respect to k for the model-generated $E(T) = 0$. That is:

$$\partial(\Delta E(T)_k)/\partial v = 0$$

Consider first an independent unlimited-capacity parallel model. For this model,

$$E(T)_{k,v} = 1/v \sum_{i=1}^{k} 1/i$$

Regarding case (a),

$$\Delta^2 E(T)_k = 1/v(\sum_{i=1}^{k+2} 1/i - \sum_{i=1}^{k+1} 1/i)$$
$$- 1/v (\sum_{i=1}^{k+1} 1/i - \sum_{i=1}^{k} 1/i)$$
$$= 1/v[1/(k + 2) - 1/(k + 1)] \neq 0$$

Turning to case (b),

$$\partial(\Delta E(T)_k)/\partial v = -1/v^2[1/(k + 1)] \neq 0$$

For each of the following models, $E(T)_k = k/v$: the standard serial model, the fixed-capacity parallel model with reallocation, and the MLC independent parallel model. Regarding case (a),

$$\Delta^2 E(T)_k = \Delta(1/v)/\Delta k = 0$$

Case (b), then, results in

$$\partial(\Delta E(T)_k)/\partial v = \partial(1/v)/\partial v = -1/v^2 \neq 0$$

Thus, impairment represented by an increase in subprocesses, additional to that occurring to encoding load increase, leads to additivity of expected total completion times for these models. Differences in $E(T)$ resulting from impairment can be represented as $[(k + g)/v] - k/v = g/v$ under the lower encoding load conditions and as $[(k + h + g)/v] - [(k + h)/v] = g/v$ under the higher encoding load conditions. Here, $g>0$ represents the additional subprocesses associated with impairment. The difference in $E(T)$ brought about by increased encoding load can be represented by h/v under either the presence or absence of impairment. The term $h>0$ denotes the added subprocesses occurring under the higher encoding load condition.

The *variances* in total completion times are identical for the standard serial model and the unlimited-capacity model with reallocation. For example, where the number of subprocesses $= k + h + g$, the predicted variance is $(k + h + g)/v^2$. In the case of the MLC independent parallel model, the predicted variance is

$$\Sigma_i^{k+h+g} 1/i^2$$

$$\cdot[k^2 + h^2 + g^2 + 2(kh + kg + hg)]/v^2$$

$$\cdot(1/\Sigma_i^{k+h+g} 1/i)^2$$

Letting the number of subprocesses vary from 1 through 4, and setting $v = 1.23$ for sake of illustration, the variances for the first two models are 0.66, 1.32, 1.98, and 2.64; corresponding values for the MLC independent parallel model are 0.66, 1.47, 2.42, and 3.47.

Computing variances in the case of self-terminating processing can be considerably more complex. Derivations pertinent to the first two models have been presented by Townsend and Ashby (1983).

Finally, the above three models do not exhaust those predicting additivity of mean latencies, given $g>0$; they simply are among the more prominent models that do so. For example, a "negative dependency" parallel model has been described by Townsend (1984). Where $k = 2$, both items are processed at rate v during the first stage. During the second stage, a fatiguelike effect sets in and the remaining item is processed at rate $2v/3$. Once again, $E(T) = k/v$, with variance now $= 2.5/v^2$.

REFERENCES

American Psychiatric Association. (1987). *Diagnostic and statistical manual of mental disorders* (3rd ed., rev.). Washington, DC: American Psychiatric Press, Inc.

Averill, J. R. (1973). Personal control over aversive stimuli and its relationship to stress. *Psychological Bulletin, 80,* 287–303.

Biederman, I., & Kaplan, R. (1970). Stimulus discriminability and S-R compatibility: Evidence for independent effects in choice reaction time. *Journal of Experimental Psychology, 86,* 434–439.

Broga, M. I., & Neufeld, R. W. J. (1981a). Evaluation of information-sequential aspects of schizophrenic performance, I: Framework and current findings. *Journal of Nervous and Mental Disease, 169,* 559–568.

Broga, M. I., & Neufeld, R. W. J. (1981b). Multivariate cognitive performance levels and response styles among paranoid and nonparanoid schizophrenics. *Journal of Abnormal Psychology, 90,* 495–509.

Carpenter, P. A., & Just, M. A. (1975). Sentence comprehension: A psycholinguistic processing model of verification. *Psychological Review, 82,* 45–73.

Cohen, J. D., & Servan-Schreiber (1992). Context, cortex, and dopamine: A connectionist approach to behavior and biology in schizophrenia. *Psychological Review, 99,* 45–77.

Cromwell, R. L. (1975). Assessment of schizophrenia. *Annual Review of Psychology, 26,* 593–619.

Dobson, D., & Neufeld, R. W. J. (1982). Paranoid-nonparnoid schizophrenic distinctions in the implementation of external conceptual constraints. *Journal of Nervous and Mental Disease, 170,* 614–621.

Edelman, G. (1986). *Neural Darwinism: The theory of neuronal group selection.* New York: Basic.

Estes, W. K. (1976). The cognitive side of probability learning. *Psychological Review, 83,* 37–64.

George, L., & Neufeld, R. W. J. (1984). Imagery and verbal aspects of schizophrenic informational performance. *British Journal of Clinical Psychology, 23,* 9–18.

George, L., & Neufeld, R. W. J. (1985). Cognition and symptomatology in schizophrenia. *Schizophrenia Bulletin, 11,* 264–285.

Hebb, D. O. (1949). *The organization of behavior.* New York: John Wiley & Sons.

Highgate-Maynard, S. (1984). *Information processing among schizophrenics: Extraction and manipulation of nonverbal stimulation.* Unpublished master's dissertation, Department of Psychology, University of Western Ontario.

Highgate-Maynard, S., & Neufeld, R. W. J. (1986). Schizophrenic memory-search performance involving nonverbal stimulus properties. *Journal of Abnormal Psychology, 95,* 67–73.

Hockley, W. E., & Murdock, B. B., Jr. (1987). A decision model for accuracy and response latency in recognition memory. *Psychological Review, 94,* 341–358.

Hoffman, R. E. (1987). Computer simulations of neural information processing and the schizophrenia/mania dichotomy. *Archieves of General Psychiatry, 44,* 178–187.

Hoffman, R. E., & Dobscha, S. K. (1989). Cortical pruning and the development of schizophrenia: A computer model. *Schizophrenia Bulletin, 15,* 477–490.

Kahneman, D. (1973). *Attention and effort.* Englewood Cliffs, NJ: Prentice-Hall, Inc.

Kraeplin, E. (1919). *Dementia praecox and paraphrenia.* (R. M. Barclay, Trans.). Edinburgh: E & S Livingston.

Link, S. W., & Heath, R. A. (1975). A sequential theory of psychological discrimination. *Psychometrika, 40,* 77–105.

Marr, D. (1982). *Vision.* San Francisco: Freeman.

Mather, J. A., Neufeld, R. W. J., Merskey, H., & Russell, N. C. (1992). Disruption of saccade production during oculomotor tracking in schizophrenia, and the use of its change across target velocity as a discriminator of the disorder. *Psychiatry Research, 43,* 93–109.

McClelland, J. L., & Rummelhart, D. E. (1986). A distributed model of memory. In J. L. McClelland & D. E. Rummelhart and the PDP Research Groups, *Parallel distributed processing—Explorations in the microstructure of cognition, Vol. 2: Psychological and biological models* (pp. 170–215). Cambridge, MA: The MIT Press.

McCormick, D., & Broekema, V. (1978). Size estimation, perceptual recognition, and cardiac rate response in acute paranoid and nonparanoid schizophrenia. *Journal of Abnormal Psychology, 87,* 385–398.

Morrison, M. S., Neufeld, R. W. J., & Lafebvre, L. A. (1988). The economy of probabilistic stress: Interplay of controlling activity and threat reduction. *British Journal of Mathematical and Statistical Psychology, 41,* 155–177.

Navon, D., & Gopher, D. (1980). Task difficulty, resources, and dual-task performance. In R. S. Nickerson (Ed.), *Attention and performance, VIII.* Hillsdale, NJ: Lawrence Erlbaum Associates.

Neufeld, R. W. J. (1977). Components of processing deficit among paranoid and nonparanoid schizophrenics. *Journal of Abnormal Psychology, 86,* 60–64.

Neufeld, R. W. J. (1978). Paranoid and nonparanoid schizophrenics' deficit in the interpretation of sentences: An information-processing approach. *Journal of Clinical Psychology, 34,* 333–339.

Neufeld, R. W. J. (1982). On decisional processes instigated by threat: Some possible implications for stress-related deviance. In R. W. J. Neufeld (Ed.), *Psychological stress and psychopathology* (pp. 240–270). New York: McGraw-Hill.

Neufeld, R. W. J. (1989b). *Stochastic models and memory-search performance in schizophrenia.* Paper presented at the Annual Meetings of the Society for Mathematical Psychology, Irvine, CA.

Neufeld, R. W. J. (1990a). Stimulus encoding in schizophrenia, and the capacity deficit hypothesis. Paper presented at the Annual Meetings of the Society of Mathematical Psychology, Toronto, Ontario, Canada.

Neufeld, R. W. J. (1990b). Morrison, Neufeld, & Lefebvre's game theoretic approach to stress and decisional control: Some further mathematical results. Research Bulletin No. 688, Department of Psychology, University of Western Ontario, London, Ontario, Canada.

Neufeld, R. W. J., & Broga, M. I. (1981). Evaluation of information-sequential aspects of schizophrenic performance, II: Methodological considerations. *Journal of Nervous and Mental Disease, 169,* 569–579.

Neufeld, R. W. J. (1991). Memory in paranoid schizophrenia. In Magaro, P. A. (Ed.), *Annual Review of Psychopathology* (pp. 31–61). New York: Sage Publications.

Neufeld, R. W. J., & Nicholson, I. R. (1991). Types of a differential and other equations essential to a servocybernetic systems approach to stress schizophrenia relations. Research Bulletin No. 698, Department of Psychology, University of Western Ontario, London, Ontario, Canada.

Neufeld, R. W. J., & Williamson, P. C. (in press). Neuropsychological correlates of positive symptoms: Delusions and hallucinations. In C. Pantelis, H. Nelson, & T. Barnes (Eds.), *The neuropsychology of schizophrenia*. London: Wiley.

Neufeld, R. W. J., Mather, J. A., Merskey, H., & Russell, N. C. (in press). Multivariate structure of eye movement dysfunction distinguishing schizophrenia. *Multivariate Experimental Clinical Research*.

Neufeld, R. W. J., & Gardner, R. C. (1990). Data aggregation in evaluating psychological constructs: Multivariate and logical deductive considerations. *Journal of Mathematical Psychology, 34*, 276–296.

Nicholson, I. R., & Neufeld, R. W. J. (1989). Forms and mechanisms of susceptibility to stress in schiozphrenia. In R. W. J. Neufeld (Ed.), *Advances in the investigation of psychological stress* (pp. 392–420). New York: John Wiley & Sons.

Nicholson, I. R., & Neufeld, R. W. J. (1992). A dynamic vulnerability perspective on stress and schizophrenia. *American Journal of Orthopsychiatry, 62*, 117–130.

Nicholson, I. R., & Neufeld, R. W. J. (in press). The classification of the schizophrenias according to symptomatology: A two-factor model. *Journal of Abnormal Psychology*.

Pachella, R. G. (1974). The interpretation of reaction time in information processing research. In B. H. Kantowitz (Ed.), *Human information processing: Tutorials in performance and cognition* (pp. 41–82). Hillsdale, NJ: Lawrence Erlbaum Associates.

Paivio, A. (1975). Perceptual comparisons through the mind's eye. *Memory and Cognition, 3*, 635–647.

Posner, M. I., & Mitchell, R. (1967). Chronometric analysis of classification. *Psychological Review, 74*, 392–409.

Price, R. H., & Eriksen, C. W. (1966). Size consistency in schizophrenia: A reanalysis. *Journal of Abnormal Psychology, 71*, 155–160.

Pylyshyn, Z. W. (1984). *Computation and cognition*. Cambridge, MA: The MIT Press.

Rummelhart, D. E., & McClelland, J. L. (1986). PDP models and general issues in cognitive science. In J. L. McClelland & D. E. Rummelhart, *Parallel distributed processing—Explorations in the microstructure of cognition, Vol. 2: Psychological and biological models* (pp. 110–149). Cambridge, MA: The MIT Press.

Schweikert, R. (1985). Separate effects of factors on speed and accuracy: Memory scanning lexical decision, and choice tasks. *Psychological Bulletin, 97*, 530–546.

Shannon, C. E., & Weaver, W. (1949). *The mathematical theory of communication*. Urbana: University of Illinois Press.

Spaulding, W. D., & Cole, J. K. (Eds.). (1983). *Nebraska symposium on mortivation, Vol. 31: Theories of schizophrenia and psychosis*. Lincoln: University of Nebraska Press.

Staddon, J. E. R. (1984) Social learning theory and the dynamics of interaction. *Psychological Review, 91*, 502–507.

Sternberg, S. (1975). Memory and scanning: New findings and current controversies. *Quarterly Journal of Experimental Psychology, 27*, 1–32.

Thompson, S. C. (1981). Will it hurt less if I can control it? A complex answer to a simple question. *Psychological Bulletin, 90*, 89–101.

Townsend, J. T. (1974). Issues and models concerning the processing of a finite number of inputs. In B. H. Kantowitz (Ed.), *Human information processing: Tutorials in performance and cognition* (pp. 133–185). Hillsdale, NJ: Lawrence Erlbaum Associates.

Townsend, J. T. (1984). Uncovering mental processes with factorial experiments. *Journal of Mathematical Psychology, 28*, 363–400.

Townsend, J. T., & Ashby, F. G. (1978). Methods of modeling capacity in simple processing systems. In J. Castellan & F. Restle (Eds.), *Cognitive theory* (Vol. 3, pp. 238–253). Hillsdale, NJ: Lawrence Erlbaum Associates.

Townsend, J. T., & Ashby, F. G. (1983). *Stochastic modelling of elementary psychological processes*. London: Cambridge University Press.

Triesman, A., & Paterson, R. (1984). Emergent features, attention, and object perception. *Journal of Experimental Psychology, 10*, 12–31.

Wallace, C. J., & Boone, S. E. (1983). Cognitive factors in the social skills of schizophrenic patients: Implications for treatment. In W. D. Spaulding & J. K. Cole (Eds.), *Nebraska Symposium on Motivation, Vol. 31: Theories of schizophrenia and psychosis* (pp. 283–318). Lincoln: University of Nebraska Press.

Wickens, C. D. (1984). Attentional resources. In R. Parasuraman & D. R. Davies (Eds.), *Varieties of attention* (pp. 95–114). New York: Academic Press.

Winters, K. C., & Neale, J. M. (1983). Delusions and delusional thinking in psychotics: A review of the literature. *Clinical Psychology Review, 3*, 227–253.

Wright, B. D. (1977). Solving measurement problems with the Rasch model. *Journal of Educational Measurement, 14*, 97–116.

12

Missing Facts and Other Lacunae in Orienting Research in Schizophrenia

ALVIN S. BERNSTEIN

Over the last 8 or 9 years orienting response research in schizophrenia has been especially fruitful. A good deal now is known about the incidence of orienting response dysfunction and some of its correlates, and something about the kind of patient who displays it. Let me note briefly just some of what has been determined before turning to what is missing or indefinite.

There is now wide agreement that about half the schizophrenic population is orienting nonresponsive to moderate innocuous stimuli, and that this is equally true of chronic and acute schizophrenics, of those long institutionalized and those in a first episode, of those on neuroleptics and those drug free (e.g., Alm, Lindstrom, & Ohman, 1984; Bernstein et al., 1982; Dawson, Nuechterlein, & Schell, 1988; Iacono, 1985; Venables & Bernstein, 1983). The dysfunction appears to involve the orienting response rather than isolated peripheral systems because it appears simultaneously in orienting response components that are independent—skin conductance and finger pulse volume responses (SCOR and FPVOR; Bernstein, Pava, Reidel, Schnur, & Lubowsky, 1985; Bernstein et al., 1981, 1988; E. Straube, personal communication, 1986), as well as in the pupillary dilation orienting response (e.g., Steinhauer & Zubin, 1982). Orienting response deficit has been reported to be associated with a family history of schizophrenia (Alm et al., 1984), and

to occur primarily in those who display long-standing evidence of emotional withdrawal and social isolation, premorbidly (Cannon & Mednick, 1988), during psychosis (Bernstein et al., 1981; Dawson et al., 1988; Straube, 1979), and during remitted periods (Ohman et al., 1989).

Although this orienting response absence was first thought to signal the absence of an orienting response–associated attentional capacity, subsequent work showed this not to be the case. If the innocuous stimuli to which schizophrenics are nonresponsive are presented at greater intensity (Bernstein, 1964, 1970; Bernstein et al., 1981; Gruzelier, Connolly, et al., 1981; Gruzelier, Eves, Connolly, & Hirsch, 1981), or if the moderate-intensity stimulus is made explicitly significant (Bernstein, Schneider, Juni, Pope, & Starkey, 1980; Bernstein & Taylor, 1976; Bernstein et al., 1985, 1988; Gruzelier & Venables, 1973; Ohman, Nordby, & d'Elia, 1986), nonresponder schizophrenics begin to show normal-like orienting responses. These findings suggest that nonresponding in these patients primarily reflects differences in allocational policy (i.e., in the decision about whether and when to engage the orienting response rather than an inability to engage it) (Bernstein, 1987).

Further studies in my laboratory examined the ability of schizophrenics to respond to designated target signals presented against noisy or silent backgrounds, and to shift orienting responses appropriately as new targets are designated and old targets discarded. Schizophrenics were able to respond as well to signals presented during background noise as to those presented during silent background, and as well when the background noise provided maximal distraction value (i.e., subjects had to respond to 1,500-Hz signals in the middle of a background noise continuously shifting within a 1,250- to 1,750-Hz range) as when the distraction was reduced (i.e., subjects had to respond to 1,500-Hz signals completely outside the range of a background noise continuously shifting within a 500- to 1,000-Hz band) (Bernstein, Riedel, Graae, Essig, Smith, & Lubowsky, unpublished study). Thus, stimulus discrimination per se did not prove to be a problem here.

In addition, schizophrenics proved as able as normal subjects to display orienting responses promptly whenever a new target signal was designated, *and* as capable as normal subjects of disengaging orienting responses promptly when a previously designated target became irrelevant (Bernstein et al., 1990). Schizophrenics thus displayed considerable flexibility in the orienting response attentional resource.

Attempts to explore the possible limits of the orienting response "normalization" produced by targeting a significant signal for patients revealed that this effect might last for only 15 to 20 presentations; after that orienting responses declined and schizophrenics again became hyporesponsive (Bernstein et al., 1985; Ohman et al., 1986). Schizophrenics seem unable to sustain orienting responses, even when an initial response is elicited. Our recent work (Bernstein et al., 1990) indicates that this is not simply a matter of loss of signal valence over time (because orienting response decline appeared despite signal reminders repeated after every 16 trials), nor is it a matter of rapid boredom or fatigue caused by repetitions of a single target (because targets were changed every 16 trials). Failure to sustain orienting response thus seems to reflect some other characteristic of schizo-

phrenia, not specifically identifiable at present.

Finally, orienting nonresponding has also been proposed by several investigators as an effective vulnerability marker for a subtype of schizophrenia characterized by social and emotional withdrawal, gradual onset, familial transmission, and poor response to treatment (e.g., Alm et al., 1984; Cannon, Mednick, & Parnas, 1990; Dawson & Nuechterlein, 1984; Holzman, 1987; Iacono, 1985).

New orienting response studies are beginning to examine the relationship between nonresponding in schizophrenia and many other factors. If the work here is sometimes contradictory, that, perhaps, is to be expected as the first steps are taken in each area. For example, Cannon et al. (1990) noted increased pregnancy and birth complications among nonresponders in the Denmark high-risk sample. There are also reports of greater third ventricle width among schizophrenic responders than among nonresponders, whether these are acute (Bartfai, Levander, Nyback, & Schallings 1987) or chronic (Schnur et al., 1989), although Cannon et al. (1988) reported greater third ventricle size among *nonresponder's* in a high-risk sample combining schizophrenics with healthy controls. Cohen, Sommer, and Hermanutz (1981) reported especially diminished cortical evoked potential N220 and frontal slow wave activity in SCOR-nonresponsive schizophrenics. Spohn (personal communication, 1989) noted a positive association between SCOR nonresponding and impaired smooth pursuit eye movement, (although Bartfai, Levander, and Sedvall (1983) reported the reverse.)

In an interesting development, Ohlund, Ohman, Alm, Ost, and Lindstrom (1990) reported more frequent births during the winter trimester among schizophrenics who are orienting nonresponders. Anne Yeager and I are studying this issue in our laboratory as well. Examining 83 schizophrenics, 81 normal controls, and 57 depressives, we have obtained only weak support for such a conclusion. Among the total samples, 42.2% of the schizophrenics, 31.6% of the depressives, and 40.7% of the normal subjects were born during the January-to-April winter trimester ($\chi_2^2 = 1.77$, $p>.30$). However, among those in each sample who were nonresponders, 47.7% of the schizophrenics were born during January to April versus 26.8% of the depressives and 26.3% of the normal controls ($\chi_2^2 = 4.92$, $p<.10$; two-tailed). (Among responders in each diagnostic group, there were again no significant differences in the incidence of winter trimester birth ($\chi_2^2<1$.)

Thus, although it *may* be associated with orienting nonresponding in schizophrenia, winter birth does not seem to be a robust factor in accounting for nonresponding. With the evidence of a greater incidence of familial schizophrenia in nonresponder schizophrenics (Alm et al., 1984), winter birth may be one of the elements contributing to the increased early stress Cannon et al. (1990) suggested may be important in the subsequent development of schizophrenia in this genetically vulnerable population.

With this brief summary to show that orienting response research is alive and productive, let me now turn to identifying several soft spots.

IS ORIENTING NONRESPONDING A STABLE TRAIT?

This question was raised when Alm, Ost, and Ohman (1987) suggested that SCOR nonresponding might not be entirely stable among their schizophrenic subjects. Instead, Ohman et al. (1989) recommended a broader measure termed "orienting hyporesponding," which combines nonresponders with others showing small responses appearing only on trials 1 or 2 (i.e., the "fast habituator" schizophrenics identified by Patterson and Venables [1978]).

It is not possible to evaluate this fully because only an abstract was published by Alm et al. (1987). However, the abstract suggests design problems that make firm conclusions difficult. For one, Alm et al. presented two successive trial series, one with 80-dB and one with 100-dB tones. Many reports (e.g., from my lab; Gruzel-

ier's work; Green & Nuechterlein, 1988) show that orienting nonresponding among schizophrenics diminishes when more intense stimuli are given, especially when these exceed 90 dB (Ohman, 1981). Thus, patients nonresponsive to 80 dB at the close of one session might be expected to respond to the 100-dB tones starting the next session, whereas those responsive to 100 dB should "switch" to nonresponder status when given 80 dB at the next test. (Ohman [personal communication, 1989] agrees that the use of mixed 80- and 100-dB tone series may make the Alm et al. results ambiguous.)

One may also question the wisdom of combining nonresponders with fast habituators. Patterson and Venables (1978, 1980) showed that fast habituators differed from nonresponders in perceptual sensitivity (the d' index) and in skin conductance level, and Spohn and Patterson (1979, p. 585) considered them "an utterly distinct electrodermal group." Furthermore, both Bernstein (1967) and Rubens and Lapidus (1978) showed that, whereas nonresponding was stable over 6 to 10 weeks, fast habituation sometimes was not. In each study, some schizophrenics habituating after an isolated trial 1 response on one test showed nonhabituating SCORs on the other. Combining nonresponders with those displaying fast habituation may therefore combine unlike groups, and actually increase measurement instability.

Furthermore, other data seem to contradict Alm et al. (1987). For example, Bernstein (1967) found that 23 of 31 orienting nonresponder schizophrenics (74%) remained nonresponsive when retested 6 to 10 weeks later, whereas 52 of 69 responder schizophrenics (75%) remained responsive on retest. These were considered conservative estimates of retest reliability because there were no controls for noise, temperature, or humidity. With such controls, Rubens and Lapidus (1978) found that all 10 (100%) of their nonresponder schizophrenics remained nonresponsive 6 weeks later, and Spohn, Coyne, Spray, and Hayes (1989) found that 49 of 56 nonresponder schizophrenics remained nonresponsive 2 weeks later (87%), with 51 of 56 (91%) remaining nonresponders 4 weeks later. Spohn et al. also noted that only 18 of 30 responder patients (60%) remained responders in 2 weeks, with the proportion dropping to 13 of 30 (43%) still responsive on second retest after 4 weeks.

A similar difference between orienting responder and nonresponder stability over time was found by Dawson (personal communication, 1989): of 22 stabilized, relatively remitted outpatients on low fluphenazine doses, 11 (50%) were skin conductance response (SCR) nonresponders and 11 were SCR responders. A year later, 7 of 11 nonresponder patients were still nonresponders, whereas only 2 of 11 responder patients were still responders. Whereas the Spohn et al. (1989) patients were retested across a variety of changes in clinical and medication state, Dawson's patients were retested in the same clinical and drug status as at initial testing. Thus, as Spohn et al. (1989) concluded, orienting response status does not seem to depend on any specific clinical or medication status.

A suggestion by Straube, Schmied, Rein, and Breyer-Pfaff (unpublished) appears to conflict with this conclusion. These authors suggested that, although some patients might shift nonresponder status, those high in emotional withdrawal never did, remaining SCOR nonresponsive on three test sessions over a period of 28 days. Thus, nonresponding is suggested as stable specifically in those schizophrenics marked clinically by withdrawal. This can only be considered suggestive because of the small sample sizes involved; the use of an overly long (1- to 5-second) latency window to define SCOR (inviting artifact as a result of the more frequent nonspecific electrodermal fluctuations found in schizophrenics, as Frith, Stevens, Johnstone, and Crow [1982] and Levinson and colleagues [Levinson & Edelberg, 1985; Levinson, Edelberg, & Bridger, 1984] demonstrated); and the use of 85-dB tones, something we found did not produce reliable nonresponding among schizophrenics (e.g., Bernstein, 1970).

The Spohn et al. (1989) and Dawson (1989) data cited above are especially interesting because they present evidence of *stable orienting nonresponder* status coupled with *unstable orienting responder* status. Given the vital role of stimulus uncertainty or "novelty" in triggering orienting response, and the simple repetition of stimuli and conditions in all studies of orienting response status over time to date, a decline in the number of responders on each test occasion is expected. It would be surprising if such repetition did not produce a growing shift toward nonresponding among those responsive on the initial testing. The negatively accelerated curve for responding over repeated testings in the Spohn et al. (1989) data is consistent with such a habituation process (Simons, Losito, Rose, & MacMillan, 1983).

Although this bias toward orienting nonresponding may artifactually impair the evidence for stable responder status, it may also serve to inflate the evidence for stability of nonresponder status. Any tendencies toward subsequent responding among initially nonresponsive subjects could be offset to some degree by the habituation effect associated with cross-testing stimulus repetition. At the close of this section, I suggest another approach to the question of the stability and generalizability of responder/nonresponder status.

The stability of orienting response status among normal subjects was briefly examined by Simons et al. (1983), who selected college students to be initially responsive or nonresponsive. They found 62% of the former and 67% of the latter retained the same status on 2-week retest. Although Simons et al. concluded "that nonresponding is a reliable phenomenon" (p. 504), these figures are slightly below those of the other labs cited, despite good environmental controls, and may suggest somewhat lessened stability among normal subjects.

Another point may be suggested from the literature. The time span over which stability is tested may also be an important factor and needs further study. All the work supporting the stability of orienting nonresponding involves intervals no longer than

6 to 10 weeks, whereas Alm et al. (1987) retested after an average of 110 days. This may suggest some break in reliability after 2 to 3 months—and not simply because longer intervals allow greater chance for change in clinical or drug status. Changes here within the 2- to 3-month period did *not* alter orienting response (Spohn et al., 1989; Zahn, Carpenter, & McGlashan, 1981).

It should be emphasized, however, that virtually every investigator in the field considers orienting nonresponding to be a stable, within-subject phenomenon over the short term (e.g., 2 to 3 months), and probably over the longer term too. This includes Ohman as well, in whose laboratory the issue of nonresponding stability was first raised (Alm et al., 1984). As Ohman pointed out (personal communication, April 1989), the finding that nonresponding is a singularly strong indicator of long-term (2-year) prognosis in first-illness schizophrenics (Ohman et al., 1989) clearly points to the stability of the nonresponding pattern.

Despite this, a review of the literature makes it plain that the issue of orienting response stability has not yet received a sufficient degree of research attention. Further work is needed, focusing on the stability of responding as well as nonresponding, and examining the normal population as well as schizophrenics and other pathological groups. In particular, such studies should seek to minimize the bias toward increased nonresponding over successive retests associated with the repetition of a single given stimulus—a bias that undermines every study of orienting response stability now available.

I suggest that two simple stimuli be used in such studies, alternating between adjacent retest sessions, rather than repeating a single stimulus across sessions. These might be a simple visual stimulus and a simple tone, in an *a-b-a-b* sequence over a total of four test sessions, spaced according to the investigator's interest in short- or long-term effects. To counterbalance for sequence, *a* could be visual for half the subjects and auditory for the other half.

Two specific benefits would be gained

from such a design. First, switching stimulus modality between adjacent testings would reduce any accumulating habituation effect that might otherwise bias later test results toward increased nonresponding. Second, investigators here assume that nonresponding in schizophrenia represents a *general* absence of orienting response to innocuous stimuli. Early on I recognized this and reported similar nonresponding patterns in schizophrenics whether auditory or visual stimuli were used (Bernstein, 1964, 1970). However, I used different samples for each modality; within-subject consistency of nonresponding across stimuli and modalities remains to be demonstrated. Furthermore, by repeating stimuli within each modality we also will be able to compare nonresponding stability across modalities.

IS ORIENTING RESPONSE DEFICIT SPECIFIC IN SCHIZOPHRENIA?

The specificity of orienting response deficit to schizophrenia has been challenged. In recent years, for example, Straube (1980) and Iacono et al. (1983, 1984) reported that SCOR nonresponding among depressives was indistinguishable from that shown by schizophrenics, and Venables (1986) and Straube (1980) speculated that orienting nonresponding might be associated with negative symptoms such as emotional and social withdrawal and loss of motivation, rather than reflecting the schizophrenic process itself. If orienting response deficit is nonspecific, much of the interest in this work is diminished; certainly, attempts to establish nonresponding as a vulnerability marker within schizophrenia would be misbegotten.

Because of this, my colleagues and I began studying schizophrenics and depressives jointly. We now have two studies—Bernstein et al. (1988) and another still in progress. Both suggest that schizophrenia *does* involve a change in orienting response activity, whereas many depressives seem to display something different.

In the earlier study (Bernstein et al.,

1988), we examined 50 Research Diagnostic Criteria (RDC)–defined schizophrenics (14 drug free at least 2 weeks), 50 depressives (20 drug free), and 50 normal controls. All received identical 1-second 1-kHz (60-dB) or 2-kHz (58-dB) tones to either the right or left ear. One subsample in each group (*ns* = 14) received simple habituation instructions and was told to do nothing but sit quietly while tones were given. The remainder of each diagnostic group was assigned a specific target signal (right ear; left ear; 1 kHz; or 2 kHz) in response to which they had to press a pedal immediately, ignoring all other tones. Cash bonuses were given for fast correct presses and penalties levied for slow or wrong presses.

Figure 12.1 displays the incidence of nonresponding in SCR and in the simultaneously recorded FPV response to initial stimuli. Under simple habituation conditions, schizophrenics revealed significantly more frequent nonresponding than normal subjects, and they did so *simultaneously* in both SCR and FPV orienting response components. When given significant target signals (press trials), schizophrenics showed a drop in nonresponding to normal levels, again *jointly* in both components. Similar findings have appeared in Gruzelier's, Straube's, and Ohman's work, as well as in my own previous work.

In depressives, results of studies by Iacono et al. (1983, 1984) and Straube (1980) were confirmed. Under habituation conditions the incidence of SCR nonresponse *is* indistinguishable from that of schizophrenics. SCR in habituation conditions only distinguishes psychiatric patients from normal subjects, not one pathology from the other. However, the data do show two ways in which depressives and schizophrenics can be distinguished as well. First, SCR does not normalize initially among depressives; nonresponding remains essentially at the same high level in response to both habituation and target (press) signals. Second, heightened nonresponsivity is specific to SCR in depressives; in FPV, depressives are similar to normal subjects in both habi-

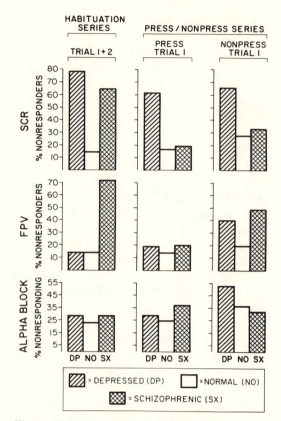

Figure 12.1. The percentage of subjects in each group who were nonresponsive in skin conductance response (SCR) and finger pulse volume (FPV) to trials 1 and 2 in the habituation series and to the initial press (and nonpress) trials in the reaction time series. (Reprinted with permission from Bernstein, A., Reidel, J., Graae, F., Seidman, D., Steele, H., Connolly, J., & Lubowsky, J. [1988]. Schizophrenia is associated with altered orienting activity, depression with electrodermal (cholinergic?) deficit and normal orienting response. *Journal of Abnormal Psychology, 97,* 3–12. Copyright 1988 by the American Psychological Association. Reprinted by permission of the publisher.)

tuation and press conditions. We found that the pattern of SCR absence coupled with FPV presence was particularly common within depression. (Clinically this was associated with high psychomotor retardation and/or with low agitation in depression, but not with depth of depression either as rated by clinicians [Hamilton scale] or by patients [Zung scale].)

What can these differences mean? SCR

and FPV response are orienting response components whose independence has been demonstrated by correlational studies (e.g., Bernstein, Taylor, Austin, Nathanson, & Scarpelli, 1971; Bernstein et al., 1981; Prout, 1967), and by cholinergic and adrenergic blockade showing SCR to be cholinergic and FPV adrenergic (Lader & Montague, 1962). The simultaneity with which these components disappear (with innocuous stimuli) and reappear (with targeted signals) among schizophrenics suggests that some shift in responding is indeed at work here. Schizophrenics often fail to allocate central processing resources as and when most normal people do. This is sustained by evidence of schizophrenic deficit in other orienting response components as well, such as the pupillary dilation response (Friedman, Hakerem, Sutton, & Fleiss, 1973; Steinhauer & Zubin, 1982), and in the evoked potential P300 response (e.g., Roth, 1977) seen by many as another orienting response component.

In depressives, the unimpaired FPV response (seen also in the results of Bruno, Myers, & Glassman, 1983) suggests that the SCR deficit does *not* involve the orienting response. This is supported by evidence that, unlike schizophrenics, depressives do not display abnormal pupillary dilation (Steinhauer & Zubin, 1982) nor a consistently deficient P300 (e.g., Thier, Axmann, & Giedke, 1986). Whatever is wrong with these depressives seems to be more specific to the SCR. Given the distinctive cholinergic mediation of the SCR, compared with the adrenergic mediation of the normally responsive pupillary and FPVOR systems, it suggests that some depressives (especially those with high retardation?) may show a specific deficit in cholinergic response rather than in orienting response.

A review of studies examining non–orienting response cholinergic responses in these patients supports such a conclusion. For example, Brown (1970) cited 11 studies reporting reduced salivation in depression, whereas four of five studies of schizophrenia found normal output. Busfield and Wechsler (1961) noted that the presence of schizophrenia among schizoaffectives "negates the diminished salivation associated with depression." Giedke and Heimann (1987) recently found joint diminution in salivary and electrodermal systems within the same depressive sample, further suggesting a hypocholinergic dimension here. With respiratory sinus arrhythmia (RSA) in the resting electrocardiogram clearly under vagal/cholinergic control, Strian, Klicpera, and Caspar (1977) found reduced variability in the resting heat rate of depressives (especially those displaying retardation), and Lovett Doust (1980) found RSA to be somewhat greater in schizophrenics (on or off medication) than in controls. Lower colon and rectal motility, both cholinergic functions, were also shown by Lechin et al. (1983) to be reduced in retarded depressives. Finally, although debate continues about whether skeletal muscle blood flow is cholinergic in humans, data here too support such a conclusion: blood flow response in the forearm muscles has been shown to be normal in schizophrenics (e.g., Kelly & Walter, 1968) but persistently diminished in depressives (e.g., Bruno et al., 1983; Kelly & Walter, 1969). The common thread through this mix of deficiencies in depressives thus seems to reflect cholinergic rather than orienting response deficits.

Our second study further extends this. Preliminary findings are based on 32 schizophrenics (18 drug free), 21 depressives (17 drug free), and 28 normal subjects. Every subject begins with a series of six 5-second 60-dB, 1-kHz tones under habituation instructions. Then each group is split into four subgroups, of whom two receive six 5-second 80-dB, 1-kHz tones, one at 1-ms and one at 250-ms rise/decay times. The other two receive six trials with a 5-second 100-dB white noise, also at either 1- or 250-ms rise/decay. This study, and two others also in progress, examine orienting response, defensive, and startle responses in each population.

Figure 12.2A shows SCR elicited by the 60-dB tones in 75% of the normals, 43% of the schizophrenics, and 33% of the depressives. On average, these subjects also displayed orienting response in the other two components: constrictive FPV and decelerative heart rate, peaking at 6 to 9 seconds after tone onset (another cholinergic response [Obrist, Wood, & Perez-Reyes, 1965]). Although there is dispute concerning the "unitary" orienting response and possible differences among orienting response components in onset and habituation characteristics (e.g., Barry, 1979), this indicates that components can occur jointly, as might be expected if they index a common central event.

The remaining 57% of the schizophrenics (labeled "60 dB SCR Nonresponders") show no SCR to 60 dB, and also no FPV response here. Some heart rate deceleration may appear, but it is smaller than that shown by schizophrenics SCR responsive to 60 dB, and, unlike the consistent deceleration shown by 60-dB responder schizophrenics, those SCR nonresponsive to 60 dB revealed great variability here. Thus, as in our previous work, many schizophrenics again show orienting response absence to moderate innocuous tones consistent over SCR and FPV response components, and, probably over heart rate response (HRR) too.

As stimulus intensity increases, within-subject intensity comparisons (Figure 12.2B) show that subjects who had been SCR responsive to 60-dB tones show greater SCR to 80 dB, and greater response still to 100-dB noise. More importantly, schizophrenics who were 60-dB SCR nonresponders begin to display SCRs to 80-dB tones, accompanying this newly apparent SCR with a newly apparent FPV response to 80 dB and with an evident HRR deceleration as well. Thus, whereas Figure 12.1 shows initial orienting response normalization across components when targeted signals are presented to schizophrenics, Figure 12.2 shows the same when more intense stimuli are used.

The addition of the 100-dB noise here allows us to see that depressives who are SCR nonresponsive but FPV responsive to 60-dB tones may actually consist of two differing subgroups. One shows the completely nonresponsive SCR we had expected to see in all such depressives. Labeled "SCR Nonresponders All Stimuli," Figure 12.2A shows that, as in Bernstein et al. (1988), these patients ($n = 8$, 38% of the depressive sample) were SCR nonreactive to 60 dB despite the presence of a vigorous FPV response here. The heart rate cholinergic orienting response deceleration is absent as well. As more intense stimuli are given (Figure 12.2B), SCR remains inactive in all instances while FPV response appears strongly in each. Furthermore, there is no apparent cholinergic heart rate deceleration either, regardless of the stimulus used. Thus, *this* subgroup strongly suggests a specific cholinergic deficit, in the absent SCR and heart rate responses under all stimulus conditions, coupled with the large FPV responses elicited under all tone conditions.

The newly apparent depressive subgroup ($n = 6$, 29% of the sample) was also "60 dB SCR Nonresponsive," but differs from the depressives SCR nonresponsive to all stimuli in two important ways: (a) given 100-dB noise, they showed a large SCR, and (b) they also displayed a 6- to 9-second heart rate deceleratory response to 80-dB tones and 100-dB noise. Given this capacity, why did these people remain SCR unresponsive to everything below 100-dB noise? Our current speculation is that the degree of cholinergic deficit in these depressives may be less severe than among those displaying absence of SCR and heart rate deceleration in all stimulus conditions. Thus, given the powerful stimulus of 100-dB noise, some response can be elicited that is not seen following 60- or 80-dB tones, or the possibly less compelling (compared to 100-dB noise) target signals used in Bernstein et al. (1988).

These studies suggest that orienting response dysfunction *is* specific to schizophrenia. SCR nonresponsiveness in many depressives is accompanied by a vigorous FPV response, which suggests that the orienting response is functional. In many such depressives there appears to be a deficit in

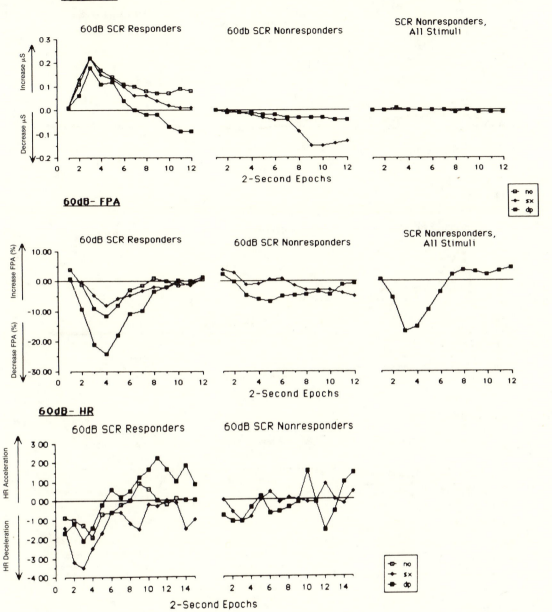

60dB- SCR

60dB SCR Responders

60db SCR Nonresponders

SCR Nonresponders, All Stimuli

60dB- FPA

60dB SCR Responders

60dB SCR Nonresponders

SCR Nonresponders, All Stimuli

60dB- HR

60dB SCR Responders

60dB SCR Nonresponders

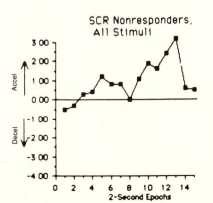

SCR Nonresponders, All Stimuli

Figure 12.2A. Consecutive 2-second epochs from stimulus onset displaying response in SCR, finger pulse amplitude (FPA), and heart rate (HR) to 60-dB tones in normal subjects ($n = 26$); schizophrenics who were SCR responsive to 60-dB tones ($n = 13$), schizophrenics SCR nonresponsive to 60-dB tones but responsive to 100-dB noise ($n = 15$); depressives SCR responsive to 60-dB tones ($n = 7$); depressives SCR nonresponsive to all stimuli ($n = 7$); and depressives SCR nonresponsive to 60-dB tones but SCR responsive to 100-dB noise ($n = 8$).

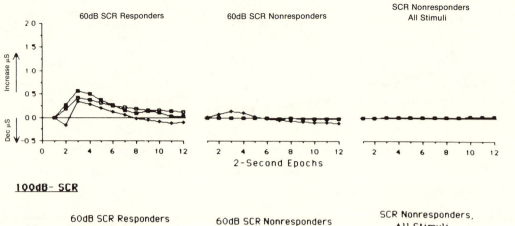

100dB- SCR

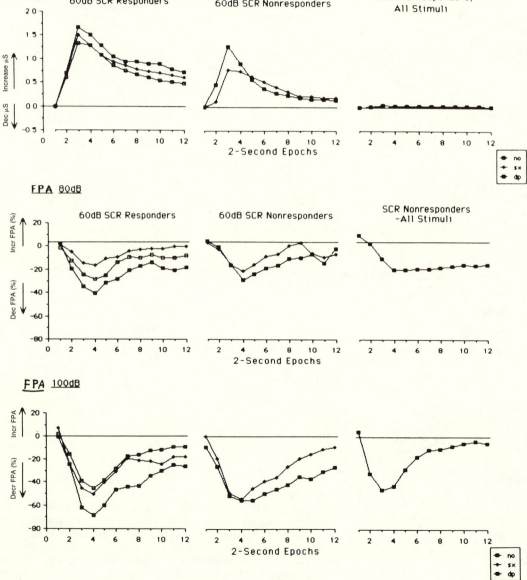

FPA 80dB

FPA 100dB

Figure 12.2B. *Legend on opposite page.*

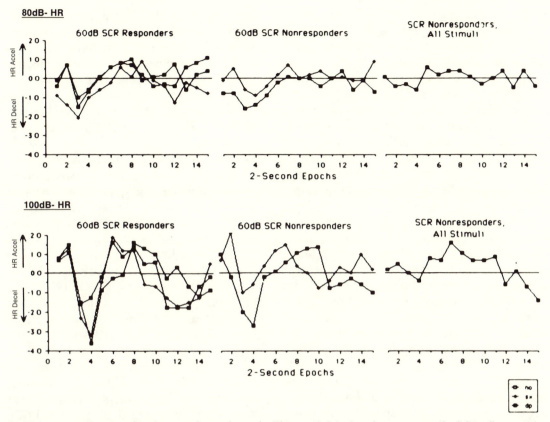

Figure 12.2B. Consecutive 2-second epochs as in Figure 12.2A showing response in SCR, finger pulse amplitude (FPA), and heart rate (HR) to 80-dB tones and to 100-dB noise among normal subjects and among subgroups of schizophrenics and depressives who were either SCR responsive to 60-dB tones, entirely SCR nonresponsive to all stimuli, or SCR nonresponsive to 60-dB tones but SCR responsive to 100-dB noise.

cholinergic response[1] that mimics an orienting response deficit because some orienting response components, such as SCOR and heart rate deceleration, are themselves cholinergically mediated. Clearly, work in

1. Others (e.g., Janowsky & Risch, 1987) have presented compelling evidence of central cholinergic hypersensitivity in depressives. The causes and consequences of such hypersensitivity can be complex (Dilsaver, 1986), and we do not yet know how to fit this presumptive peripheral deficit to it. However, two other laboratories have also concluded that their data suggest cholinergic hypofunction in depression. First, from their electrodermal data, Ward and Doerr (1986) suggested reduced peripheral cholinergic function as a "homeostatic adaptation" to increased central cholinergic sensitivity, but noted that it is unknown whether any direct relationship exists between central and autonomic nervous system cholinergic systems. Second, although Bruno et al. (1983) specified a central cholinergic deficit, their data are peripheral (finger pulse constriction, forearm muscle blood flow, and cardiac pre-ejection period), and the locus for such deficit is still uncertain.

this area is only beginning. Clearly too, work will have to be done in other laboratories besides mine to establish validity.

IF ORIENTING RESPONSE DEFICIENCY IS IMPORTANT IN SCHIZOPHRENIA, WHY DOES PROGNOSTIC SIGNIFICANCE SEEM TO ATTACH ONLY TO ORIENTING RESPONSE EXCESS?

Psychophysiological research is often cited with regard to its prognostic value in two specific areas: (a) ability to predict future onset of schizophrenia in the high-risk children of schizophrenic parents, and (b) ability to predict clinical response to treatment among adult schizophrenics. In each, the findings appear to conflict with any claim that it is an *absence* of orienting response that is associated with schizophrenia, because the prognostic relationships emphasize hyperactive autonomic response and orienting response activity.

The pioneering work with regard to high-risk children, that of Mednick and Schulsinger (1968), reported that high-risk children who later became schizophrenic identified themselves years earlier by displaying larger SCRs with faster latency and recovery to "irritating" loud noise. Although the Mednick group later noted the relationship to be more complex (applicable essentially to male offspring, and influenced by the presence or absence of an intact family and of sociopathy in the biological father), and despite the fact that differences in SCR recovery and latency did not appear in other laboratories, Prentky, Salzman, and Klein (1981) and van Dyke, Rosenthal, and Rasmussen (1974) did confirm the presence of larger-than-normal SCRs to 95- to 96-dB noise in such subjects.

In reply, I would note that it is often overlooked that this excessive SCR has been consistently reported in response not to orienting response stimuli but to "unpleasant" loud noise, likely to trigger defensive responses rather than orienting responses. Whereas orienting responses are intake facilitative, defensive responses are likely to be associated with an attenuation of information intake (Graham, 1979; Sokolov, 1963). Thus, it may perhaps be an excessive sensitivity to unpleasant stimuli and a resultant protective *reduction* of intake that marks these high-risk subjects (see Bernstein, 1987, for a discussion of the need for study of the defensive response in schizophrenia).

Furthermore, it now appears that the role of orienting response deficit as a prognosticator here may have been too long overlooked. Some studies (i.e., Erlenmeyer-Kimling et al., 1984; Kugelmass, Marcus & Schmueli, 1985) not only failed to confirm the presence of excessive SCRs in high-risk children, but actually reported some trends toward electrodermal *hyporesponsiveness*. Because these were nonsignificant differences, they were, understandably, given

less weight than the apparently more robust fact of SCR excess. Dawson and Nuechterlein (1987) did speculate, however, that these findings might point to "two electrodermal subgroups of high risk subjects" (p. 48), one hyperresponsive and the other hyporesponsive. This has received confirmation in the latest reports from the Mednick group.

Cannon and Mednick (1988) have now reported that orienting hyporesponsiveness detected among high-risk adolescents in 1962 did predict the appearance of schizophrenia as adults in 1972. Working with the subsample of high-risk subjects ($N = 66$) who received diagnoses of schizophrenia ($n = 15$), schizotypal personality ($n = 28$), or no mental illness ($n = 23$) in 1972, they found that 7 of the 15 schizophrenics (47%) had been hyporesponsive in adolescence. Of the remaining 51 high-risk subjects, only 9 (18%) had been hyporesponsive in 1962 ($\chi^2 = 5.52$, $p < .02$). (No data were presented for the incidence of earlier hyporesponding among the schizotypals versus those with "not mental illness" in 1972). Furthermore, Cannon and Mednick (1988) noted that hyporesponders in 1962 were characterized by negative symptoms (e.g., lacking spontaneity, isolated, silent, nonresponsive to praise) both as adolescents (based on school records) and as young adult schizophrenics (based on clinical interviews).

Based on such findings, Cannon et al. (1990) now conclude that there are two routes to (different subtypes of) schizophrenia. One is associated with hyporesponsive orienting response and is characterized by essentially negative symptoms,—for example, decreased drive and absence of social and emotional engagement, both in children and in adult schizophrenics. The other is associated with electrodermal hyperactivity and displays more positive-type behavior disturbances premorbidly and more positive symptoms as schizophrenics.

The Mednick group has always made it plain (e.g., Mednick et al., 1978) that SCR hyperactivity predicted only that type of schizophrenia marked by florid hallucinatory and delusional symptoms. Because this electrodermal characteristic was thus associated with one type of schizophrenia, it remained possible that a different one might identify another subtype. It now appears that orienting hyporesponding might occupy a place beside that of electrodermal hyperactivity as a predictor of schizophrenia in a high-risk population, the difference between them reflecting essentially the subtype of schizophrenia involved.

Much the same point can be made with regard to use of the orienting response to predict clinical response to treatment. The frequently cited studies by Frith, Stevens, Johnstone, and Crow (1979) and Zahn et al. (1981) both found that schizophrenics who displayed overly frequent orienting responses showed poor response to either drug or "psychosocial" treatment. Straube, Schied, Rein, and Breyer-Pfaff (1987) recently reconfirmed this, noting that a more favorable outcome to drug treatment was shown by their orienting nonresponders.

In evaluating this work one must, once again, pay close attention to the nature of the patient sample studied. Frith et al. (1979) used Schneiderian criteria to establish diagnosis. Their sample was actively hallucinatory and delusional, with little evidence of negative symptoms. Zahn et al. (1981) studied acute schizophrenics with "flagrant symptomatology" who generally lacked deficit symptoms. Their patients were chosen to have relatively good prognoses: most had remitted from earlier episodes and showed good work and social histories in remission. Straube, Scheid, Rein, and Breyer-Pfaff (1987) worked with acute paranoid schizophrenics, primarily in a first hospitalization, all of whom showed "successful vocational integration" for at least 3 months preceding hospitalization.

Thus, all three studies reporting that excessive orienting response predict poor treatment outcome in schizophrenia studied a similar subtype, one with good premorbid functioning and episodic, remitting periods of psychosis characterized by florid Schneiderian symptoms. Excessive orienting response might thus predict poor treatment

response only for this subtype, much as excessive electrodermal reactivity predicted the subsequent appearance of a similar subtype of schizophrenia in high-risk children. Schneider's (1982) work serves to confirm this. Studying a chronic population, largely with negative symptoms, he found that patients displaying *greater* electrodermal response showed better clinical response than did nonresponders.

Whereas some decrease in electrodermal/autonomic reactivity may offer a positive prognostic sign among florid, hyperalert schizophrenics, signs of *increased* reactivity may do so among patients who are withdrawn and isolated. As Bernstein (1987) noted, overreactive orienting responses may provide an index of poor prognosis with regard to florid, remitting forms of schizophrenia, marking both high-risk children most likely to slide into schizophrenia and adult patients least likely to slide out of an existing episode. The work of Cannon and Mednick (1988) and Schneider (1982) now suggests that deficient orienting responses may similarly index poor prognosis with regard to forms of schizophrenia marked by strong negative symptoms. Admittedly, less evidence is available here at present, and more study is needed. In addition, it may be unwise to approach schizophrenia as a simple dichotomy—positive subgroups versus negative ones—but this is discussed below.

Additional gaps exist in the current outcome/prognosis literature. As Ohman et al. (1989) noted, outcome in schizophrenia must be considered in multidimensional terms. Yet the work considered above focused solely on active psychotic symptoms. Looking at broader indices of posthospital social and occupational adjustment, Ohman et al. (1989) found poorer outcome here was associated with *orienting response deficit* during the preceding hospitalization, rather than with excess. A study by Straube, Wagner, Foerster, and Heimann (1987) emphasized the importance of outcome criterion. The relationship they found between hyperactive orienting response and poor outcome held when total Brief Psychiatric Rating

Scale (BPRS) score or Thought Disorder score was the criterion measure, but showed no reliable differences based on orienting response activity when outcome was defined in terms of any other BPRS syndrome.

The length of time given to follow-up must also be considered. Most existing work is based on short-term follow-up: 4 weeks in the case of Frith et al. (1979) and Straube, Scheid, Rein, and Breyer-Pfaff (1987), 2 to 3 months for Zahn et al. (1981), and about 6 months for Schneider (1982). Ohman et al. (1989) moved toward longer term study. Over a 2-year period, they found the relationship between orienting response deficit and poor social–occupational outcome to be stronger the second year than the first. A complex interaction between follow-up period and criterion is indicated by the increased robustness in the relationship between orienting response deficit and social performance in the second year of Ohman's study, whereas Straube, Wagner, Foerster, and Heimann (1987) noted a weakening over time of the relationship between orienting response excess and outcome measures based essentially on psychotic behavior: orienting response excess predicted greater hospital stay over 4 weeks but showed no significant relationship with "relapse" at either 9-month or 2-year periods. Indeed, one may suspect a second-order interaction as well involving Schizophrenia Subtype × Criteria × Follow-up Period.

The orienting response literature dealing with prognosis has made some case for a relationship between hyperresponsiveness and a Schneiderian psychosis, and has just begun to make a case relating orienting response deficit to a negative-symptom, Kraepelinian psychosis, but has not so far considered these interactive effects.

DOES ORIENTING NONRESPONDING APPEAR ONLY IN PATIENTS WITH STRONG NEGATIVE SYMPTOMS?

It is now widely concluded that orienting nonresponding appears in those schizo-
phrenics who show primarily negative symptoms (e.g., Venables, 1983; Zahn, 1986). Indeed, as noted earlier, some writers (Straube, 1980; Venables 1983) speculate that nonresponding may be tied more basically to negative features than to any specific schizophrenic process, and may appear in schizophrenia or in depression only to the extent that these are accompanied by negative symptoms. I think such conclusions probably oversimplify a more complex relationship.

A respectable literature now exists to support a role for negative symptoms in the equation with orienting response deficit. A simple listing of some of this evidence might cite Straube (1979), Bernstein et al. (1981), and Dawson et al. (1988), noting a heightening of BPRS emotional withdrawal and blunted affect together with reduced excitement among nonresponder schizophrenics; Cannon and Mednick (1988) reporting heightened negative features in hyporesponders, both premorbidly and during psychosis; the finding by Ohman et al. (1989) that orienting response–deficient schizophrenics showed diminished social contacts; the reports by Simons (1981) and Bernstein and Riedel (1987) that college students high in Chapman Scale Anhedonia were hyporesponsive whereas those high in Perceptual Aberration (a more positive feature) were not; and Venables et al. (1978; personal communications, 1988, 1989) reporting that Mauritian children SCOR nonresponsive at age 3 (especially among males) were more socially withdrawn, showed less constructive play, and could be characterized as "preschizophrenic" by age 6½.

Although negative symptoms are part of the relationship, it is doubtful that they are all of it. For example, that listing fails to acknowledge several other findings. Alm et al. (1984) reported that their orienting-non-responsive schizophrenics differed from responders only in showing heightened *positive* symptoms such as "delusional mood" and "commenting voices." The studies by Straube (1979), Bernstein et al. (1981), and Dawson et al. (1988) actually reported a positive–negative mix, with increased conceptual disorganization, loading on a positive BPRS factor (Guy, 1976), as prominent as the negative symptoms. Green, Nuechterlein, and Satz (1987) and Spohn et al. (unpublished) reported that nonresponders tended to be higher than responders in both positive and negative symptoms, concluding that nonresponders were simply more severely ill overall. In any case, the use of RDC and *Diagnostic and Statistical Manual of Mental Disorders,* third edition (DSM-III; American Psychiatric Association, 1980) criteria in most studies means that, when strong negative symptoms are reported, they must coexist with at least that appreciable minimum of positive symptoms needed to satisfy the criteria for schizophrenia.

Orienting response–deficient schizophrenics thus appear to show a mixed symptom pattern, dominated perhaps by heightened emotional withdrawal and conceptual disorganization. Several other laboratories have independently identified this same pattern, emphasizing the importance of a joint increase in conceptual disorganization and emotional withdrawal. Using a variety of scales, these findings announce a relationship between this specific symptom pattern and electrodermal nonresponsiveness in chronic female psychiatric patients (Fenz & Steffy, 1968), altered cerebral blood flow in schizophrenia (Franzen & Ingvar, 1975a, 1975b), and impaired performance in tests of reaction time, word similarities, vocabulary, and ataxia (Schooler & Goldberg, 1972). Using multivariate techniques, Overall and Hollister (1982) defined a "thinking disorder prototype" based on high BPRS scores in conceptual disorganization, emotional withdrawal, and blunted affect, and termed this a "Withdrawn–Disorganized" subtype. This mirrors the BPRS pattern my colleagues and I found to characterize the nonresponsive schizophrenics (Bernstein et al., 1981), and overlaps the findings of Straube (1979) and Dawson et al. (1988) as well.

Orienting response deficiency does not seem to be associated simply with negative symptoms. Rather, it may be a characteristic of those schizophrenics who display a more complex symptom pattern cross-cutting the positive–negative dichotomy. In this regard, Kay, Opler, and Lindemayer (1988) recently made an interesting point that might be useful in further attempts to define the correlates of positive and negative symptoms. Although the precise relationship between positive and negative symptoms is still in dispute, Kay et al. found that each correlated with measures of overall severity of psychopathology, and suggested that, if one partialled out the variance due to global severity, a clearer picture might emerge of the specific correlates of residual positive and negative features. It now seems wise to begin looking more closely for such mixed symptom patterns, perhaps starting with the Withdrawn–Disorganized group.

WHAT DOES IT COST THE NONRESPONDER SCHIZOPHRENIC TO BE NONRESPONSIVE?

Two years ago I noted that we could give no clear answer to this question (Bernstein, 1987). Unfortunately, we are no closer to one today.

From its beginnings in Soviet laboratories, the orienting response has been shown to be associated with increased sensory sensitivity and information intake and improved processing and storage (Sokolov, 1963, 1966, 1969). As our appreciation of the complexities of attentional processes has grown, Western laboratories have begun to focus on complexities in the relationship of the orienting response to these processes. For example, there are considerations of preattentional/automatic versus attentional/voluntary orienting responses (e.g., Maltzman, 1979); the precise role of stimulus significance and priority of access to the limited-capacity orienting response–associated processor (e.g., Bernstein, 1979, 1981; O'Gorman, 1979); and stimulus-related orienting responses, looking back to the eliciting information, versus anticipatory orienting responses, looking ahead to expected information (e.g., Spinks & Siddle, 1985).

The most widely held current conception of the orienting response links it to a call for a high-level, limited-capacity information processor (Ohman, 1979). The "limited capacity" refers to the finite space available to any given information source at any given time. Because of this, when more than one informative input requires this processor, they can only be handled sequentially. In recent years, Dawson and his colleagues have borrowed the secondary reaction time task from cognitive psychologists (Posner & Boies, 1971) to test the relationship between the orienting response and this limited-capacity resource. Siddle and his associates have begun similar work.

In essence this paradigm provides subjects with a primary task, attending to irregularly presented orienting response stimuli, and with a secondary task, a series of reaction time stimuli presented either temporally remote from any orienting response stimulus or at selected brief intervals following such stimuli. If the orienting response stimulus is allocated all or part of the limited-capacity resource, less will be available to process any reaction time signal that overlaps, resulting in a slowing of reaction time in comparison with that to signals that are separate from the orienting response. Studies to date indicate that the orienting response *is* associated with allocation of space in this limited-capacity processor (Dawson & Filion, 1989; Dawson, Schell, Beers, & Kelly, 1982; Dawson, Schell, & Munro, 1985; Filion, Dawson, & Schell, 1986; Packer & Siddle, 1989; Siddle & Packer, 1987).[2] Dawson et al. (1982) and

Dawson and Filion (1989) also reported a positive correlation between SCOR amplitude and the degree of limited-capacity allocation, concluding that large SCOR responders devote greater processing capacity to significant environmental stimuli than do small responders, and that their processing may begin, and be completed, more rapidly.

With this background one might expect schizophrenics who are orienting nonresponders to show reduced stimulus detection, discrimination, reaction time, and the like. Although there are studies supporting such a conclusion, there are others that do not. In the first category, Straube (1979) found deficient auditory intake among schizophrenic nonresponders only; Gruzelier and Venables 91974) found poor perceptual resolution in tests of two-flash threshold among nonresponder patients; and Houlihan (1975) found better word recognition among schizophrenics who had displayed decelerative HRR to pretest stimuli than among those who showed heart rate acceleration here.

In contrast, Straube, Maier, Lemcke, and Germer (unpublished study) failed to replicate Straube (1979); Gruzelier and Hammond (1978) also reported orienting responders were poorer than nonresponders in tone discrimination; Patterson and Venables (1980) found poorer perceptual sensitivity in both nonresponders and normally habituating responder patients than in normal subjects or fast habituators; and Bernstein et al. (1985) and Ohman et al. (1986) both reported that the sharp drop in autonomic orienting response incidence shown by schizophrenics to imperative reaction time stimuli on repeated presentations was not accompanied by a change in reaction times vis-à-vis normal controls. Similar findings have been reported with (possible) cortical evoked potential orienting response components. Roth, Pfefferbaum, Horvath, and Kopell (1980) and Steinhauer and Zubin (1982) noted that schizophrenics continued

---

2. A still mysterious glitch has appeared within this relationship. Dawson et al. (1985) and Filion et al. (1986) have found that, if subjects are presented with orienting response tones to which to attend (task relevant) and others to be ignored (task irrelevant), the latter unexpectedly reveal a stronger allocation of limited-capacity processors, although only at 50 to 150 ms following stimulus onset. This happens despite the occurrence of a larger SCOR to the task-relevant tones. Filion, Dawson, Schell, and Hazlett (1991) suggested that this is due to the physical similarity of the task-irrelevant stimulus to the relevant signal, and have shown that this unexpected call for processing space following the irrelevant stimulus disappears if relevant

and irrelevant stimuli are presented to different modalities.

to display diminished P300 even on trials in which reaction time or stimulus counting performance was matched to those of normal subjects. Kemali et al. (1988) found that schizophrenics continued to display reduced late positive components despite nonsignificant differences from normal subjects in reaction time and errors.

These results will not support any coherent conclusion. It is not uncommon to find weak concordance between behavioral performance and psychophysiological data (see Spinks & Siddle, 1983), but the continuing ambiguity here regarding the functional meaning of orienting response deficit in schizophrenia is unsettling. One problem may lie in the use of designs that place too little load on information-processing capacities. Limited-capacity resources are allocated only when the simple, preattentional processors are not adequate to the task (Ohman, 1979). Orienting response studies have so far imposed slight demands on information-processing capacity. As a consequence, more or less automatic behavioral responses may continue at little cost, even without accompanying orienting responses. Perhaps this may be related to the evidence of Nuechterlein (1985) that decreased perceptual sensitivity (the d' measure of signal detection theory) provides a robust indicator of vulnerability for schizophrenia only if measured in tasks placing heavy demands on information processing. The possibility of a similar distinction should be probed with the orienting response.

It is surprising that so few attempts have been made to learn the meaning of orienting response loss in schizophrenia, or to explore, for example, the relationship between orienting response deficit and altered d' or beta (the response criterion index). Some studies have explored the relationship between autonomic lability and d' and beta among normal subjects (e.g., Crider & Augenbraun, 1975; Hastrup, 1979; Munro & Dawson, 1985; Sostek, 1978), but not that between orienting response and these indices. One reason may be the belief that orienting response by definition, must habituate rapidly, thereby failing to provide data

over the long sequence of trials needed to evaluate d'/beta. If so, a mistake exists for two reasons. First orienting nonresponding appears to be a stable characteristic of a subgroup of schizophrenic patients. Thus, responder versus nonresponder subgroup comparisons could be made, analogous to that between labile and stable subjects in the general population. Further, orienting response activity readily can be extended over trials by using more complex significant signals. In fact, Bernstein and Taylor (1979) and Bernstein (1981) challenged the notion that orienting response *must* habituate. If orienting response is keyed to stimulus uncertainty, it should not decline over trials if uncertainty is maintained, despite the occurrence of familiarity involving the physical stimulus elements. For example, Bernstein and Taylor (1979) used trials each consisting of three different tones. By varying the sequence unpredictably within each trial, thereby varying, and sustaining, the information value of each tone in each trial, we found no orienting response habituation over the eight trials run. Graham, Putnam, and Leavitt (1975) also found sustained orienting response over many trials by varying the relationship between a lead stimulus and the following startle stimulus unpredictably over trials.

It is important to begin studies aimed at answering questions about the meaning of orienting nonresponding in schizophrenia; the relationship with d' and beta may be a good place to begin.

HAS ORIENTING NONRESPONDING ALREADY BEEN ESTABLISHED AS A VULNERABILITY MARKER FOR SCHIZOPHRENIA?

With irrefutable evidence of a major genetic role in schizophrenia, interest has focused in recent years on attempts to define trait or vulnerability markers that would, among other things, identify affected individuals before schizophrenia was clinically evident. Several reviewers, Dawson and Nuechterlein (1984) and Iacono (1985) among them, consider orienting nonresponding to be one of a likely handful of candidates here.

There is evidence to support such a view. The orienting nonresponding of schizophrenia does not depend on neuroleptic medication, nor is it affected by changes in clinical status (i.e., remission, relapse); it appears often in those patients whose schizophrenia is likely to have a genetic origin, and has appeared years premorbidly in the biological offspring of schizophrenics, especially those who tended to become schizophrenics themselves, as well as among students psychometrically defined as displaying a likely heightened risk for schizophrenia. Much of this information has been reviewed elsewhere (Bernstein, 1991) and is not again reviewed here.

To firmly establish status as a vulnerability marker, two further characteristics must also be displayed. First, a heightened incidence of orienting response deficit should also appear in the blood relatives of nonresponder schizophrenics who are not themselves schizophrenic, to show that such deficit does follow a specifically defined genetic track. Second, many of the ostensible "normal" subjects who display such an orienting response deficit should also be seen to display signs of schizophrenia spectrum disorder more frequently than these are seen in the general population, to show that the marker does tag the pathology, and is not secondary to treatment or institutionalization. To the best of my knowledge, no one has attempted to gather data in either area so far.

Orienting response research in schizophrenia is alive and vigorous after 20-odd years, and as the current work exploring orienting response deficit in relation to such things as computerized tomography scan brain changes, smooth pursuit eye movement deficit, season of birth, and frequency of birth complications indicate, it is expanding into new areas. The course of such study should not be haphazard or unexamined, however. It is necessary to call attention periodically to soft spots so that, as the crest of new work moves on, it never gets too far from solid ground.

ACKNOWLEDGMENT

This chapter was prepared with the support of National Institutes of Mental Health grant MH28594.

REFERENCES

Alm, T., Lindstrom, L., Ost, L.-G., & Ohman, A. (1984). Electrodermal nonresponding in schizophrenia: Relationships to attentional, clinical, biochemical, computed tomographical, and genetic factors. *International Journal of Psychophysiology, 1,* 195–208.

Alm, T., Ost, L.-G., & Ohman, A. (1987). The stability of electrodermal orienting responses in schizophrenic patients [abstract]. *Psychophysiology, 24,* 576.

American Psychiatric Association. (1980). *Diagnostic and statistical manual of mental disorders* (3rd ed.). Washington, DC: American Psychiatric Press, Inc.

Barry, R. (1979). A factor-analytic examination of the unitary OR concept. *Biological Psychology, 8,* 161–178.

Bartfai, A., Levander, S., Nyback, H., & Schalling, D. (1987). Skin conductance nonresponding and nonhabituation in schizophrenic patients. *Acta Psychiatrica Scandinavica, 75,* 321–329.

Bartfai, A., Levander, S., & Sedvall, G. (1983). Smooth pursuit eye movement, clinical symptoms, CSF metabolites, and skin conductance habituation in schizophrenic patients. *Biological Psychiatry, 18,* 971–987.

Bernstein, A. (1964). The galvanic skin response orienting reflex among chronic schizophrenics. *Psychonomic Science 1,* 391–392.

Bernstein, A. (1967) The orienting reflex as a research tool in the study of psychotic populations. In I. Ruttkay-Nedecky, L. Ciganek, V. Zikmund, & E. Kellerova (Eds.), *Mechanisms of orienting reaction in man* (pp. 257–266). Bratislava: Slovak Academy of Science.

Bernstein, A. (1970). The phasic electrodermal orienting response in chronic schizophrenics: Response to auditory signals of varying intensity. *Journal of Abnormal Psychology, 75,* 146–156.

Bernstein, A. (1979). The orienting reflex as novelty and significance detector: A reply to O'Gorman. *Psychophysiology, 16,* 263–273.

Bernstein, A. (1981). The orienting response and stimulus significance: Further comments. *Biological Psychology, 12,* 171–185.

Bernstein, A. (1987). Orienting response research in schizophrenia: Where we have come and where we might go. *Schizophrenia Bulletin, 13,* 623–641.

Bernstein, A. (1991). The autonomic orienting response as a possible vulnerability marker in schizophrenia. In H. Hafner, W. Gattaz (Eds.), *Search for the causes of schizophrenia* (pp. 321–341). New York: Springer-Verlag.

Bernstein, A., Frith, C., Gruzelier, J., Patterson, T., Straube, E., Venables, P., & Zahn, T. (1982). An analysis of the skin conductance orienting response in samples of American, British, and German schizophrenics. *Biological Psychology, 14,* 155–211.

Bernstein, A., Pava, J., Riedel, J., Schnur, D., & Lubowsky, J. (1985). A limiting factor in the "normalization" of schizophrenic orienting response dysfunction. *Schizophrenia Bulletin, 11,* 230–254.

Bernstein, A., & Riedel, J. (1987). Psychophysiological response patterns in college students with high physical anhedonia: Scores appear to reflect schizotypy rather than depression. *Biological Psychiatry, 22,* 829–847.

Bernstein, A., Riedel, J., Graae, F., Seidman, D., Steele, H., Connolly, J., & Lubowsky, J. (1988). Schizophrenia is associated with altered orienting activity, depression with electrodermal (cholinergic?) deficit and normal orienting response. *Journal of Abnormal Psychology, 97,* 3–12.

Bernstein, A., Riedel, J., Graae, F., Seidman, D., Steele, H., Lubowsky, J., & Margolis, R. (1990). The effect of prolonged stimulus repetition with repeated switching of target status on the orienting response in schizophrenia and depression. *Journal of Nervous and Mental Disease, 178,* 96–104.

Bernstein, A., Schneider, S., Juni, S., Pope, A., & Starkey, P. (1980). The effect of stimulus significance on the electrodermal response in chronic schizophrenia. *Journal of Abnormal Psychology, 89,* 93–97.

Bernstein, A., & Taylor, K. (1976). Stimulus significance and the phasic electrodermal orienting response in schizophrenic and nonschizophrenic adolescents. In D. Siva Sankar (Ed.), *Mental health in children* (pp. 251–280). Westbury, NY: PJD Publications.

Bernstein, A., & Taylor, K. (1979). The interaction of stimulus information with potential stimulus significance in eliciting the skin conductance orienting response. In H. Kimmel, E. van Olst, & J. Orlebeke (eds.), *The orienting reflex in humans* (pp. 499–519). Hillsdale, NJ: Lawrence Erlbaum Associates.

Bernstein, A., Taylor, K., Austin, B., Nathanson, M., & Scarpelli, A. (1971). The orienting response and apparent movement toward or away from the observer. *Journal of Experimental Psychology, 87,* 37–45.

Bernstein, A., Taylor, K., Starkey, P., Juni, S., Lubowsky, J., & Paley, H. (1981). Bilateral skin conductance, finger pulse volume, and EEG orienting response to tones of differing intensities in chronic schizophrenics and controls. *Journal of Nervous and Mental Disease, 169,* 513–528.

Brown, C. (1970). The parotid puzzle: A review of the literature on human salivation and its applications to psychophysiology. *Psychophysiology, 7,* 66–85.

Bruno, R., Myers, S., & Glassman, A. (1983). A correlational study of cardiovascular autonomic functioning and unipolar depression. *Biological Psychiatry, 18,* 227–235.

Busfield, B., & Wechsler, H. (1961). Studies of salivation in depression: I. A comparison of salivation rates in depressed, schizoaffective depressed, nondepressed hospitalized, and in normal controls. *Archives of General Psychiatry, 4,* 10–15.

Cannon, T., Fuhrman, M., Mednick, S., Machon, R., Parnas, J., & Schulsinger, F. (1988). Third ventricle enlargement and reduced electrodermal responsiveness. *Psychophysiology, 25,* 153–156.

Cannon, T., & Mednick, S. (1988). *Autonomic nervous system antecedents of positive and negative symptoms in schizophrenia.* Paper presented at the meeting of the Society for Psychophysiological Research, San Francisco.

Cannon, T., Mednick, S., & Parnas, J. (1990). Two pathways to schizophrenia in children at risk. In L. Robins, & M. Rutter (Eds.), *Straight and devious pathways from childhood to adulthood* (pp. 328–350). Cambridge, England: Cambridge University Press.

Cohen, R., Sommer, W., Hermanutz, M. (1981). Auditory event-related potentials in chronic schizophrenics. Advances in Biological Psychiatry 6, 180–185.

Crider, A., & Augenbraun, C. (1975). Auditory vigilance correlates of electrodermal response habituation speed. *Psychophysiology, 12,* 36–40.

Dawson, M., & Filion, D. (1989). Is elicitation of the autonomic orienting response associated with allocation of processing resources? *Psychophysiology, 26,* 560–572.

Dawson, M., & Nuechterlein, K. (1984). Psychophysiological dysfunctions in the developmental course of schizophrenic disorders. *Schizophrenia Bulletin, 10,* 204–232.

Dawson, M., & Nuechterlein, K. (1987). The role of autonomic dysfunction within a vulnerability-stress model of schizophrenic disorders. In D. Magnusson, & A. Ohman,

(Eds.), *Psychopathology: An interactional perspective* (pp. 41–57). New York: Academic Press.

Dawson, M., Nuechterlein, K., & Schell, A. (1988). *Symptomatic correlates of electrodermal responsiveness in recent-onset schizophrenia.* Paper presented at the meeting of the Society for Psychophysiological Research, San Francisco.

Dawson, M., Schell, A., Beers, J., & Kelly, A. (1982). Allocation of cognitive processing capacity during human autonomic classical conditioning. *Journal of Experimental Psychology: General, 111,* 273–295.

Dawson, M., Schell, A., & Munro, L. (1985). *Autonomic orienting, electrodermal lability, and the allocation of processing resources.* Paper presented at the meeting of the Society for Psychophysiological Research, Houston.

Dilsaver, S. (1986). Cholinergic-monoamine systems, depression, and panic. *Biological Psychiatry, 21,* 571–573.

Erlenmeyer-Kimling, L., Marcuse, Y., Cornblatt, B., Friedman, D., Rainer, J., & Rutschmann, J. (1984). The New York high-risk project. In N. Watt, E. Anthony, L. Wynne, & J. Rolf (Eds.), *Children at risk for schizophrenia: A longitudinal perspective* (pp. 169–189). New York: Cambridge University Press.

Fenz, W., & Steffy, R. (1968). Electrodermal arousal of chronically ill psychiatric patients undergoing intensive behavior treatment. *Psychosomatic Medicine, 30,* 423–436.

Filion, D., Dawson, M., & Schell, A. (1986). *Autonomic orienting and the allocation of processing resources.* Paper presented at the meeting of the Society for Psychophysiological Research, Montreal.

Filion, D., Dawson, M., Schell, A., & Hazlett, E. (1991). *The relationship between skin conductance orienting and the allocation of processing resources: Generality of a dissociation effect. Psychophysiology, 28,* 410–425.

Franzen, G., & Ingvar, D. (1975a). Abnormal distribution of cerebral activity in chronic schizophrenia. *Journal of Psychiatric Research, 12,* 199–214.

Franzen, G., & Ingvar, D. (1975b). Absence of activation of frontal structures during psychological testing of chronic schizophrenics. *Journal of Neurology, Neurosurgery and Psychiatry, 38,* 1027–1032.

Friedman, D., Hakerem, G., Sutton, S., & Fleiss, J. (1973). Effect of stimulus uncertainty on the pupillary dilation response and the vertex evoked potential. *Electroencephalography and Clinical Neurophysiology, 34,* 475–484.

Frith, C., Stevens, M., Johnstone, E., & Crow, T. (1982). Skin conductance habituation during acute episodes of schizophrenia: Qualitative differences from anxious and depressed patients. *Psychological Medicine, 12,* 575–583.

Frith, C., Stevens, M., Johnstone, E., & Crow, T. (1979). Skin conductive responsivity during acute episodes of schizophrenia as a predictor of symptomatic improvement. *Psychological Medicine, 9,* 101–106.

Giedke, H., Heimann, H. (1987). Psychophysiological aspects of depressive syndromes. *Pharmacopsychiatry, 20,* 177–180.

Graham, F. (1979). Distinguishing among orienting, defense, and startle reflexes. In H. Kimmel, E. van Olst, & J. Orlebeke (Eds.), *The orienting reflex in humans.* (pp. 137–167). Hillsdale, NJ: Lawrence Erlbaum Associates.

Graham, F., Putnam, L. & Leavitt, L. (1975). Lead-stimulus effects on human cardiac orienting and blink reflexes. *Journal of Experimental Psychology: Human Perception and Performance, 104,* 161–169.

Green, M., & Nuechterlein, K. (1988). Neuroleptic effects on electrodermal responding to soft tones and loud noises in schizophrenia. *Psychiatry Research, 24,* 79–86.

Green, M., Nuecherlein, K., & Satz, P. (1988). Electrodermal activity and symptomatology in schizophrenia. In P. Harvey & W. Walker (Eds.), *Positive and negative symptoms in psychosis* (pp. 243–257). Hillsdale, N.J.: Lawrence Erlbaum.

Gruzelier, J., Connolly, J., Eves, F., Hirsch, S., Zaki, S., Weller, M., & Yorkston, N. (1981). Effect of propranolol and phenothiazines on electrodermal orienting and habituation in schizophrenia. *Psychological Medicine, 11,* 93–108.

Gruzelier, J., Eves, F., Connolly, J., & Hirsch, S. (1981). Habituation, sensitization, and dishabituation in the electrodermal system of consecutive drug-free admissions for schizophrenia. *Biological Psychology, 12,* 187–209.

Gruzelier, J., & Hammond, N. (1978). The effect of chlorpromazine upon physiological, endocrine, and information processing in schizophrenia. *Journal of Psychiatric Research, 14,* 167–182.

Gruzelier, J., & Venables, P. (1973). Skin conductance responses to tones with and without attentional significance in schizophrenic and nonschizophrenic patients. *Neuropsychology, 11,* 221–230.

Gruzelier, J., & Venables, P. (1974). Bimodality and lateral asymmetry of skin conductance orienting activity in schizophrenics: Replication and evidence of lateral asymmetry in patients with depression and disorders of personality. *Biological Psychiatry, 8,* 55–73.

Guy, W. (1976) *ECDEU assessment manual for psychopharmacology* (pp. 160–161). Bethesda MD: National Institute of Mental Health.

Hastrup, J. (1979). Effects of electrodermal lability and introversion on vigilance decrement. *Psychophysiology, 16,* 302–310.

Holzman, P. (1987). Recent studies of psychophysiology in schizophrenia. *Schizophrenia Bulletin, 13,* 49–76.

Houlihan, J. (1975). Visual word recognition and automatic responsivity of schizophrenic patients. *JSAS Catalog of Selected Documents in Psychology, 5,* 195 (ms #865).

Iacono, W. (1985). Psychophysiological markers of psychopathology in chronic schizophrenia. *Canadian Journal of Psychology, 26,* 96–112.

Iacono, W., Lykken, D., Haroian, K., Peloquin, L., Valentine, R., & Tuason, V. (1984). Electrodermal activity in euthymic patients with affective disorders: One-year retest stability and the effects of stimulus intensity and significance. *Journal of Abnormal Psychology, 93,* 304–311.

Iacono, W., Lykken, D., Peloquin, L., Lumry, A., Valentine, R., & Tuason, V. (1983). Electrodermal activity in euthymic unipolar and bipolar affective disorders. *Archives of General Psychiatry, 40,* 557–565.

Janowsky, D., & Risch, S. (1987). Role of acetylcholine mechanisms in the affective disorders. In H. Meltzer (Ed.), *Psychopharmacology: The 3rd generation of progress* (pp. 527–533). New York: Raven Press.

Kay, S., Opler, L., & Lindenmayer, J.-P. (1988). Reliability and validity of the Positive and Negative Syndrome Scale for schizophrenia. *Psychiatry Research, 23,* 99–110.

Kelly, D., & Walter, C. (1968). The relationship between clinical diagnosis and anxiety, assessed by forearm blood flow and other measurements. *British Journal of Psychiatry, 114,* 611–626.

Kelly, D., & Walter, C. (1969). A clinical and physiological relationship between anxiety and depression. *British Journal of Psychiatry, 115,* 401–406.

Kemali, D., Galderisi, S., Maj, M., Mucci, A., Cesarelli, M., & D'Ambria, L. (1988). Event-related potentials in schizophrenic patients: Clinical and neurophysiological correlates. *Research Communications in Psychology, Psychiatry and Behavior 13,* 3–16.

Kugelmass, S., Marcus, J., & Schmueli, J. (1985). Psychophysiological reactivity in high risk children. *Schizophrenia Bulletin, 11,* 66–73.

Lader, M., & Montague, J. (1962). The psychogalvanic reflex: A pharmacological study of the peripheral mechanisms. *Journal of Neurology, Neurosurgery and Psychiatry, 25,* 126–133.

Lechin, F., van der Dijs, B., Acosta, E., Gomez, F., Lechin, E., & Arocha, L. (1983). Distal colon motility and clinical parameters in depression. *Journal of Affective Disorders, 5,* 19–26.

Levinson, D., & Edelberg, R. (1985). Scoring criteria for response latency and habituation in electrodermal research: A critique. *Psychophysiology, 22,* 417–426.

Levinson, D., Edelberg, R., & Bridger, W. (1984). The orienting response in schizophrenia: Proposed resolution of a controversy. *Biological Psychology, 19,* 489–507.

Lovett Doust, J. (1980). Sinus tachycardia and abnormal cardiac rate variation in schizophrenia. *Neuropsychobiology, 6,* 305–312.

Maltzman, I. (1979). Orienting reflexes and classical conditioning in humans. In H. Kimmel, E. van Olst, & J. Orlebeke (Eds.), *The orienting reflex in humans* (pp. 323–352). Hillsdale NJ: Lawrence Erlbaum Associates.

Mednick, S., & Schulsinger, F. (1968). Some premorbid characteristics related to breakdown in children with schizophrenic mothers. In D. Rosenthal, & S. Kety (Eds.), *Transmission of schizophrenia* (pp. 267–291). New York: Pergamon.

Mednick, S., Schulsinger, F., Teasdale, T., Schulsinger, H., Venables, P., & Rock, D. (1978). Schizophrenia in high risk children: Sex differences in predisposing factors. In G. Serban (Ed.), *Cognitive defects in the development of mental illness* (pp. 169–197). New York: Brunner/Mazel.

Munro, L., & Dawson, M. (1985). *Electrodermal lability and rapid performance decrement in a degraded stimulus continuous performance test.* Paper presented at the meeting of the Society for Psychophysiological, Research, Houston.

Nuechterlein, K. (1985). Converging evidence for vigilance deficit as a vulnerability indicator for schizophrenic disorders. In M. Alpert (Ed.), *Controversies in schizophrenia* (pp. 175–198). New York: Guilford Press.

Obrist, P., Wood, D., & Perez-Reyes, M. (1965). Heart rate during conditioning in humans: Effects of CS intensities, vagal blockade, and adrenergic block of vasomotor activity. *Journal of Experimental Psychology, 70,* 32–42.

O'Gorman, J. (1979). The orienting reflex: Novelty or significance detector? *Psychophysiology 16,* 253–262.

Ohlund, L., Ohman, A., Alm, T., Ost, L.-G., & Lindstrom, L. (1990). Season of birth and electrodermal unresponsiveness in male schizophrenics. *Biological Psychiatry, 27,* 328–340.

Ohman, A. (1979). The orienting response, attention, and learning: An information-processing perspective. In H. Kimmel, E. van Olst, J. Orlebeke (Eds.), *The orienting reflex in humans* (pp. 443–471). Hillsdale, NJ: Lawrence Erlbaum Associates.

Ohman, A. (1981). Electrodermal activity and vulnerability to schizophrenia: A review. *Biological Psychology, 12,* 87–145.

Ohman, A., Nordby, H., & d'Elia, G. (1986). Orienting and schizophrenia: Stimulus significance attention, and distraction in a signalled reaction time task. *Journal of Abnormal Psychology, 95,* 326–334.

Ohman, A., Ohlund, L., Alm, T., Wieselgren, I.-M., Ost, L.-G., & Lindstrom, L. (1989). Electrodermal nonresponding, premorbid adjustment, and symptomatology as predictors of long term social functioning in schizophrenics. *Journal of Abnormal Psychology, 98,* 426–435.

Overall, J., & Hollister, L. (1982). Decision rules for phenomenological classification of psychiatric patients. *Journal of Consulting and Clinical Psychology 50,* 535–545.

Packer, J., & Siddle, D. (1989). Stimulus miscuing, electrodermal activity, and the allocation of processing resources. *Psychophysiology, 26,* 192–200.

Patterson, T., & Venables, P. (1978). Bilateral skin conductance and skin potential in schizophrenic and normal subjects: The identification of the fast habituator group of schizophrenics. *Psychophysiology, 15,* 556–560.

Patterson, T., & Venables, P. (1980). Auditory vigilance: Normals compared to chronic schizophrenic subgroups defined by skin conductance variables. *Psychiatry Research, 2,* 107–112.

Posner, M., & Boies, S. (1971). Components of attention. *Psychological Review 78,* 391–408.

Prentky, R., Salzman, L., & Klein, R. (1981). Habituation and conditioning of skin conductance responses in children at risk. *Schizophrenia Bulletin, 7,* 281–291.

Prout, B. (1967). Independence of the galvanic skin reflex from the vasoconstrictor reflex in man. *Journal of Neurology, Neurosurgery and Psychiatry, 30,* 319–324.

Roth, W. (1977). Late event-related potentials and psychopathology. *Schizophrenia Bulletin, 3,* 105–120.

Roth, W., Pfeferbaum, A., Horvath, T., & Kopell, B. (1980). P 300 and reaction time in schizophrenics and controls. In K. Kornhuber, & L. Deecke (Eds.), *Progress in brain research, motor and sensory processes of the brain: Electrical potentials, behavior, and clinical use* (pp. 522–525). Amsterdam: Elsevier.

Rubens, R., & Lapidus, L. (1978). Schizophrenic patterns of arousal and stimulus barrier functioning. *Journal of Abnormal Psychology, 87,* 199–211.

Schneider, S. (1982). Electrodermal activity and therapeutic response to neuroleptic treatment in chronic inpatients. *Psychological Medicine, 12,* 607–613.

Schnur, D., Bernstein, A., Mukherjee, S., Loh, J., Degreef, G., & Riedel, J. (1989). The autonomic orienting response and CT scan findings in schizophrenia. *Schizophrenia Research, 2,* 449–455.

Schooler, N., & Goldberg, S. (1972). Performance tests in a study of phenothiazines in schizophrenia: Caveats and conclusions. *Psychopharmacology, 24,* 87–98.

Siddle, D., & Packer, J. (1987). Stimulus omission and dishabituation of the electrodermal orienting response: The allocation of processing resources. *Psychophysiology, 24,* 181–190.

Simons, R. (1981). Electrodermal and cardiac orienting in psychometrically defined high risk subjects. *Psychiatry Research, 4,* 347–356.

Simons, R., Losito, B., Rose, S., & MacMillan, F. Electrodermal nonresponding among college undergraduates. Temporal stability situation specificity, and relationship to heart rate change. *Psychophysiology, 20,* 498–506.

Sokolov, E. (1963). *Perception and the conditioned reflex.* New York: Pergamon.

Sokolov, E. (1966). Orienting reflex as information regulator. In A. Leontiev, A. Luria, & A. Smirnov (Eds.). *Psychological research in the USSR* (Vol. 1, pp. 334–360). Moscow: Progress Publishers.

Sokolov, E. (1969). The modeling properties of the nervous system. In M. Coles & I. Maltzman (Eds.), *Handbook of contemporary Soviet psychology* (pp. 671–704). New York: Basic Books.

Sostek, A. (1978). Effects of electrodermal lability and payoff instructions on vigilance performance. *Psychophysiology, 15,* 561–568.

Spinks, J., & Siddle, D. (1983). The functional significance of the orienting response. In D. Siddle (Ed.), *Orienting and habituation: Perspectives in human research* (pp. 237–314). New York: John Wiley & Sons.

Spinks, J., & Siddle, D. (1985). The effects of anticipated information on skin conductance and cardiac activity. *Biological Psychology, 20,* 39–50.

Spohn, H., Coyne, L., Spray, J., & Hayes, K. (1989). Skin conductance orienting response in chronic schizophrenics: The role of neuroleptics. *Journal of Abnormal Psychology, 98,* 478–486.

Spohn, H., & Patterson, T. (1979). Recent studies of psychophysiology in schizophrenia. *Schizophrenia Bulletin,* 581–611.

Steinhauer, S., & Zubin, J. (1982). Vulnerability to schizophrenia: Information processing in the pupil and event-related potential. In E. Usdin, & I. Hanin (Eds.), *Biological markers in psychiatry and neurology* (pp. 371–385). New York: Pergamon.

Straube, E. (1979). On the meaning of electrodermal nonresponding in schizophrenia. *Journal of Nervous and Mental Disease 167,* 601–611.

Straube, E. (1980). Reduced reactivity and psychopathology: Examples from research in schizophrenia. In M. Kakkou, D. Lehman, & J. Angst (Eds.), *Functional status of the brain* (pp. 291–307). Amsterdam: Elsevier.

Straube, E., Schied, H.-W., Rein, W., & Breyer-Pfaff, U. (1987). Autonomic nervous system differences as predictors of short-term outcome in schizophrenics. *Pharmacopsychiatry, 20,* 105–110.

Straube, E., Wagner, W., Foerster, K., & Heimann, H. (1987). *Findings significant with respect to short- and medium-term outcome in schizophrenia.* Paper presented at the meeting of the Society for Psychophysiolgical Research, Amsterdam.

Strian, F., Klicpera, C. & Caspar, F. (1977). Autonomic activation and endogenous depression. *Archiv fur Psychiatrie und Nervenkranken 223,* 203–218.

Thier, P., Axmann, D., & Giedke, H. (1986). Slow brain potentials and psychomotor retardation in depression. *Electroencephalography and Clinical Neurophysiology, 63,* 570–581.

van Dyke, J., Rosenthal, D., & Rasmussen, P. (1974). Electrodermal functioning in adopted away offspring of schizophrenics. *Journal of Psychiatric Research, 10,* 199–215.

Venables, P. (1983). Cerebral mechanisms, autonomic responsiveness, and attention in schizophrenia. In W. Spaulding & J. Cole (Eds.), *Nebraska symposium on motivation, Vol. 31: Theories of schizophrenia and psychoses* (pp. 47–91). Lincoln: University of Nebraska Press.

Venables, P. (1986). Psychophysiology and psychiatry. In R. Rosenberg, F. Schulsinger, & E. Stromgren (Eds.). *Psychiatry and its related disciplines:* The next 25 years (pp. 79–96). Geneva: World Psychiatric Association.

Venables, P., & Bernstein, A. (1983). The orienting response and psychopathology: Schizophrenia. In D. Siddle (Ed.), *Orienting and habituation: Perspectives in human research* (pp. 475–504). New York: John Wiley & Sons.

Venables, P., Mednick, S., Schulsinger, F., Raman, A., Bell, D., Dalais, J., & Fletcher, R. (1978). Screening for risk of mental illness. In G. Serban (Ed.), *Cognitive defects in the development of mental illness* (pp. 273–303). New York: Brunner/Mazel.

Ward, N., & Doerr, H. (1986). Skin conductance: A potentially sensitive and specific marker for depression. *Journal of Nervous and Mental Disease 174,* 553–559.

Zahn, T. (1986). Psychophysiological approaches to psychopathology. In M. Coles, E. Donchin, & S. Porges (Eds.), *Psychophysiology* (pp. 508–610). New York: Guilford Press.

Zahn, T., Carpenter, W., McGlashan, T. (1981). Autonomic nervous system activity in acute schizophrenia. *Archives of General Psychiatry, 38,* 260–266.

Part IV

CLINICAL SYMPTOMS, COURSE, AND TREATMENT OUTCOMES

13

Social Self and the Schizophrenic Process: Theory and Research

SEYMOUR ROSENBERG

There is incredible diversity in the meaning and use of the term "social self," and of the related terms "identity" and "ego." I hope to convey the meaning of these terms as they are used in our work to probe the role of the social self in the schizophrenic process, first by offering a brief overview of the historical roots of the concept of social self.

Although philosophers have pondered the psychological nature of self for several centuries, it was William James (1890) who first conceptualized the self within the context of a modern, empirically oriented psychology. The concept of social self or, more correctly, that of social selves was born when James enunciated his famous statement: "Properly speaking, *a man has as many social selves as there are individuals who recognize him*" (James, 1890, p. 294). James made a person's social selves a major constituent of the person's total self.

Less than a decade later another American psychologist, James Baldwin (1897/1973), laid out a theory of the development of self in childhood, in which he argued that all of the self is essentially a social self—the product of a person's particular interpersonal and cultural milieu. The views I have about me and the views I have about others that I know, that I can imagine, and that are fictional or mythical all comprise my social self, according to Baldwin. He would dub my view of me "ego," and my view of others "alter." Neither Baldwin nor James had much to say about psychopathology of the self. Baldwin discussed briefly the interplay between heredity and the social norms of a particular community in determining whose self is "socially fit" and whose self is "socially unfit" (Baldwin, 1897, pp. 71–81).

Baldwin's writings have been all but obscured by contemporary historiographers. Nevertheless, it was his and James's ideas about social self that were further developed by two prominent and influential figures in social psychology and sociology: Charles Cooley (1902) and George Herbert Mead (1934).

Cooley and Mead have also had a discernible influence in social psychiatry. The preeminence that Cooley and Mead gave to social and cultural factors in the development and maintenance of self became an important tributary in Harry Stack Sullivan's (1953) interpersonal conceptions of psychiatry. For Sullivan (1924), psychiatry was concerned with "interpersonal situations through which persons manifest mental health or mental disorder" (Sullivan, 1953, p. 18). Somewhat more radically, Laing (1960, 1961) construed self within a social system, and psychosis as anomalies in the interpersonal arrangements within such systems. Not obviously influenced by early American social psychology, but worth mentioning in the context of the history of social self, are Adler and post-Freudian psychoanalysts such as Erikson, Horney, and Kohut.

This historical exegesis is necessarily brief and limited to the seminal thinkers in the field. However, their ideas stimulated a rich and provocative body of thought and writing about the composition of the social self, about its anomalies, about the social and cultural factors that determine the development of social self in childhood and adolescence, and about how social conditions and life's exigencies might affect the functioning and psychiatric status of the person with (or without) anomalies of social self.

From this broad-ranging social psychology of self and psychopathology, my colleagues, Michael Gara and Bertram Cohen, and I have extracted for study the nature of the social self in schizophrenia. By social self, I refer to the system of beliefs that a person holds about self and about others—essentially Baldwin's definition of social self. Social psychiatrists have sometimes given disturbances of this social self etiological significance, as when they are attributed directly to early family experiences. Sometimes these disturbances are viewed as a complex derivative of biological/genetic factors and social development.

Conjectures about the nature and etiological significance of social self in schizophrenia have relied by and large on a clinically based and discursive methodology. There has been no empirical methodology for studying the social self comparable in rigor to the methods available for measuring neurobiological, sensorimotor, and cognitive correlates of psychopathology. The first part of this chapter is taken up with the description of a research method for studying social self in schizophrenia, a method that has evolved from laboratory studies of social self and personal identity in nonclinical populations (e.g., Rosenberg, 1988; Rosenberg & Gara, 1985). Two studies of social self in schizophrenia are then summarized that reveal certain anomalies of the social self (Gara, Rosenberg, & Mueller, 1989) and about the probable role of the patient identity in stabilizing the patient's personal and social functioning (Robey, Cohen, & Gara, 1989). The substantive questions in these studies were framed within a theoretical conception of the role of identity resources in the schizophrenic process (Gara, Rosenberg, & Cohen, 1987).

Although definitive answers to questions about etiology remain elusive (and perhaps always will when judged by exacting logical and experimental standards), mappings of social self with an explicit research methodology may prove useful in sorting out various pathologies of the social self. Such measurable pathologies in social self, like other measurable psychological and biological deviations, may not tell us about etiology, but such information may be valuable in the further development of a social psychological theory of psychopathology—and, in turn, to an improved prognosis and treatment of such disorders. I will address these possibilities in the concluding section of this chapter.

METHODOLOGY

The broad distinction between *habitual self* and *accommodating self* (Baldwin, 1897/1973, p. 34; Breakwell, 1986, pp. 80–96) is useful as a first cut in studying the social self. Habitual self refers to the relatively enduring views one has of self and others. Habitual self acts to assimilate one's everyday experience of self and others to these established conceptions. Accommodating self refers to perceptions of self and others that are stimulated by new, unique, or transient social and personal conditions. These perceptions may (or may not) reshape the habitual self. This chapter is concerned primarily with the content and organization of habitual social self in schizophrenic patients.[1] For simplicity, I will refer to habit-

1. Elsewhere, my colleagues and I have described the schizophrenic break in terms of a habitual self that is negated and hence is no longer available for assimilating everyday experiences (Gara et al., 1987). In our theoretical analysis of this process, the accommodating self now consists of a flood of inchoate perceptions of self and other, as described by several writers (e.g., Docherty, VanKammen, Siris, & Marder, 1978; Herz, 1984; Schneider, 1959). In these terms, the "psychotic resolution" is the person's attempt to assimilate these fragmented perceptions of self and other by constructing a new habitual self. Models for this new self "are usually based on global stereotypes, or organized delusions, with perhaps fragments of features and enact-

ual social self as social self in the rest of this chapter.

To obtain an inventory of the content of a person's social self, we use a ''free-response'' format that allows individuals to use their own vocabulary to describe the physical characteristics, the personality traits, the attitudes, the competencies, and so on that they habitually see in themselves and others. They are also asked to describe, in their own terms, how self and others make them feel. The advantages of this open-ended format over a fixed list of traits and feelings composed by an investigator are that the open-ended approach neither imposes conceptual categories that are not salient to the subject nor slights categories that are salient. Also, the open-ended format, although idiographic, offers no impediments to analyses that reveal nomothetic properties of social self.

George Kelly (1955) and other personal construct theorists since (e.g., Adams-Webber, 1979; Bannister & Mair, 1968; Bonarius, Holland, & Rosenberg, 1981; Mancuso & Adams-Webber, 1982) have long advocated free-response instruments to obtain and interpret a person's views of self and others. The rationale for such instruments and the way they are analyzed is to be found in the basic tenets of personal construct theory. The free-response instruments used by personal construct theorists are exemplified by the repertory grids methods originally devised by Kelly (1955), and the variations subsequently introduced by other investigators. The free-response methods described in this chapter for the study of social self, albeit different in format from the repertory grid, are consistent with Kelly's personal construct theory.

Classes and Patterns of Attributes

The attributes that a person variously associates with self and others can be summarized in a two-way matrix. The example

shown in Table 13.1 is of a hypothetical person who described self (''me'') and nine others using the seven attributes shown as columns. A cell entry of one means that the person attributed the content of the given column to the person in the given row. This hypothetical example, although miniature in size, illustrates certain key organizational features that are commonly found in real data.

First, the example in Table 13.1 illustrates some basic relationships among attributes. Note that *intelligent* and *articulate* go together in a person whether or not other attributes are also associated with the person. *Intelligent* and *articulate* are thus said to constitute a set or class of attributes. *Sad* and *shy* constitute another class for the same reason. An asymmetrical relationship also exists among certain classes of attributes; for example, the attribution of *intelligent* and *articulate* to a person implies *outgoing,* but not vice versa. *Outgoing* is in a class by itself.

Similar patterns exist among ego and alters. For example, Brother, Cousin, and Friend constitute a class of alters in that the person gives them all the same two attributes, *kind* and *outgoing,* and only these two attributes. Father is not in this class of alters but subsumes it in that he is also *kind* and *outgoing,* as well as having characteristics that they do not have. Mother also subsumes Brother, Cousin, and Friend. Still other such asymmetrical relationships exist in this example—that is, relationships where the attributes possessed by one person imply their presence in another person, but not vice versa.

A theoretical model (De Boeck & Rosenberg, 1988) and a computer-based algorithm (De Boeck, 1986) recently developed for analyzing two-way matrices make it possible to identify classes and the asymmetrical relations among them in large, empirically derived matrices of social self. A visual search for classes and the relations among them is generally not feasible in actual data matrices, matrices that inevitably also contain a certain amount of measurement error. The

ments from the premorbid identity.'' (Gara et al., 1987, p. 272).

Table 13.1. Hypothetical Example of a Persons × Attributes Matrix

Persons	Attributes						
	Intelligent	Articulate	Outgoing	Kind	Sad	Shy	Sensuous
Teacher	1	1	1				
Brother			1	1			
Girlfriend			1	1			1
Mother	1	1	1	1			
Cousin			1	1			
Friend			1	1			
Casual friend					1	1	1
Father			1	1	1	1	
Me	1	1	1	1	1	1	
Neighbor							1
Acquaintance					1	1	

algorithm is dubbed HICLAS (an acronym for *hi*erarchical *clas*ses).

Figure 13.1 is a graphic representation of the HICLAS analysis of the hypothetical example in Table 13.1. Four of the ego and alter classes are bottom classes in the hierarchy: Teacher; Brother, Cousin, Friend; Acquaintance; and Neighbor. The remaining classes are superordinate classes. A superordinate class is distinguished from a bottom class in that it subsumes two or more lower ordered classes. Any given arrow in Figure 13.1 denotes the fact that a lower class with the arrow leading to it is subsumed by all higher classes from which the arrow originates, either directly, or indirectly through another superordinate class.

There are several superordinate classes in this example. Me is a superordinate class that encompasses other superordinate classes, such as Mother and Father. Since Mother and Father, in turn, subsume the bottom classes containing Teacher, Brother, Cousin, Friend, and Acquaintance, Me also subsumes these bottom classes.

On the attribute side, there is only one superordinate class: *outgoing*. The other attributes are all in bottom classes. In actual data, the attribute structure can be as intricate as that for ego and alters.

The vertical zigzag lines connect attribute classes to ego and alter classes. I will use an example to interpret how the zigzag lines

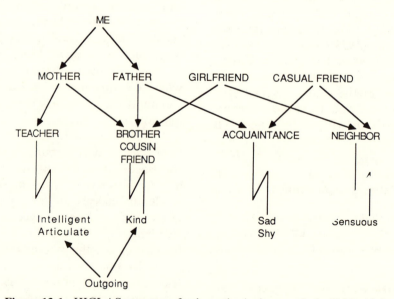

Figure 13.1. HICLAS structure for hypothetical example in Table 13.1.

connect attributes with people. The left arrow from *outgoing* points to *intelligent, articulate,* which then connect, via the leftmost zigzag line, to Teacher and its superordinates, Mother and Self. This tracing means that *intelligent, articulate,* and *outgoing* are associated with Teacher, Mother, and Self. This also corresponds to the cell entries in Table 13.1. In fact, Figure 13.1 is an exact model of all the data in Table 13.1, which is to say that it is possible to recreate Table 13.1 exactly from Figure 13.1.

Elaboration of Ego and Alters

What is the psychological significance of the location of ego and alters in a structure of hierarchical classes? To answer this question, I need to introduce the psychological concept of "elaboration" of an ego or alter element. Elaboration refers to the full set of ways in which such an element is habitually experienced. There are several indices of elaboration that are defined by the location of an element in a hierarchical structure.

One index of elaboration is the hierarchical level of the element in the structure. Thus, in the example, Me is highly elaborated in that it subsumes a number of alters in the structure. Another, related index of elaboration is the relative number of attribute classes associated with the element. This index can differentiate elements at the same hierarchical level. For example, by this index Father is more elaborated than Casual Friend in that Father has three attribute classes associated with him (kind; outgoing; sad, shy) and Casual Friend has two (sad, shy; sensuous). A third index of elaboration of an ego or alter element within a given hierarchical level is the number of other elements in its class; thus, members of a class that contains many elements are more elaborated than members of a class that contains few elements. For example, by this index elements in the bottom class consisting of Brother, Cousin, and Friend are more elaborated than elements in the other bottom classes. The hypothetical example was designed to be congruent with what one might intuitively expect: the more

elaborated elements of a person's social self are ego and the significant alters in the person's life.

The utility of these indices of elaboration was tested in an empirical study of a sample of college students in which ego and alters were classified as either elaborated or unelaborated (Gara, 1990). It was found that elaborated alters were the significant and important people in the subjects' lives, whereas unelaborated alters consisted of disliked or superficially known people. Of special interest was the finding that ego was elaborated in all but one of the college students in this study. These and other findings (Rosenberg, 1988, 1989) attest to the psychological significance of indices of elaboration as measured properties of a HICLAS structure.[2] We make extensive use of the various indices of elaboration that can be gleaned from a HICLAS structure in our studies of social self and identity in schizophrenia.

STUDY 1: SOCIAL SELF IN SCHIZOPHRENIA

Following Bleuler (1950/1911, p. 143), clinicians have observed that the fragmentation or loss of a sense of self is a salient feature of the phenomenology of schizophrenic patients. How does this loss of a sense of self show up in a mapping of the social self of a schizophrenic patient? Specifically, is ego less elaborated in a sample of schizophren-

2. The notion of a hierarchical set–theoretical organization among ego and alters and among their attributes has long been part of the theoretical discourse about social self, but theory-driven algorithms have been lacking (e.g., D'Andrade, 1976; Epstein, 1973; Kelly, 1955; Kihlstrom & Cantor, 1984; McCall & Simmons, 1966; Stryker & Serpe, 1982). Algorithms for hierarchical clustering, which is *not* a hierarchical classes model, have been available and have been used for some time now to cluster attributes in terms of their co-occurrence patterns in two-way matrices. Analogously, persons can also be clustered with hierarchical clustering in terms of attributes they do or do not share. However, these are not set-theoretical representations of the kind described in this paper because they are based on the simplifying assumption that the relation between any two attributes (or persons) is symmetrical, and this precludes the representation of a superset–subset relation between clusters.

Table 13.2. Demographic Data for the Two Groups and Chronicity Data for the Schizophrenic Subjects

	Average age	Average years education	Chronicity patient sample		
			Age of first hospitalization	Number of hospital admissions	Total months in hospital
Schizophrenic sample	25.5 (20–35)[a]	14.5 (13–18)	22.5 (18–33)	2 (0–6)	4.5 (0–26)
Normal sample	24.5 (20–29)	15.0 (13–18)	NA	NA	NA

[a] Range of individual values given in parentheses.

Reprinted with permission from Gara, M. A., Rosenberg, S., & Mueller, D. R. (1989). The perception of self and other in schizophrenia. *International Journal of Personal Construct Psychology, 2*, 253–270.

ics than in a comparable sample of normal subjects? Are there other features of the social self that differentiate schizophrenics from normals?

To answer these questions, a subset of patients from a dissertation study (Mueller, 1977) was selected for reanalysis (Gara et al., 1989). The selected patients were those that retrospectively met the criteria of the *Diagnostic and Statistical Manual of Mental Disorders,* third edition, revised (American Psychiatric Association, 1987) for schizophrenia. Eight (3 male, 5 female) of the 11 patients in the original study met these criteria—criteria more stringent than the New Haven Schizophrenia Index (Astrachan et al., 1972) used in the original study. At the time of the study, all the patients were in treatment either at the Community Mental Health Center of the (then) Rutgers Medical School or with a private psychiatrist, and all were taking antipsychotic medication. Data on social self were obtained from the patients after the acute psychotic phase had remitted.

Eleven normal control subjects (six male, five female) were recruited both from the staff of the Mental Health Center and from the college student population of Rutgers University. None of these subjects reported any history of severe psychopathology. Demographic data for the normal and schizophrenic samples and information about chronicity in the schizophrenic sample are summarized in Table 13.2.

Each subject was asked to describe 34 people from his or her life, including members of the nuclear family, significant members of the extended family, and nonfamily friends or acquaintances.[3] In addition, each subject described Me Now. A free-response vocabulary of attributes was obtained for each subject by first asking him or her to describe each of these persons with five to 10 traits. A composite list of traits, with duplicates removed, constituted the subject's free-response trait vocabulary. Similarly, a separate feeling vocabulary was constructed for each subject by first asking him or her to describe how each of the persons made him or her feel and then making a composite list of these feeling terms. Subjects then described Me Now and each of their 34 other people with their own composite trait vocabulary and their own composite feeling vocabulary. These descriptions yielded a two-way matrix of 35 persons by *a* attributes (traits and feelings). The number of attributes depended on how many terms a subject had generated. (The range of *a* for the schizophrenic sample was 74 to 139; that for the normal sample was 97 to 206.)

Before I describe overall differences be-

3. Laboratory studies of person perception using a free-response format (Rosenberg, 1977, p. 193) show that an individual's recurrent perceptual and affective categories in person perception are elicited in his or her description of 30 to 35 persons, when the majority of them are significant others. Moreover, the co-occurrence patterns among these categories as estimated from those 30 to 35 persons correlate at .90 with the co-occurrence patterns estimated from a sample almost triple that size. This information guided the selection of a parsimonious sample of others in the two laboratory studies described in this paper.

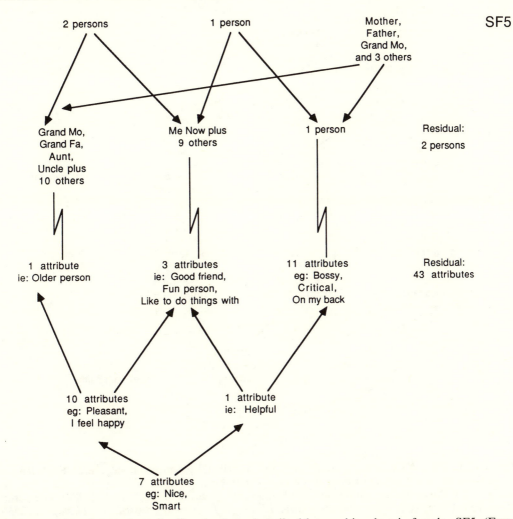

Figure 13.2. HICLAS structure of self and others described by a schizophrenic female, SF5. (From Rosenberg, S., & Gara, M. A. (1993). Disorders of self in schizophrenia. *European Review of Applied Psychology, 42,* 141–150. Based on data from Gara, M. A., Rosenberg, S., & Mueller, D. R. [1989]. The perception of self and other in schizophrenia. *International Journal of Personal Construct Psychology, 2,* 253–270.)

tween the two groups, it may be of interest to show the main features of the HICLAS structure for one of the schizophrenic patients and one of the normal controls.

Figure 13.2 represents the social self of a schizophrenic female (SF5) who described her ego and alter elements with 76 attributes (50 traits, 26 feelings). The subject in Figure 13.3 is a normal male (NM2) who described his ego and alters with 117 attributes (74 traits, 43 feelings). Because of space limitations and to permit the main features of the structure to be seen clearly, only a few representative trait and feeling terms in each

class are shown in the figures. However, the format in these figures is the same as that of the hypothetical example shown in Figure 13.1. That is, the upper part of each figure shows the ego and alter classes and the relationships among them; the lower part shows the trait and feeling classes and their relationships. The vertical zigzag lines connect attributes to people.

HICLAS also identifies ego and alter elements as "residuals" when and if the traits and feelings associated with them are thinly scattered across several classes, and hence cannot be placed reliably anywhere in the

NM2

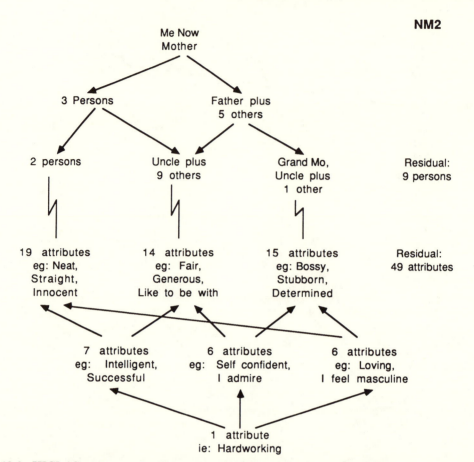

Figure 13.3. HICLAS structure of self and others described by a normal male, NM2. (From Rosenberg, S., & Gara, M. A. [1993]. Disorders of self in schizophrenia. *European Review of Applied Psychology*, *42*, 141–150. Based on data from Gara, M. A., Rosenberg, S., & Mueller, D. R. [1989]. The perception of self and other in schizophrenia. *International Journal of Personal Construct Psychology*, *2*, 253–270.)

structure. For SF5, two persons are "residual." (HICLAS also identifies traits and feelings as "residuals" when and if they are thinly scattered over ego and alter elements.)

The diagrams in Figures 13.2 and 13.3 summarize a considerable amount of information about the social self of each of the two persons. They reveal, for example, the degree of elaboration with which the subjects view various persons in their lives; with whom they identify and do not identify; which persons are liked, which are disliked, and which the subjects feel ambivalent about; and so on. However, the feature that is most relevant to this study is the relative location of Me Now.

For SF5, Me Now is in a bottom class. By

criteria established in studies of nonclinical populations for classifying elements as elaborated or unelaborated (Gara, 1990), Me Now and other members of this bottom class would be classified as unelaborated. In contrast, the location of Me Now in NM2's structure is in a superordinate class, along with Mother, both of whom would be classified as elaborated.

Half of the schizophrenic sample had an unelaborated Me Now, whereas none of the subjects in the normal sample had an unelaborated Me Now. The difference between the two groups is statistically significant (contingency $\chi_1^2 = 6.97$, $p < .01$). The extremely high ratio of elaborated Me Nows to unelaborated Me Nows in the normal sample (11:0) is apparently very reliable.

Earlier in the chapter, I cited another study of the social self of college students in which it was found that only one of the 14 students in that sample had an unelaborated Me Now (Gara, 1990). The second study to be described in this paper corroborates the reliability of the effect found for the schizophrenic sample in this study, albeit in a somewhat different way. As a methodological note, I should add that previous comparisons of the two groups in this study using hierarchical clustering (which is not a hierarchical classes model; see footnote 2) did not detect the differences just described (Mueller, 1977).

The finding that some schizophrenics have poorly elaborated views of themselves is consistent with the idea that a person with insufficient diversity in his or her self-concept may be at considerable risk for psychosis (Gara et al., 1987). That is, such a person can be viewed as having few psychological resources for handling challenges to self-definition that he or she may encounter in life. Self-fragmentation and conceptual disorganization may develop in such persons when interpersonal or other challenges to identity become especially intense. Additional studies are needed to probe into why some patients show this effect and others do not.

There are two other differences that we found between the two groups in this study. One is the overall goodness of fit of the structure—that is, how well the diagram can reproduce the actual data matrix.[4] A

structural representation with relatively high goodness of fit reflects relatively more regularity in the subject's assignment of a class of attributes, as a class, to self and others—or, in other words, it reflects social stereotypy. Structures from the schizophrenic sample averaged higher in goodness of fit than those from the normal group. This difference may be a labile one, however, depending on when social self data are obtained from a patient. If it were possible to obtain such data during an acute psychotic episode (and it may be, albeit with a different methodology), one would expect goodness of fit to drop dramatically to a level below that of normal subjects. A result consistent with this conjecture has been obtained using the Rep Grid (Bannister & Salmon, 1966; McPherson, Armstrong, & Heather, 1975).

Finally, another difference between the two groups in this study is in the average number of attributes they generated spontaneously (per se, a nonstructural variable). Schizophrenic patients generated fewer traits and feelings than did the normal controls. We do not give this variable much psychological significance. It may be that the difference between the two groups reflects an attention problem in the patients when describing self and others. We were concerned, however, that the differences we found for elaboration of ego and for goodness of fit were somehow a consequence of the difference in the number of attributes. Statistical analyses ruled out this possibility (Gara et al., 1989).

STUDY 2: THE IDENTITY SYSTEM

The idea that each of us has a number of social roles and that attached to each of these roles is a set of characteristics is a common one in psychology and sociology,

---

4. The HICLAS algorithm provides successive structures of increasing rank or dimensionality. Rank refers to the maximum number of bottom classes in the structure and is analogous to the "dimension" of the structure. For each rank, HICLAS calculates the goodness of fit of the structure—that is, how closely the structure represents the data matrix. In this study, structures of rank greater than 3 do not change the picture dramatically, although the goodness of fit (necessarily) continues to improve after rank 3, usually in very small increments.

For SF5 (Figure 13.2), the overall goodness of fit is 0.71, which means that this structure accounts for 71% of her attributes in the two-way matrix. For NM2 (Figure 13.3), the overall goodness of fit is .50. The structures in both figures are of rank 3. For the hypothetical example (Figure 13.1), the overall goodness of fit is 1.00—the structure accounts for 100% of the entries

in Table 13.1.

HICLAS also gives goodness of fit for each of the ego and alter elements. These values are not used in the present study. As an example, however, the goodness of fit of SF5's Mother is 0.79, which means that the location of Mother in her structure accounts for 79% of the trait and feeling attributions that SF5 made about her mother.

a notion readily traceable to James's (1890) social selves. That is, there are shared cultural beliefs about the attributes associated with social roles such as professor, mother, and daughter. Society also gives us other social identities, such as our nationality, ethnicity, religion, political affiliation, and mental health status.

At the psychological level, social roles and social identities are personal identities elaborated by each of us within seemingly broad societal constraints. It is these idiographic views that each of us has of the self in our various identities that are the subject matter of the second study. Moreover, our identities range beyond social roles and social identities to include idiosyncratic clusters of attributes not associated with any particular social role or social identity. That is, each of us also labels aspects of self in terms of our hobbies, our interests, our possessions, and so on. Identities such as "gourmet cook," "hiker," "owner of a Porsche," and "heavy smoker" may be highly elaborated in certain persons and illustrate something of the potpourri of tags with which persons label their identities.

In psychological terms, an identity is a subjectively experienced amalgam of personal characteristics, feelings, values, images, and intentions. The various identities of a person, their psychological content, and interrelationships are referred to as the person's identity structure. A person's identity structure is part of the person's social self—more specifically, it is a part of

ego, a substantial part. In effect, ego itself is a related set of elements, each labeled as one of the person's identities.

We were motivated to take a close look at the nature of identity structure in psychopathology by the results of the first study and by theoretical analyses—ours and others—in which serious disturbances of the ego are implicated in schizophrenia. The empirical methods for doing this were already at hand from our previous work on the social self. I will illustrate with an example.

Table 13.3 depicts a set of work-related identities of a hypothetical academic psychologist. The rows in Table 13.3 are the identities as this psychologist labeled them and the columns are seven of the attributes she variously associated with them. For example, she characterized herself as *demanding* and *articulate* when she thought of herself as an Undergraduate Teacher, as a Professor, and as a Psychologist, but not so in any other work-related identities.

The HICLAS analysis of this hypothetical example is shown in Figure 13.4. The identities are hierarchical, with Psychologist as the most elaborated identity, subsuming as it does Professor, Researcher, Undergraduate Teacher, Graduate Teacher, Reviewer, and Scholar. The psychological validity of representing a person's identity structure as hierarchical and of characterizing certain identities as more elaborated than others has been demonstrated in several diverse nonclinical popu-

Table 13.3. Hypothetical Example of the Identities × Attributes of an Academic Psychologist

	Demanding	Articulate	Interdisciplinary	Judgmental	Curious	Speculative	Prescient
Undergraduate teacher	1	1		1			
Graduate teacher			1	1			
Reviewer			1	1			
Scholar					1	1	
Professor	1	1	1	1			
Researcher		1		1	1	1	
Professional in community			1	1			1
Meditator					1	1	1
Psychologist	1	1	1	1	1	1	
Occultist							1

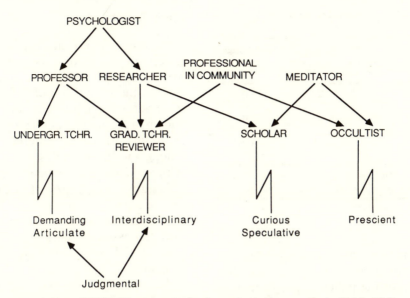

Figure 13.4. HICLAS structure for hypothetical example in Table 13.3.

lations, including professional women, retirees, and college students (Grubb, 1986; Joseph, 1985; Ogilvie, 1987; Rosenberg & Gara, 1985).

The study we devised is an investigation of the identity structure of a sample of schizophrenics (Robey et al., 1989). This study included as controls both a matched normal group and a clinically depressed group. Comparisons among the three groups focused on possible differences in degree of elaboration of the overall identity structure, as measured by the proportion of identities located in superordinate classes. Put another way, is the relatively unelaborated ego of some schizophrenic patients that we observed in the first study also present in another psychiatric group?

We also had another, intriguing question that motivated this study on identity structure. Elsewhere, we had theorized that a schizophrenic patient with a weakened ego is particularly vulnerable to developing a strong (i.e., elaborated) "patient identity." This patient identity now provides the person with a habitual view of self by which to assimilate everyday experiences of self (Gara et al., 1987). Paradoxically, then, we predicted that a strong patient identity, like any strong identity, would return the patient to a less psychotic level of functioning. The

question, then, is: Is the degree of elaboration of a patient identity positively correlated with an independent assessment of personal and social functioning?

Participant Characteristics and Methodology

The two clinical groups were inpatients either at the University of Medicine and Dentistry of New Jersey's Community Mental Health Center or at the Carrier Foundation. Both groups were on medication at the time of the study. The diagnosis of both clinical groups was based on the Research Diagnostic Criteria (Spitzer, Endicott, & Robins, 1975). The normal controls were a sample of evening-division students at Rutgers University, selected from this particular student population so as to be close in age to the patients. Demographic data for the three groups are summarized in Table 13.4.

Each subject was seen individually for several sessions. In the first session, a structured interview, the subject was asked to list as comprehensively as possible the sources of his or her identities by considering family relationships, other important interpersonal relationships (e.g., friends, coworkers, supervisors), occupational roles,

Table 13.4. Demographic Data for the Three Groups[a]

	No. of subjects	Average age	Average years education
Schizophrenic sample	10	27.0	13.0
Depressed sample	10	32.0	13.0
Normal sample	10	25.5	14.0

[a] Each sample contained an equal number of men and women.
Reprinted by permission from Roby, K. L., Cohen, B. D., & Gara, M. A. (1989). Self-structure in schizophrenia. *Journal of Abnormal Psychology, 98,* 436–442.

group affiliations, hobbies and interests, special personal physical conditions, ethnicity, and, for the patients, problems precipitating hospitalization. From this list of identities, the investigator selected the most important (as rated by the subject) for further description by the subject in subsequent sessions. Also included by the investigator in this list of identities were "myself as I usually am" and "my ideal self," and, for the patients, "myself as psychiatric patient." The total list of identities ranged in number from 15 to 21.

In the second session, a free-response vocabulary of attributes was devised for each subject by first asking him or her to describe self in each identity as fully as possible. When the identity to be described was self in relationship with another person, the identity was phrased so that it was clear to the subject that the referent was self and not the other person (e.g., "how I am with my father," "how I am with my mother"). A composite list of the 60 attributes most frequently used by a subject constituted that subject's vocabulary.

In subsequent sessions, each subject was asked to rate each identity with the 60 attributes. The resulting matrix of data (Identities × Attributes) was analyzed with HICLAS. The identity structure of one of the schizophrenic patients is shown in Figure 13.5. The figure shows all the identities in his protocol as well as all but the residual attributes he used to describe these identities.

Study Results

Comparisons were made among the three groups in the relative elaboration of their identity structure, using as an index of elaboration the proportion of identities located in superordinate classes. For the patient shown in Figure 13.5, this proportion is 0.31 (5 of 16). An overall difference was found among the groups ($F_{2,27} = 5.62$, $p<.01$), with schizophrenic patients showing a significantly lower degree of elaboration than that of normal subjects ($t_{18} = 2.71$, $p<.01$) or of depressed patients ($t_{18} = 3.01$, $p<.01$). The depressed patients show the same degree of elaboration as that of the normal subjects.

This result corroborates the basic finding from the first study—that is, that ego is relatively less elaborated among the schizophrenic patients when compared to a nonclinical group. The present study also reveals a similar finding when these patients are compared to another major psychiatric group. The data on which comparisons were based in this study are different and more substantial than those in the first study. In the first study, ego was represented by one globally phrased element, Me Now, and its elaboration was measured relative to alters. In the present study each subject's ego was represented by at least 15 separate identities, and the elaboration of the identity structure per se was used to compare the groups.

Is it possible that the significantly lower elaboration of identity structure in the schizophrenic group is simply part of a general "cognitive deficit" and not unique to self-perception? This question was anticipated in the original experimental design by scheduling separate sessions in which each subject described 10 persons they knew. The question of cognitive deficit, rephrased in terms of these data, is whether the alter structure shows the same pattern of differences in elaboration as the identity structure. The answer is an unambiguous no. That is, no significant differences in elaboration of alter structure attributable to diagnostic group were found. Moreover, the

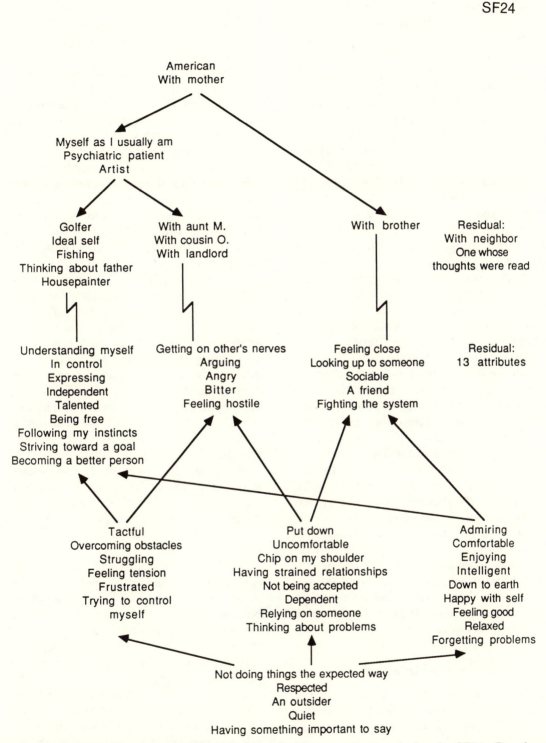

Figure 13.5. HICLAS structure of identities described by a schizophrenic female, SF24. (Based on data from Robey, K. L., Cohen, B. D., & Gara, M. A. [1989]. Self-structure in schizophrenia. *Journal of Abnormal Psychology, 98,* 436–442.)

mean elaboration of the alter structure in the schizophrenic sample fell in an intermediate position between the normals and the depressed patients.

The last finding I will present from this study addresses the question of whether the elaboration of the psychiatric patient identity is related to the patient's everyday functioning. Functioning was measured using the Global Assessment Scale (GAS) (Endicott, Spitzer, Fleiss, & Cohen, 1976).

The results are shown in Figure 13.6. The top scatterplot summarizes the results obtained from the schizophrenic group, and the bottom scatterplot the results from the depressed group. Each patient's rating on the GAS (horizontal axis) is plotted against the elaboration measure used for the patient identity (vertical axis). Low ratings on the GAS scale indicate limited personal and social functioning; the more normal the functioning, the higher the GAS rating.

The scatterplot for the schizophrenic group shows that, the more elaborated the patient identity, the more normal the rating of personal and social functioning. The correlation for this scatterplot is significant ($r_8 = 0.74$, $p < .01$). No such pattern can be seen in the scatterplot for the clinically depressed group. The correlation for the depressed group is not significant ($r_8 = 0.25$, $p < .10$). If we remove the outlier at the left of the plot for the depressed group (an apparent high suicidal risk), the correlation is further reduced ($r_7 = 0.08$, $p < .10$).[5] A recent replication with another sample of clinically depressed patients confirms the absence of a relationship between patient identity and personal and social functioning (M. Gara, personal communication).

Patient Identity in Schizophrenics

Why is there a difference between the schizophrenic patient and the depressed patient on the apparent role of the patient iden-

tity in psychological functioning? Social support for a psychiatric patient identity is certainly not limited to schizophrenic patients. The mental health system, for example, includes socially prescribed roles for clinicians, support staff, and patients alike, regardless of the psychiatric diagnosis. Indeed, a prescribed patient role is not unique to the mental health system. A patient identity that is supported by a variety of external sources may become elaborated by a person with a chronic illness, psychiatric or not. However, it is the psychiatric patient with rudimentary or fragmented identity resources for whom the patient identity is most likely to have a stabilizing effect. The study summarized above shows that it is the schizophrenic patient, but not the depressed patient, whose identity structure is less elaborated relative to that of normal subjects. Thus, a person undergoing a schizophrenic episode is vulnerable to incorporating the patient role into his or her personal identity, since any identity, however negative, serves to organize experience more effectively than does no identity (Erikson, 1956; Schafer, 1984). The patient identity is a "sick cure," as it were. Finally, the differences among schizophrenic patients in their development of a patient identity, and, hence, in their everyday functioning, may be an index of a more general difference among them in their ability to develop and maintain other stabilizing identities.

Medication may also play an important role in the development of a patient identity. Antipsychotic medication prevents schizophrenic relapse for two reasons that interact. First, antipsychotic medication per se inhibits psychosis, perhaps by selectively "turning down the volume" in the sensory pathways, thereby directly constricting the experiential field that the patient must sort out and organize conceptually. Antipsychotic medication also reduces motor output and thereby indirectly reduces the patient's experiential field. Second, the very real effects of antipsychotic medication become salient ingredients in the building of a patient identity. That is, certain medication

---

5. No significant correlations with GAS ratings were found for any of the other four identities present in or added to the identity list of all patients: "myself as I usually am," "my ideal self," "myself when I am with my mother," and "myself when I am with my father."

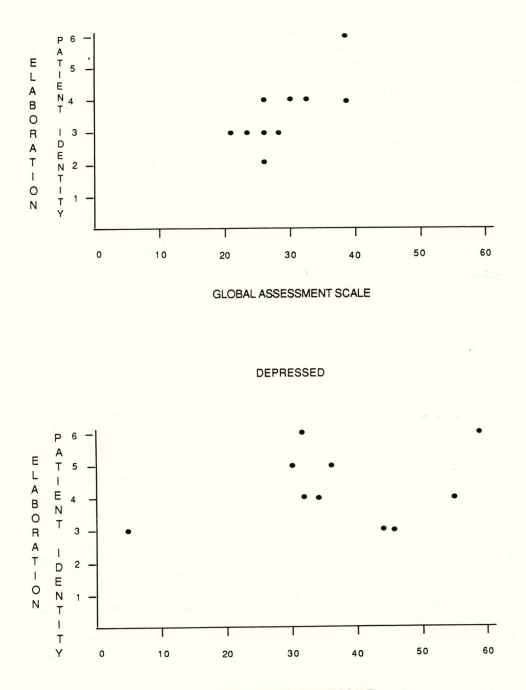

Figure 13.6. Scatterplot of identity structure versus Global Assessment Scale values for the schizophrenic sample and the depressed sample. (Based on data from Robey, K. L., Cohen, B. D., & Gara, M. A. [1989]. Self structure in schizophrenia. *Journal of Abnormal Psychology, 98,* 436–442.)

produces both a psychophysical and a purely psychological effect, both of which support a patient identity for a person whose major identities have been invalidated or for whom identities were diffuse to begin with. Thus, the specific effects of neuroleptics and their effects on identity combine to produce a total antipsychotic effect that is at least as great as the sum of these two separate effects.

There are several new and intriguing research questions that can be raised within this formulation. Do other psychoactive agents (e.g., antianxiety medications, antidepressants) fail to produce an antipsychotic effect because they lack certain neurobehavioral effects, and hence are not potent enough to shape an *elaborated* patient identity in schizophrenic patients? Do changes in the structural characteristics of the patient identity precede, follow, or accompany noncompliance with medication and the onset of psychotic symptoms? If the former, it may be possible to predict noncompliance and/or decompensation by measuring structural changes in identity over time. Can schizophrenic persons with identity resources beyond the patient self be safely taken off medication or have its dose substantially reduced if these resources are socially supported? These questions may be tractable using the empirical methods that have been described in this chapter.

CONCLUSIONS AND IMPLICATIONS

Within the present theoretical framework, the primary goal in the treatment of schizophrenia should be to foster the elaboration of new nonpatient identities and/or to transform invalidated or disowned identities to better suit life circumstances. Vocational rehabilitation, interpersonal skills training, family therapy, behavior therapy, and individual psychotherapy can make explicit the goal of building or rebuilding elaborated identities. Identity assessment techniques developed especially for clinical application may be useful for an identity-oriented approach to treatment and for evaluating outcome. The use of antipsychotic medication

probably makes psychological treatment more feasible and its goals more realizable than ever before. However, the analysis offered at the end of the previous section also suggests that medication has a role in shaping beliefs about self as patient, and therefore may warrant close monitoring.

The focus on the structure, functioning, and dysfunctioning of personal identity may also have merit in integrating a variety of important biological and genetic findings regarding schizophrenia. Most biologically based explanations of schizophrenia need clear theoretical links between the purported biological/genetic anomaly and the variety of specific behavioral symptoms that get the person diagnosed as schizophrenic in the first place (Haracz, 1985; Neale, Oltmanns & Harvey, 1985; Sarbin & Mancuso, 1980; Wing, 1978). Given that somatic deficits may, in many social contexts, profoundly retard the development of adequate identity resources, they are usually considered to be more fundamentally etiological in the development of the disorder. Nonetheless, the link to actual symptoms may be mediated, at least in part, by the social consequences of such somatic deficits for the anomolous development of personal identity.

In more general terms, constitutional features as well as elements in the social/interpersonal context recombine at each developmental phase to create new biological and social elements—including new features of personal identity—that then, in turn, help determine whether identity elaboration is promoted, obstructed, or unchanged in successive phases. The impact of a somatic anomaly on the beliefs and conduct of the person and significant others cannot be ascertained without knowledge of the community and of the interpersonal context in which that anomaly is embedded.

ACKNOWLEDGMENTS

This chapter was written while I was a Fellow in the Center for the Critical Analysis of Contemporary Culture, Rutgers University. I am grateful for the support provided by the Center in the writing of this paper. The research was supported in part by National Science Foundation Grant BNS-86-15937 to Seymour Rosenberg and in part by National Institute of Mental Health Grant MH42935 to Michael A. Gara. I also want to acknowledge Drs. Michael Gara, Bertram Cohen, and David Mueller, all of whom gave impetus to the application of social psychological theory and research to psychopathology. The expertise in schizophrenia that they shared with me did much to enhance my understanding of this disorder.

REFERENCES

Adams-Webber, J. R. (1979). *Personal construct theory*. New York: John Wiley & Sons.

American Psychiatric Association. (1987). *Diagnostic and statistical manual of mental disorders* (3rd ed., rev.). Washington, DC: American Psychiatric Press, Inc.

Astrachan, B. M., Harrow, M., Adler, D., Brauer, L., Schwartz, A., & Tucker, G. (1972). A checklist for the diagnosis of schizophrenia. *British Journal of Psychiatry, 121,* 529–539.

Baldwin, J. M. (1897). *Social and ethical interpretations in mental development*. New York: Macmillan. (Second edition reprinted 1973, New York: Arno Press)

Bannister, D., & Mair, J. M. M. (1968). *The evaluation of personal constructs*. London: Academic Press.

Bannister, D., & Salmon, P. (1966). Schizophrenic thought disorder: Specific or diffuse? *British Journal of Medical Psychology, 39,* 215–219.

Bleuler, E. (1950). *Dementia praecox, or the group of schizophrenias* (J. Zisk, Trans.). New York: International Universities Press. (Original work published 1911)

Bonarius, H., Holland, R., & Rosenberg, S. (Eds.). (1981). *Personal construct psychology: Recent advances in theory and practice*. London: Macmillian.

Breakwell, G. M. (1986). *Coping with threatened identities*. London: Methuen.

Cooley, C. H. (1902). *Human nature and the social order*. New York: Scribner's.

D'Andrade, R. G. (1976). A propositional analysis of the U.S. American beliefs about illness. In K. H. Basso & H. A. Selby (Eds.), *Meaning in anthropology* (pp. 155–180). Albuquerque: University of New Mexico Press.

De Boeck, P. (1986, October). *HICLAS Computer Program: Version 1.0*. Leuven, Belgium: Katholieke Universiteit Leuven, Psychology Department.

De Boeck, P., & Rosenberg, S. (1988). Hierarchical classes: Model and data analysis. *Psychometrika, 53,* 361–381.

Docherty, J. P., VanKammen, D. P., Siris, S. G., & Marder, S. R. (1978). Stages of onset of schizophrenic psychosis. *American Journal of Psychiatry, 135,* 420–426.

Endicott, J., Spitzer, R. L., Fleiss, J. L., & Cohen, J. (1976). The Global Assessment Scale: A procedure for measuring overall severity of psychiatric disturbance. *Archives of General Psychiatry, 33,* 766–771.

Epstein, S. (1973). The self-concept revisited: Or a theory of a theory. *American Psychologist, 28,* 404–416.

Erikson, E. H. (1956). The problem of ego identity. *Journal of the American Psychoanalytic Association, 4,* 56–121.

Gara, M. A. (1990). A set-theoretical model of person perception. *Multivariate Behavioral Research, 25,* 275–293.

Gara, M. A., Rosenberg, S., & Cohen, B. D. (1987). Personal identity and the schizophrenic process: An integration. *Psychiatry, 50,* 267–279.

Gara, M. A., Rosenberg, S., & Mueller, D. R. (1989). The perception of self and other in schizophrenia. *International Journal of Personal Construct Psychology, 2,* 253–270.

Grubb, P. D. (1986). *The self as a multiplicity: An empirical analysis of identity structure theory*. Unpublished doctoral dissertation, Rutgers University, New Brunswick, NJ.

Haracz, J. L. (1985). Neural plasticity in schizophrenia. *Schizophrenia Bulletin, 11,* 191–229.

Herz, M. I. (1984). Recognizing and preventing relapse in patients with schizophrenia. *Hospital and Community Psychiatry, 35,* 344–349.

James, W. (1890). *Principles of psychology*. New York: Holt.

Joseph, C. (1985). *Identity patterns of professional women*. Unpublished master's thesis, Rutgers University, New Brunswick, NJ.

Kelly, G. A. (1955). *The psychology of personal constructs*. New York: Norton.

Kihlstrom, J. F., & Cantor, N. (1984). Mental representations of the self. In L. Berkowitz (Ed.), *Advances in experimental social psychology* (Vol. 17, pp. 1–47). New York: Academic Press.

Laing, R. D. (1960). *The divided self*. London: Tavistock Publications.

Laing, R. D. (1961). *Self and others*. London: Tavistock Publications.

Mancuso, J. C., & Adams-Webber, J. R. (Eds.).

(1982). *The construing person.* New York: Praeger.

McCall, G. J., & Simmons, J. L. (1966). *Identities and interactions.* New York: Free Press.

McPherson, F. M., Armstrong, J., & Heather, B. B. (1975). Psychological construing "difficulty" and thought disorder. *British Journal of Medical Psychology, 48,* 303–315.

Mead, G. H. (1934). *Mind, self, and society.* Chicago: University of Chicago Press.

Mueller, D. R. (1977). *Parent-self and family-nonfamily differentiation in the person perceptions of good-premorbid schizophrenics.* Unpublished doctoral dissertation, Rutgers University, New Brunswick, NJ.

Neale, J. M., Oltmanns, T. F., & Harvey, P. D. (1985). The need to relate cognitive deficits to specific behavioral referents of schizophrenia. *Schizophrenia Bulletin, 11,* 286–291.

Ogilvie, D. M. (1987). Life satisfaction and identity structure in late middle-aged men and women. *Psychology and Aging, 2,* 217–224.

Robey, K. L., Cohen, B. D., & Gara, M. A. (1989). Self structure in schizophrenia. *Journal of Abnormal Psychology, 98,* 436–442.

Rosenberg, S. (1977). New approaches to the analysis of personal constructs in person perception. In J. K. Cole & A. W. Landfield (Eds.), *Nebraska symposium on motivation* (Vol. 24, pp. 174–242). Lincoln: University of Nebraska Press.

Rosenberg, S. (1988). Self and others: Studies in social personality and autobiography. In L. Berkowitz (Ed.), *Advances in experimental social psychology* (Vol. 21, pp. 57–95). New York: Academic Press.

Rosenberg, S. (1989). A study of personality in literary autobiography: An analysis of Thomas Wolfe's *Look Homeward, Angel. Journal of Personality and Social Psychology, 56,* 416–430.

Rosenberg, S., & Gara, M. A. (1985). The multiplicity of personal identity. In P. Shaver (Ed.), *Review of personality and social psychology* (Vol. 6, pp. 87–113). Beverly Hills, CA: Sage.

Rosenberg, S., & Gara, M. A. (1993). Disorders of self in schizophrenia. *European Review of Applied Psychology, 42,* 141–150.

Sarbin, T. R., & Mancuso, J. C. (1980). *Schizophrenia: Medical diagnosis or moral verdict?* New York: Pergamon.

Schafer, R. (1984). The pursuit of failure and the idealization of unhappiness. *American Psychologist, 39,* 398–405.

Schneider, K. (1959). *Clinical psychopathology.* New York: Grune & Stratton.

Spitzer, R. L., Endicott, J., & Robins, E. (1975). *Research Diagnostic Criteria (RDC).* New York: Biometrics Research, New York State Psychiatric Institute.

Stryker, S., & Serpe, R. T. (1982). Commitment, identity salience, and role behavior: Theory and research example. In W. Ickes & E. Knowles (Eds.), *Personality, roles and social behavior* (pp. 199–218). New York: Springer-Verlag.

Sullivan, H. S. (1924). Schizophrenia: Its conservative and malignant features. *American Journal of Psychiatry, 4,* 77–91.

Sullivan, H. S. (1953). *The interpersonal theory of psychiatry.* New York: Norton.

Wing, J. K. (1978). The social context of schizophrenia. *American Journal of Psychiatry, 135,* 1333–1339.

14

Deficit–Negative and Positive Symptoms During the Acute and Posthospital Phases of Schizophrenia: A Longitudinal Study

NEAL S. RUBIN AND MARTIN HARROW

The present longitudinal research seeks to further our understanding of the role of *deficit–negative* and *positive* symptoms in the lives of young adult schizophrenic and other psychiatric patients. The current follow-up study examines the *course* of symptomatology in the postacute, posthospital period of a large sample of early, young schizophrenic and other psychotic patients. Goals of this follow-up research program are to use longitudinal data on course and outcome to evaluate current theoretical proposals regarding etiology, diagnosis, and prognosis that are associated with the positive–negative symptom distinction.

Over the years, a variety of different views of schizophrenia have been proposed (Strauss, Carpenter, & Bartko, 1974; Wynne, Cromwell, & Matthysse, 1978; Zubin & Spring, 1977). Both recently and historically, theorists have sought the central elements and subtypes in the diagnosis of schizophrenia. At times in the past, the attention of both researchers and clinicians has been drawn to the most flagrant and dramatic symptoms—hallucinations, delusions, and formal thought disorder—as the principal components of schizophrenia. More recently, investigators' interests have shifted from these florid *reality distortions* or *positive symptoms* to the examination of *negative symptoms* associated with schizo-

phrenia, such as poverty of speech and flat affect, and *deficit–negative* symptoms such as psychomotor retardation and concrete thinking.

Hence there has been a transformation in conceptualizations of schizophrenia. After Kraepelin's (1919) seminal formulation of dementia praecox as an early-onset dementia marked by a deteriorating clinical course, deficit symptoms have been de-emphasized and positive symptoms have become pre-eminent in the definition of schizophrenia (Pogue-Geile & Zubin, 1988). Investigators have searched for signs pathognomonic of "nuclear" schizophrenia (Carpenter & Stephens, 1979). It has been proposed that a population of nuclear or "true" schizophrenic patients with an unremitting, downhill course may be distinguished from other psychotic or "schizophreniform" patients (Langfeldt, 1937; Schneider, 1959). Currently, negative symptoms are proposed to represent the persistent, stable constellation of symptoms that may cull nuclear schizophrenic patients from a larger population of psychiatric patients. Negative symptoms have become the most recent attempt to define specific symptoms pathognomonic of schizophrenia (Crow, 1980). This suggests that the study of deficit–negative symptoms has major implications both diagnostically and prognostically in the study of major mental disorders.

As a result, recent theorizing on schizophrenia has seen an increasingly pivotal role for negative and deficit–negative symptoms (Andreasen, 1979a, 1979b; Crow, 1980; Pogue-Geile & Harrow, 1985; Strauss et al., 1974). Major hypotheses about these symptoms propose that they are predictably stable and that they are associated prognostically with a deteriorating clinical course. In contrast, current hypotheses about positive symptoms predict a fluctuating clinical course and suggest that they are relatively unimportant prognostically (Andreasen & Olsen, 1982; Strauss et al., 1974). However, fundamental questions still remain regarding both the course of negative symptoms and the relationship between negative and positive symptoms in schizophrenia compared to other functional disorders (Andreasen, Flaum, Swayze, Tyrell, & Arndt, 1990). Research, and in particular longitudinal research, is essential in order to further knowledge on the course of negative and deficit symptoms.

Recent findings on the outcome of schizophrenia have also contributed to the increasing interest in negative symptoms. Modern investigators conducting systematic, longitudinal follow-up studies have raised questions about traditional concepts of a necessarily poor-outcome schizophrenia (M. Bleuler, 1978). Schizophrenia has been portrayed as having a multiplicity of courses, with investigators differing on whether the outcome of this disorder remains pessimistic (Harrow, Grinker, Silverstein, & Holzman, 1978). Schizophrenic outcome also has been described as overlapping with the types of outcome found in other disorders (Strauss & Carpenter, 1972, 1974, 1977). While these studies have contributed to enriching our understanding of the potential variability of outcome in schizophrenia and other major mental disorders, they concomitantly underscore the need to develop diagnostic criteria to distinguish Kraepelinian or nuclear schizophrenia from major affective and other psychotic disorders. Further longitudinal research on the

role of negative and positive symptoms in the course of patients' lives in the extended posthospital period would appear essential to addressing these major questions.

In order to examine proposals regarding deficit–negative and positive symptoms in schizophrenia, the present longitudinal follow-up study addressed the following empirical questions:

1. Do positive symptoms present during the acute, inpatient hospitalization diminish in the early postacute period?
2. Do deficit–negative symptoms tend to persist from the acute to the early postacute phase of disorder?
3. Do severe positive symptoms show traitlike characteristics, in terms of patients experiencing the most severe positive symptoms at index hospitalization, and continuing to experience the most severe positive symptoms when followed up 2 years later, during the postacute period?
4. Do deficit symptoms show traitlike characteristics, in terms of patients exhibiting the most severe deficits in performance during the acute phase, and continuing to experience the most severe deficits relative to other patients when followed up 2 years later, during the postacute period?
5. Do deficit–negative symptoms present in schizophrenics and in other psychotic patients after the acute phase (at a 2-year follow-up) diminish as these patients move even further from the acute phase to the extended posthospital period (i.e., when they are followed up 4 to 5 years after the acute phase of hospitalization)?
6. Does the severity of deficit–negative symptoms during the early postacute phase predict subsequent symptom severity at the second follow-up, approximately 2.5 years later, in the extended posthospital period?

METHOD

Sample Selection

The present research is part of the Chicago Followup Study, a multidisciplinary, prospective, longitudinal study of major mental disorders, focusing on negative symptoms, thought disorder, psychosis, and posthospital adjustment, being conducted at Michael Reese Hospital and Medical Center and the University of Illinois College of Medicine (Grinker & Harrow, 1987; Harrow, Carone, & Westermeyer, 1985; Harrow & Marengo, 1986; Pogue-Geile & Harrow, 1985; Rubin, Harrow, & Pogue-Geile, 1987). Subjects in the study (N = 189) were admissions to either a private hospital, Michael Reese Hospital (MRH) or to a public hospital, the Illinois State Psychiatric Institute. The patient population in the present research was diagnosed using Research Diagnostic Criteria, and is comprised of 62 schizophrenics, 55 other psychotic patients, and 72 depressed, nonpsychotic patients. The other psychotic patients included 24 manic patients, 22 psychotic depressive patients, and 9 patients with other types of psychotic disorders. The present research report is divided into two sections. The first part of the research report, assessing issues about positive and deficit–negative symptoms as patients emerged from the acute phase, is based on a subsample of 76 relatively early patients all of whom had either no or only one previous hospital admission. This subsample included 27 schizophrenics. The second part of the research report is based on the full sample of 189 patients. Diagnoses were based on a detailed interview summarized in the patients' charts, on the Schedule for Affective Disorders and Schizophrenia (SADS) (Spitzer & Endicott, 1978), and on the Schizophrenia State Interview, a semi-structured, tape-recorded interview (Grinker & Harrow, 1987). Patients diagnosed with schizoaffective disorders were not included in these studies because of current theoretical questions regarding whether these patients are part of the schizophrenic patient group or whether schizoaffectives represent another psychotic disorder, distinct from schizophrenia. Patients were selected for the present study if they consented to inpatient and follow-up interviews and if they did not exhibit organic brain dysfunction.

Following assessment at the acute, inpatient phase, patients were studied prospectively in a systematic manner. Two follow-up interviews were conducted over the following intervals. At approximately 2 years after index hospitalization, a first follow-up interview was conducted. A second follow-up interview was administered approximately 4.5 to 5 years after index hospitalization. As indicated earlier, the current report is divided into two parts. The first part of this research report presents results on the early course and potential changes in deficit-negative symptoms and positive symptoms for a subsample of 76 patients as they moved from the acute inpatient phase to the 2-year follow-up. The second part of the research report presents the results on deficit-negative symptoms for the larger sample of 189 patients as they moved from the 2-year follow-up (which can be seen as representing the early posthospital period) to the 4.5- to 5-year follow-up (which can be seen as representing a somewhat more extended posthospital period). The follow-up interviews consisted of the SADS; a series of cognitive and performance tests; a structured interview focusing on health, social, work, and family functioning; and several paper-and-pencil questionnaires. This comprehensive battery provides data to assess social, instrumental, and cognitive functioning, symptomatology, medication and other treatments, and rehospitalization rates.

The current sample is comprised of consecutive admissions, within a defined age range, who constitute a young, early-course group of patients. Age at index hospitalization ranged from 18 to 32 years. This made it possible to assess patients relatively early in the course of their disorder, prior to the potential effects of chronic treatment and years of dysfunctioning. Subjects were typically in their early course of illness, with 52% being first-admission patients.

At the first follow-up, the mean age for

this young, early-course sample was 25.1 years. Fifty-one percent of the patients were male and 72% of the patients had never been married. The mean number of years of education was 13.6. An estimate of intellectual functioning (age corrected, scaled), derived from the Information Subtest of the Wechsler Adult Intelligence Scale (WAIS) (Wechsler, 1955), was 11.6, which places the mean of this sample within the average range of intelligence. The subjects were predominantly Caucasian (78%). The mean parental social class as calculated by the Hollingshead–Redlich Two Factor Index of Social Position (Hollingshead & Redlich, 1958) was 3.0, which places this sample within the middle range of social classes. The mean duration of index hospitalization was 3.6 months.

Instruments

Framework for assessing deficit–negative symptoms. Negative symptoms in general have been defined as involving an absence of normal functioning, impoverished thinking or behavior, or a deficit or defect state (Chapman & Chapman, 1973; Fish, 1962). There are several different ways to assess such deficits. Frequently such deficits are assessed by careful behavioral observations, in situations in which the patient is being interviewed. Another traditional way of assessing deficit behavior is by performance in controlled test-taking situations. The present investigators have used both of these assessment techniques in previous research (Harrow, Marengo, Pogue-Geile, & Pawelski, 1987; Pogue-Geile & Harrow, 1984, 1985). In the present research we have measured patients' deficit–negative symptoms by their performance in a standardized testing situation. The following deficit–negative symptoms were assessed for each subject at each time period.

Concrete Thinking. One symptom area involving a potential deficit or loss of normal functions is the abstract–concrete dimension. The abstract–concrete dimension refers to the ability to generalize beyond a specific situation to a more general frame-

work. The lack of ability to abstract, or a deficit in this area, has been a central feature of a number of conceptualizations of schizophrenia (Benjamin, 1944; Harrow, Adler & Hanf, 1974; Vygotsky, 1962). Goldstein (1944) noted that concrete thinking represents the inability of a person to think independently of that which is superficial. In the instance of proverb interpretation, as used in this study, this deficit symptom would refer to a response using words and ideas literally contained in the proverb and a difficulty in moving beyond the specific stimuli and translating the phrase into a more symbolic, generalized form. In order to assess concrete thinking, the Gorham Proverbs test was administered and rated according to a scoring system utilized previously (Harrow et al., 1974; Marengo, Harrow, & Rogers, 1980). In this system each proverb is divided into two ''legs'' and each leg is rated as concrete, abstract, or abstract correct. On any one proverb, a concrete thinking score of 0, 1, or 2 is possible depending on whether the responses to neither, one, or both of the legs of the proverb are concrete. For example, when asked to interpret the proverb ''Don't swap horses when crossing a stream,'' one patient replied, ''The difficult times are not the time to lose faith.'' This interpretation, which is *not* concrete, received a score of 0 on concreteness because, while not necessarily correct, the response represents an abstraction regarding both legs of the proverb. A second patient replied, ''Because you might get wet.'' This interpretation received a score of 2 because the response to each leg of the proverb is concrete (Marengo et al., 1980). Therefore, an elevated score would be suggestive of a diminished ability to abstract. Satisfactory inter-rater reliability has been demonstrated on this scale for rating concreteness ($r = .95$).

Psychomotor Speed. The literature on ''defect states'' in schizophrenia identifies certain characteristic negative symptoms. European investigators (Crow, 1980; Huber, Gross, Schuttler, & Linz, 1980) have suggested loss of energy, direction, drive, initiative, and perseverance as significant components of the schizophrenic defect state. Psychomotor performance has been defined by many as one type of negative symptom, or deficit symptom. Investigations in the United States by Pogue-Geile and Harrow (1984), and by others, have indicated that psychomotor speed may be a sensitive index of deficit–negative symptoms. The performance measure of psychomotor speed we have used is the Digit Symbol Substitution Test (DSST) of the WAIS. Wechsler (1939) noted that, in addition to speed and accuracy, performance on this test is influenced by the individual's ability to concentrate, to apply himself or herself, and to persist in his or her effort. Overall, the DSST may be viewed as a measure of psychomotor speed and mental efficiency, and it appears to capture a type of negative symptom, or an aspect of the deficit or defect state, mentioned above. For the present study the DSST of the WAIS was administered to subjects at the acute phase during index hospitalization and at each follow-up under the standard conditions outlined by Wechsler (1955, 1981). Age-corrected, scaled scores on the Digit Symbol were computed. Scores on this measure that fell below the "low average" range of intelligence were considered indicative of substantial difficulty in psychomotor performance. Depressed psychomotor speed scores were viewed as suggestive of this type of deficit–negative symptom.

Framework for assessing positive symptoms.

Psychotic Symptoms. Florid psychotic symptoms (e.g., delusions and hallucinations) are viewed by almost everyone as among the cardinal positive symptoms (Strauss et al., 1974). Delusions and hallucinations were assessed during index hospitalization and in follow-up interviews with the SADS (Spitzer & Endicott, 1978). Each type of psychotic symptom in the current research was rated on a 3-point scale in which 1 = absence of symptom, 2 = weak or sporadic symptom, and 3 = definite presence of symptom (Harrow et al., 1985). Inquiries regarding specific types of delusions (persecutory, nihilistic, somatic, etc.) and hallucinations (auditory, visual, olfactory, etc.) were made with all subjects. Ratings were based on the presence or absence of the symptoms within the *month* prior to the interview. Other research of ours in this area has found satisfactory reliability for these ratings.

Positive Thought Disorder. The significance of bizarre–idiosyncratic thinking, or positive thought disorder, has received extensive attention (E. Bleuler, 1950; Harrow & Marengo, 1986). In the present study, positive formal thought disorder (Andreasen, 1979b; Fish, 1962) was indexed by a composite measure of bizarre–idiosyncratic thinking described previously (Harrow & Quinlan, 1985). Three separate measures of bizarre–idiosyncratic thinking were used: the Gorham Proverbs Test (Gorham, 1956), the Comprehension Subtest of the WAIS (Wechsler, 1955), and the Goldstein–Scheerer Object Sorting Test (Goldstein & Scheerer, 1941). A detailed scoring manual for bizarreness on the Proverbs Test and the WAIS is available (Marengo, Harrow, & Rogers, et al., 1980). The scoring system for the Object Sorting Test has also been detailed and is available (Harrow, Rattenbury, Marengo, & King, 1988). Interrater reliability for the scoring of this construct from these three tests ranges from .67 to .91. Assessment of the internal consistency of these measures has been demonstrated (e.g., a Cronbach Alpha of .87 for the scoring from the Gorham Proverbs). Significant intercorrelations among the three measures ranged from $r = .53$ to $r = .65$. The composite measure of positive thought disorder, utilized in this research, was derived from the highest or most pathological score on the three ratings. Utilizing this composite measure of positive thought disorder, diagnostic groups have been successfully differentiated in previous research (Harrow & Marengo, 1986; Harrow, Marengo, & McDonald, 1986; Harrow & Quinlan, 1985).

Table 14.1. Course of Positive Symptoms from the Acute Phase to the 2-Year Follow-up

Positive symptoms	Schizophrenic (n = 27)		Other-psychotic (n = 22)		Nonpsychotic depressed (n = 27)	
	Acute phase	2-Year follow-up	Acute phase	2-Year follow-up	Acute phase	2-Year follow-up
Psychosis[a] (percent)	88	56	77	14	11	18
Positive thought disorder (mean ± SD)	5.53 ± 6.27	3.50 ± 3.60	2.25 ± 2.94	1.80 ± 2.81	3.44 ± 2.84	2.12 ± 2.12

[a] Only full psychotic symptoms were included, with some of the other-psychotic patients only showing minor signs of psychosis anmd thus not included as fully psychotic.

RESULTS ON EARLY COURSE OF POSITIVE AND DEFICIT–NEGATIVE SYMPTOMS

Positive Symptoms

Table 14.1 presents the mean scores for positive symptoms for the acute phase and for the 2-year follow-up. Two-way analyses of variance (ANOVAS) (Diagnostic Group × Phase of Disorder or Time Period) were performed. The analyses indicated that the schizophrenics showed psychotic symptoms more frequently than the other diagnostic groups ($p<.05$). In addition, both hallucinations and delusions showed significant reductions (p values $<.05$) between the acute phase and the 2-year follow-up for the schizophrenic and for the other psychotic patients. In regard to the persistence or recurrence of psychosis, fewer of the schizophrenics tended to show a reduction in psychosis after the acute phase than the other psychotic patients.

A two-way repeated-measures ANOVA (Diagnostic Group × Phase of Disorder or Time Period) for positive thought disorder (bizarre–idiosyncratic thinking) indicated a significant main effect for diagnosis ($p<.05$). The means for all diagnostic groups showed a trend toward reduced thought disorder as patients emerged from the most acute phase of their disorder, although the effect did not reach statistical significance. These results are in general accord with other recent results of ours in this area (Harrow et al., 1986).

In summary, consistent with theoretical expectations, positive symptoms, or reality distortions, tended to show reductions after the more acute phase of hospitalization, with hallucinations and delusions declining significantly and positive thought disorder also showing a decline, although the results in this area were not significant.

Deficit–Negative Symptoms

Table 14.2 reports the mean scores on deficit–negative symptoms for each diagnostic group at the acute phase and at the 2-year follow-up. A repeated-measures ANOVA for concrete thinking revealed significant main effects for both diagnosis ($p<.05$) and phase of disorder or time period ($p<.001$). There was no significant interaction. The significant main effect for phase of disorder or time period was a consequence of a significant remission of concrete thinking for all groups as patients moved from the acute phase to the early posthospital period. Post hoc Newman–Keuls tests at follow-up found that schizophrenic patients showed significantly more concrete thinking than the nonpsychotic depressive patients ($p<.05$).

The results of the repeated-measures ANOVA for psychomotor retardation from index hospitalization to the first follow-up also showed significant main effects for both diagnosis ($p<.001$) and phase of disorder ($p<.001$). Again, there was no significant interaction. Each group improved significantly in their psychomotor speed performance. Schizophrenic patients exhibited significantly more psychomotor retardation than both the nonpsychotic de-

Table 14.2. Course of Deficit–Negative Symptoms from the Acute Phase to the 2-Year Follow-up

Deficit–negative symptoms	Schizophrenic (n = 27)				Other-psychotic (n = 22)				Nonpsychotic depressed (n = 27)			
	Acute phase		2-Year follow-up		Acute phase		2-Year follow-up		Acute phase		2-Year follow-up	
	Mean	SD	Mean	SD	Mean	SD	Mean	SD	Mean	SD	Mean	SD
Psychomotor speed[a]	7.17	(2.08)	8.59	(2.60)	9.56	(2.03)	11.10	(2.36)	10.41	(3.24)	11.37	(3.55)
Concrete thinking[b]	8.52	(7.71)	4.96	(6.10)	6.50	(5.88)	3.16	(4.54)	2.58	(2.94)	1.24	(1.96)

[a] Lower scores indicate poorer psychomotor performance.
[b] Higher scores indicate less rich (more concrete) thinking.

pressed and the other psychotic patients at follow-up according to post hoc Newman–Keuls analyses ($p<.05$). In summary, deficit–negative symptoms showed significant *improvement* in all groups as patients emerged from the acute phase. Although deficit–negative symptoms were generally more frequent in schizophrenic patients than other patient groups, their reduction after the acute phase occurred in *each* type of disorder, suggesting that factors associated with the acute phase have an influence in their appearance at that time.

Stability over Time

When the longitudinal data are viewed from one aspect, by comparing the symptom levels of the diagnostic groups at the acute phase with the levels at the 2-year follow-up, important results are found concerning the improvement, or even recovery from symptoms, for some patients after the acute phase. Seen from a different aspect, the longitudinal nature of symptoms may be further clarified by assessing the relative consistency of symptoms over time within individuals. Such an analysis would evaluate, for example, whether those schizophrenic patients who tend to have slower psychomotor speed at index hospitalization will continue to rank as relatively slow at the postacute period 2 years later, despite the overall improvement of mean scores for these patients.

Table 14.3 presents the Pearson product–moment correlations of acute phase versus 2-year follow-up scores for each positive and deficit–negative symptom for (a) the entire patient sample and (b) schizophrenic patients evaluated separately. When the total sample of patients is studied as a group, among positive symptoms only hallucinations are significantly associated from the acute phase to the 2-year follow-up ($p<.001$). In contrast, for the total sample, each deficit–negative symptom showed a significant correlation from index hospitalization to the postacute phase ($p<.001$). In addition, when the schizophrenics are studied separately, concrete thinking was stable across time ($p<.001$), and psychomotor speed was relatively stable across time ($p<.06$). Thus, when the issue of the stability of acute-phase symptoms for the sample as a whole is evaluated, deficit–negative symptoms do show relatively high stability over time. The picture is more mixed for

Table 14.3. Within-Person Stability of Symptom Status from the Acute Phase to the 2-Year Follow-up

	Combined patient sample (n = 76)	Schizophrenics only (n = 27)
Positive symptoms		
Delusions	.05	− .21
Hallucinations	.37***	.30
Positive thought disorder	.03	− .18
Deficit–negative symptoms		
Psychomotor speed	.65***	.33
Concrete thinking	.64***	.54***

[a] Pearson product–moment correlations; ***, $p < .001$.

psychotic symptoms, with acute-phase hallucinations showing stability over time but acute-phase delusions and thought disorders *not* showing such stability. When the schizophrenics were studied separately, the stability over time of their acute-phase deficit–negative symptoms was also greater than the stability of their acute-phase positive symptoms. For the schizophrenics, acute-phase hallucinations did not show a significant correlation with their scores at the 2-year follow-up, although there is a trend in that direction. Because the schizophrenic sample as a group tends to experience a considerable degree of psychotic symptoms at the acute phase, with all of these patients showing at least some psychotic symptoms at that point, the skewed nature of the data on psychotic symptoms for the schizophrenics would make a high correlation between *acute*-phase psychosis and later psychosis less likely.

Treatment Effects

Within group comparisons were also conducted for each positive and deficit–negative symptom at the 2-year follow-up in order to determine whether patients receiving medication, psychotherapy, or both, exhibited fewer symptoms at follow-up than those not receiving these treatment modalities. Results did not suggest a relationship between type of treatment and the level of symptomatology. Within both the schizophrenic and the major depressive (nonpsychotic) patient groups, no significant differences were found for the impact of treatment interventions. In general, the course of positive and deficit–negative symptoms in this patient sample does not appear to have been significantly related to these treatment interventions. However, caution should be employed in interpreting the efficacy of medication and psychotherapy, because patients were not assigned to these treatment conditions on a random basis, with poorer functioning patients often being assigned to particular treatments because of their clinical conditions. A study with random assignment of patients to different treatment conditions is desirable to assess these factors adequately.

Implications of Early Postacute-Phase Results

To date, there have been few empirical longitudinal studies of the key hypotheses concerning positive and deficit–negative symptoms in schizophrenia, despite their importance to theory about this disorder. Our results on these issues are consistent with theory concerning the tendency of positive symptoms to show a reduction as schizophrenics emerge from the acute phase. However, a number of schizophrenics still showed psychosis at the 2-year follow-up, although usually at a less flagrant and less intense level. The results are also consistent with theory in showing some degree of instability in positive symptoms as schizophrenics moved from the acute phase to the 2-year follow-up. Other results we have recently reported indicate more stability of positive symptoms during the more extended posthospital period for schizophrenics (Harrow & Marengo, 1986; Harrow et al., 1985).

Contrary to some views of schizophrenia, we found that deficit–negative symptoms also improved as these patients emerged from the acute phase. This result may imply that, in addition to the possibility of a schizophrenic defect state over time, acute-phase disturbance is also associated with deficit–negative symptoms during early stages of the disorder. Although some might have hypothesized that deficit–negative symptoms do not diminish after the acute phase in schizophrenia, the rate of reduction of two types of deficit–negative symptoms, concrete thinking, or impoverishment in cognitive–conceptual areas, and psychomotor deficits, was about equal for both schizophrenics and other disorders. As many would have predicted, these deficit–negative symptoms generally tended to be more frequent in schizophrenics than in patients with other types of psychotic disorders and in depressives. These deficit–negative symptoms were not specific to schizophrenia, appearing in all types of disorders. However, they were more frequent in schizophrenics both at the acute phase and at the 2-year follow-up.

Our findings in this first phase of the research are based on a young, early-course sample who were assessed at the acute phase and then reassessed 2 years after hospitalization. From this viewpoint, the reduction of deficit–negative symptoms that we found after the most acute phase could still be an aspect of a disease process that, when studied over a considerably longer period, will reveal further declines in performance and behavior, and a Kraepelinian course. This is an empirical question to be addressed in our longitudinal analyses to follow.

Although these deficit–negative symptoms tend to show a reduction after hospitalization, the within-person stability of deficit–negative symptoms was quite high, in contrast to positive symptoms. This means, for example, that patients who performed with very slow psychomotor speed at the acute phase were likely to improve their performance somewhat by the 2-year follow-up, but would nonetheless tend to perform slowly at that time relative to the other patients in the postacute period. This finding is consistent with theory, and could suggest that some types of deficit–negative symptoms may represent important, stable, traitlike features of schizophrenic patients both while hospitalized and during partial remission after hospital discharge.

These results raise several intriguing questions about deficit–negative symptoms and positive symptoms. The issues include questions about the course over time of deficit–negative symptoms. Among these issues are questions about (a) whether deficit–negative symptoms are stable over a longer period of time and persist into the more extended posthospital period for schizophrenics, and (b) whether schizophrenics continue to show a higher frequency of these symptoms over time than do other psychotic and nonpsychotic patients. The next phase of our research was designed to answer these questions with a more extended follow-up.

RESULTS FROM THE MORE EXTENDED POSTHOSPITAL PERIOD

The second phase of our research focused on the course of deficit–negative symptoms as patients moved from the 2-year follow-up to the extended posthospital period, 4.5 years after hospitalization. One of the goals of the second follow-up was to assess whether deficit–negative symptoms are stable over time or whether patients continue to improve over time as they move further from the acute phase. Our methodology remained parallel to that in the first phase of the research because our procedures involved assessment with the same instruments. We extended our patient sample for each diagnostic group in order to include a larger number of patients in our follow-up sample. Thus the patient population for this second phase of the research included the full sample of 189 patients outlined earlier in the method section. Comparisons of our samples in each phase of the research yielded no significant differences with respect to key sociodemographic factors.

A one-way ANOVA was used to assess group differences in deficit–negative symptoms across all diagnoses at each follow-up. We used the Newman–Keuls Test to analyze differences between diagnostic groups. To assess diagnostic differences in the prevalence of symptoms over time, chi-square analyses were used that compared the presence of symptoms across groups at each follow-up. The derivation of this index has been described previously. A rating of definite deficit symptoms refers to the presence of *severe* symptomatology.

Deficit–Negative Symptoms at the 2-Year Follow-up: Diagnostic Differences

Table 14.4 reports the data concerning whether schizophrenic patients tend to exhibit more deficit–negative symptoms than the other diagnostic groups at the 2-year follow-up. In the analysis (Table 14.4) of the

Table 14.4. Course of Deficit–Negative Symptoms from the 2-Year Follow-up to the Extended Posthospital Phase (4.5-Year Follow-up)

| Deficit–negative symptoms | Schizophrenic (n = 62) | | | | Other-psychotic (n = 55) | | | | Nonpsychotic depressed (n = 72) | | | |
| | 2-Year follow-up | | 4.5-Year follow-up | | 2-Year follow-up | | 4.5-Year follow-up | | 2-Year follow-up | | 4.5-Year follow-up | |
	Mean	SD	Mean	SD	Mean	SD	Mean	SD	Mean	SD	Mean	SD
Psychomotor speed[a]	9.0	(2.8)	9.5	(2.8)	10.6	(3.1)	11.1	(2.6)	12.2	(3.5)	12.0	(3.5)
Concrete thinking[b]	4.2	(5.5)	6.3	(6.8)	2.8	(3.6)	3.0	(4.5)	1.7	(2.5)	1.4	(2.7)

[a] Lower scores indicate poorer psychomotor performance.
[b] Higher scores indicate less rich (more concrete) thinking.

mean scores for symptom *severity* on psychomotor speed, the data indicated significant diagnostic differences ($p < .001$). An a posteriori analysis for diagnostic differences suggests that the performance of schizophrenic patients differed significantly from each of the other groups ($p < .05$). The other-psychotic patient group also exhibited slower psychomotor speed than the nonpsychotic depressed patient group.

Examining the data from a different aspect, in terms of the *prevalence* of slowed psychomotor speed, or the percentage of patients with psychomotor deficits, significant diagnostic differences emerged ($p < .001$). Forty-seven percent of the schizophrenic patients exhibited a deficit in psychomotor speed at the 2-year follow-up. Although a performance deficit was also found for a few select depressed, nonpsychotic patients (12%), the differences between the schizophrenics and the depressives were striking.

Looking at the other deficit symptom assessed, concrete thinking involving a cognitive–conceptual deficit, the results indicate diagnostic differences in symptom severity at the 2-year follow-up ($p < .05$). These results, derived from Table 14.4, indicate that schizophrenic patients exhibited more severe concrete thinking than other-psychotic and depressed patients ($p < .05$).

Again, looking at the data from a different aspect in terms of the percentage of patients with concrete thinking, significant diagnostic differences emerged ($p < .01$), with 33% of the schizophrenic patients exhibiting concrete thinking at the 2-year follow-up. The sample of nonschizophrenic patients

who exhibited psychotic symptoms at index hospitalization also included a higher percentage of patients with concrete thinking at the 2-year follow-up than did the nonpsychotic depressives. Only select nonpsychotic depressed patients (10%) showed this type of deficit symptom. Thus, although there is evidence of this symptom among occasional depressed patients, this type of deficit symptom was relatively infrequent among the nonpsychotic depressives at the 2-year follow-up. It was only slightly more in evidence among the nonpsychotic depressives than would be expected among a population of normal subjects.

The above results are interesting in light of questions about the specificity of deficit symptoms to schizophrenia. The data indicate that, at the first, 2-year follow-up, deficit–negative symptoms are more severe and prevalent among schizophrenic patients. However, there is also evidence of these symptoms among other-psychotic patients and to a lesser degree in select nonpsychotic, depressed patients. Therefore, it will be of interest in analyzing symptom status at the second, 4.5-year follow-up to see whether deficit symptoms continue to show reductions over time in the nonschizophrenic patients, and especially in the nonpsychotic depressives. Such results may indicate that these symptoms become even more specific to schizophrenia over time.

Deficit–Negative Symptoms at the 4.5-Year Follow-up

The results from Table 14.4 indicate that the higher prevalence of poorer psychomotor functioning that was found among schizophrenic patients at the 2-year follow-up was also found among this diagnostic group at the 4.5-year follow-up. The data from both the schizophrenics and the other-psychotic patients indicate a slight improvement in psychomotor functioning as these patients moved from the 2-year to the 4.5-year follow-up. Whereas 34% of the nonschizophrenic psychotic patients showed deficits at the 2-year follow-up, only 16% showed a deficit in this area at the 4.5-year follow-up. The nonpsychotic patients, who had shown less difficulty in psychomotor speed at the 2-year follow-up than the other groups, again did not show much difficulty in this area at the 4.5-year follow-up.

The results for the other deficit symptom assessed, concrete thinking, are also presented in Table 14.4. These results indicate that, at the 4.5-year follow-up, the schizophrenics were significantly more concrete in their thought processes than the other diagnostic groups ($p<.05$). In addition, there was also a trend for more concrete thinking by the schizophrenics at the 4.5-year follow-up than they had shown at the 2-year follow-up.

Overall, the results on concrete thinking can be applied to theoretical formulations regarding deficit and negative symptoms. Theory regarding deficit symptoms has proposed that these symptoms are a characteristic of many or all schizophrenics and that they are associated with poor overall functioning and possibly even a Kraepelinian course. The current data indicating a trend toward increased concrete thinking in schizophrenics at the 4.5-year follow-up

suggest the possibility of a decline in performance that is linked to difficulty with cognitive processes for schizophrenics. The results might suggest that concrete thinking would play an important role as an aspect of poor outcome or even nuclear schizophrenia. These results will have to be further clarified by investigating additional changes over time for the schizophrenics.

Stability of Individual Differences in Symptoms over Time

Whereas some symptoms show a limited reduction from the postacute to the more extended posthospital period, the longitudinal nature of symptoms may be further clarified by assessing the relative consistency or stability of symptoms over time within individuals. Such an analysis would evaluate, for example, whether schizophrenic patients who perform with severely slowed psychomotor speed at the 2-year follow-up will continue, 2.5 years later, to rank as relatively slow. Table 14.5 presents correlations for each deficit–negative symptom over time.

The results in Table 14.5 provide evidence of the stability of individual differences in deficit–negative symptoms over time. The correlation for psychomotor speed scores over time is strongly positive and consistent when looking at the scores of the entire patient population ($p<.001$). Table 14.5 also presents the correlation coefficients among schizophrenic patients only. These results indicate the stability of psychomotor speed performance over time for the schizophrenics ($p<.001$).

Separate analyses of the other two patient groups also follow this pattern of strongly positive and consistent correlations at each time comparison ($p<.001$). These results suggest that individual differences in psychomotor speed performance are relatively stable across follow-ups in the entire patient sample and in each diagnostic group. Those schizophrenics who show this deficit at the 2-year follow-up continue to show the deficit at the 4.5-year follow-up. Thus, in spite of any improvement in performance over

Table 14.5. Within-Person Stability of Deficit-Negative Symptom Status from the 2-Year Follow-up to the Extended Posthospital Phase (4.5-Year Follow-up)[a]

	Combined patient sample ($n = 189$)	Schizophrenics only ($n = 62$)
Psychomotor speed	.79***	.79***
Concrete thinking	.47***	.63***

[a] Pearson product–moment correlations; ***, $p < .001$.

time, most patients who exhibited severely slowed psychomotor speed at the 2-year follow-up continued to perform slowly relative to others in their group and in the combined group sample at the 4.5-year follow-up.

Results for the deficit symptom concrete thinking also indicate some stability over time of individual differences. Correlations at each time comparison for concrete thinking are positive and significant for the entire sample and within the schizophrenic patient group ($p<.001$) (Table 14.5). Unlike the results for slowed psychomotor speed, this pattern of results did not hold for the other two patient groups. Thus, the correlations for concrete thinking from the 2-year to the 4.5-year follow-up did not reach significance in the other-psychotic group or in the sample of nonpsychotic depressives. Overall, in regard to concrete thinking, the three patient groups did not improve as they moved from the 2-year to the 4.5-year follow-up, and the schizophrenics even showed a tendency to become more concrete over time.

In this sample, the relative stability of individual differences for both types of deficit symptoms during the extended posthospital period is consistent with some theoretical expectations. For the schizophrenics, both types of deficit–negative symptoms appear stable regardless of whether they persist or show some reduction over time. This pattern holds for psychomotor speed in the other patient groups as well.

These results need to be considered in relationship to the relative persistence of symptomatology. Schizophrenic patients improved as they emerged from the most acute phase. After these patients emerged from the most acute phase, there were no further significant reductions in symptoms status. There did appear to be significant stability in the severity of their deficit symptoms. This overall pattern suggests that for schizophrenics there is persistence and stability for these symptoms in the posthospital period. Those schizophrenics who showed deficits in each of the two areas assessed at the 2-year follow-up continued to show the deficits 2.5 years later. When these results

are combined with the data presented earlier indicating relatively high correlations between scores at the acute phase and scores at the first, 2-year follow-up, our results would indicate strong traitlike characteristics for the schizophrenics for both deficit symptoms assessed. The characteristics of these symptoms fit some theoretical proposals regarding the nature of the course of deficit–negative symptoms.

DISCUSSION

The results would appear to support recent calls for a critical reappraisal of fundamental theoretical proposals regarding positive and negative symptoms and their role in schizophrenia (Andreasen et al., 1990). Since the time over 15 years ago when Strauss and colleagues (1974) proposed this avenue of research, there has been an increasing momentum to come to a better understanding of the implications of the positive versus negative symptom distinction both theoretically, in terms of the etiology of schizophrenia (Crow, 1980), and clinically, in terms of the treatment choices associated with the schizophrenias (Carpenter, Heinrichs, & Wagman, 1988). In some respects, the results of the current investigation on the course of deficit–negative and positive symptoms during the acute period and during the posthospital lives of early-course, young adult schizophrenic patients are consistent with aspects of emerging theory. At the same time, in other areas, our current research raises questions about theoretical assumptions regarding positive and deficit–negative symptoms. The following discussion summarizes some of these trends.

Positive Symptoms: Do They Persist during the Early Posthospital Phase?

Our initial investigation focused on a subsample of our larger follow-up sample (those with only one or no previous hospitalizations) in order to assess symptom status during the early postacute period, from index hospitalization to a first follow-up approximately 2 years later. Results regarding positive psychotic symptoms indicated a significant reduction from acute hospitalization to the first follow-up. This pattern of change in symptom status was found among both schizophrenic patients and other nonschizophrenic patients who were psychotic at the time of index hospitalization. Given that traditional theory proposes that positive symptoms improve after the most acute phase, these results during the early postacute hospital period would appear to support this aspect of theory.

In regard to our data on positive symptoms, and the overall reduction as patients emerged from the most acute phase, a number of theorists have proposed that positive symptoms fluctuate over time. However, some have gone one step further. Thus it has been proposed that schizophrenics are *vulnerable* to episodes, and that in between these episodes they return to their premorbid state (Zubin & Spring, 1977).

The current data on positive symptoms are not in agreement with this type of vulnerability formulation. For schizophrenics, the results show a significant decline in psychoses after the most acute phase, and indicate that some schizophrenics show no overt signs of psychosis after they emerge from the acute period and enter into the posthospital period, whereas others (over 50% of the current sample) show clear signs of psychosis during this period. In this respect, although not all schizophrenics show persistent psychosis, a substantial percentage show at least some persistence. Among those schizophrenics whose psychosis persisted into the posthospital period, it was our impression that their psychosis was less flagrant than it had been during the more acute period of hospitalization.

Overall, in regard to positive symptoms, the data on psychosis for the present sample of schizophrenics do not fit Zubin and Spring's vulnerability theory of schizophrenia. The current data could be viewed as fitting a theory in which schizophrenics are vulnerable not just to episodes of psychosis, but rather to persisting psychosis, although in less flagrant form than at the acute phase, for at least a moderate percentage of the

schizophrenics. An alternate, but related, view would be in terms of active versus inactive phases of psychosis, rather than only of acute versus nonacute phases. In this view, an active phase of psychosis could consist of either (a) flagrant acute episodes, or (b) for some schizophrenics, less flagrant but still active periods of psychoses, or of reality distortions, with these periods of psychosis or reality distortions lasting for some time.

In addition, the data for the other psychotic patients also should be considered. These data would suggest that schizophrenics are not the only patients who show signs of psychosis after the most acute phase of hospitalization. There was a significant overall decline in psychosis after the acute phase for the other psychotic patients, and *fewer of these patients* than the schizophrenics showed evidence of psychosis during the posthospital period. However, a small subgroup of other psychotic patients showed at least some signs of psychosis during the posthospital phase. The great majority of these other psychotics had concurrent affective syndromes at the *acute* phase of hospitalization. A key issue for these patients is whether their posthospital psychosis is associated with new episodes of disorder, perhaps affective disorder, or whether it is persistent over time. The data indicating such a subgroup of other psychotic patients with posthospital psychosis clearly show that their acute-phase psychosis is not just a one-time event. Rather, these are patients who are vulnerable either to subsequent psychosis or to subsequent more general disorders in which psychosis is often one component of their illness. It would seem important that there be further study of these other psychotic patients with regard to subsequent psychosis in future follow-ups to investigate both (a) whether their subsequent psychosis is persistent or recurrent and (b) what other features accompany their psychoses.

Deficit—Negative Symptoms: Do They Persist over Time?

Our results with regard to deficit—negative symptoms did not fit some aspects of current theory. First, deficit–negative symptoms were not specific to schizophrenia. These deficit symptoms were more frequent among schizophrenic patients, but were also present among other psychotic and depressed, nonpsychotic patients. Second, we also found a significant remission of deficit–negative symptoms in each diagnostic group during the first 2 years after index hospitalization. These results are not in accord with some theoretical expectations. They raise several questions with regard to why deficit symptom status would change over time. Most prominent among these questions is whether the presence of prominent deficit symptoms for these patients represents a by-product of acute psychopathological turmoil or whether their performance deficits are best characterized as traitlike features of their life functioning.

One avenue we explored to address this conceptual dilemma was to investigate the within-person stability of positive and deficit–negative symptoms between index hospitalization and the first, 2-year follow-up. Our results were consistent with theory. Thus, deficit–negative symptoms correlated significantly over time within the combined patient sample and showed relatively high correlations over time for the schizophrenic patient group when analyzed separately. Seen from one viewpoint, during the early postacute phase, patients exhibiting severe deficits in performance at the acute phase may improve their performance as they emerge from this phase of disorder. However, these patients with more severe deficits at the acute phase will nevertheless remain more severe 2 years later relative to other patients. The results lend support to proposals that these deficits are traitlike phenomena that will characterize a patient's functioning over a long period, or over the course of their disorder.

Given our findings regarding deficit–negative symptoms showing some reduction or some remission after the acute phase of hospitalization, we also embarked on a second avenue of exploring the course of deficit symptoms over time. Patients were administered a second follow-up interview 4.5 years after their index hospitalization. We were particularly interested to examine whether the remission of deficit–negative symptoms in the early postacute period continued through the extended posthospital phase.

Our results were more consistent with theoretical expectations in that, among our follow-up sample, deficit symptoms tended to persist from the first to the second follow-up interview. As schizophrenic and other formerly psychotic patients move further from the acute phase of their disorder, deficit–negative symptoms do not continue to diminish in the way that they had diminished as patients emerged from the acute phase and entered the first 2 years of the posthospital phase. This suggests that, for those patients whose deficits do not diminish within a year or two after hospitalization, the probability increases that these deficits will remain as an aspect of their posthospital adjustment. In addition, the results regarding the within-person stability of deficit symptoms, as patients moved from the first to the second follow-up, paralleled the results obtained earlier as patients emerged from the acute phase. Patients experiencing more severe psychopathology in this area tend to continue experiencing more severe problems (relative to other patients) over time. Overall, at least two factors representing both statelike and traitlike features appear salient to understanding the onset and longitudinal course of deficit symptoms over time.

A Two-Factor Formulation Regarding Deficit–Negative Symptoms

Theoretical views regarding positive and deficit–negative symptoms have attempted to shed light on the characteristic distinctions between these symptom types. Our findings indicate that a by-product of these efforts could have been the creation of constructs that may be inaccurately unidimensional within themselves. For example, with regard to deficit–negative symptoms, at least two factors appear to have emerged from our research that contribute to the onset and course of these symptoms in the lives of the patients we have assessed from the acute phase of index hospitalization to a period approximately 4.5 to 5 years later. These two factors, representing statelike features and traitlike features, may operate independently or may interact in such a way that they find expression in these forms of psychopathology.

Our results indicating a diminishing of deficit symptoms among schizophrenic and other patients during the early postacute period raised the possibility that some deficits in certain patients may result from or be a product or by-product of the tumultuousness of an acute period of disorder. This would involve *statelike* features that are in operation in regard to deficit—negative symptoms. Thus, some components of the deficits in performance may be viewed as reactions to other aspects of acute turmoil, and especially to acute psychosis. A reduction in deficit symptoms as patients emerged from the acute phase was true for the nonpsychotic patients as well as the schizophrenics and other psychotic patients. Thus, the data indicating improvement for the nonpsychotic patients would suggest that the major factor during the acute phase is not *just* psychosis, but includes other factors common to the acute phase experienced by a wide range of patients. These features have been enumerated in detail (Harrow & Quinlan, 1985) and include such features of acute disturbance as cognitive arousal, several emotional turmoil, and increased emotional intensity, factors that are present in acutely disturbed psychotic as well as nonpsychotic patients.

Our data reveal the longitudinal severity of deficit symptoms, and the tendency for deficit symptoms to show a relatively high correlation over time, persisting in many of the patients in our follow-up sample. These results suggest the likelihood that there are also *traitlike* features that are influential in their symptom picture. In other words, these deficits are not *just* temporary products of the acute phase; rather, they may be characteristic of individuals who are vulnerable to other forms of severe psychopathol-

ogy. These traitlike features may be present for many years, and possibly, for some schizophrenics, throughout the rest of their lives.

Evaluated from a different viewpoint, the data indicate more psychopathological scores for the *schizophrenics* on these two deficit symptoms at both the most acute phase and the two successive posthospital assessments. Neither these deficit symptoms nor any other symptoms are unique to schizophrenia alone. These deficit symptoms cut across a wide variety of different types of disorders. However, the schizophrenics' more pathological scores on these deficit symptoms, especially at the acute phase, would indicate the importance of disorder-specific factors, such as the presence of schizophrenia, with the schizophrenic disorder being linked to statelike factors, some of which persist over time in a traitlike manner.

Additional support for this two-factor hypothesis will be sought in our ongoing longitudinal studies. Further longitudinal studies not only of the course of symptomatology but also of the prognostic utility of these symptom categories in relation to diverse aspects of life functioning would appear important for helping to clarify emerging theoretical models of schizophrenic psychopathology.

ACKNOWLEDGMENTS

This research was supported in part by grant MH26341 from the National Institute of Mental Health, Bethesda, MD, and by research grants from the John D. and Catherine T. MacArthur Foundation, and from the Four Winds Research Fund.

REFERENCES

Andreasen, N. C. (1979a). Affective flattening and the criteria for schizophrenia. *American Journal of Psychiatry, 36,* 944–946.
Andreasen, N. C. (1979b). The clinical assessment of thought, language, and communication disorders: I. The definition of terms and

evaluation of their reliability. *Archives of General Psychiatry, 36,* 1315–1321.

Andreasen, N. C., Flaum, M., Swayze, V. W., Tyrell, G., & Arndt, S. (1990). Positive and negative symptoms in schizophrenia: A critical reappraisal. *Archives of General Psychiatry, 47,* 615–621.

Andreasen, N. C., & Olsen, S. (1982). Negative vs. positive schizophrenia. *Archives of General Psychiatry, 39,* 789–794.

Benjamin, J. D. (1944). A method for distinguishing and evaluating formal thinking disorders in schizophrenia. In J. S. Kasanin (Ed.), *Language and thought in schizophrenia* (pp. 65–90). New York: John Wiley & Sons.

Bleuler, E. (1950). *Dementia praecox, or the group of schizophrenias* (J. Zisk, Trans.). New York: International Universities Press. (Original work published 1911)

Bleuler, M. (1978). *The schizophrenic disorders: Long-term patient and family studies* (S. M. Clemens, Trans.). New Haven, CT: Yale University Press.

Carpenter, W. T., Heinrichs, P. W., & Wagman, A. M. I. (1988). Deficit and nondeficit forms of schizophrenia: The concept. *American Journal of Psychiatry, 145,* 578–583.

Carpenter, W. T., & Stephens, J. H. (1979). An attempted integration of information relevant to schizophrenic subtypes. *Schizophrenia Bulletin, 5,* 490–506.

Chapman, L. J., & Chapman, J. P. (1973). *Disordered thought in schizophrenia.* New York: Appleton-Century-Crofts.

Crow, T. (1980). Molecular pathology of schizophrenia: More than one disease process? *British Medical Journal, 280,* 1–9.

Fish, F. J. (1962). *Schizophrenia.* Baltimore: Williams & Wilkins.

Goldstein, K. (1944). Methodological approach to the study of schizophrenic thought disorder. In J. S. Kasanin (Ed.), *Language and thought in schizophrenia.* New York: W. W. Norton.

Goldstein, K., & Scheerer, M. (1941). Abstract and concrete behavior, experimental study with special tests. *Psychological Monographs, 53.*

Gorham, D. R. (1956). *Clinical manual for the Proverbs Test.* Missoula, MT: Psychological Test Specialists.

Grinker, R. R., Sr. & Harrow, M. (Eds.). (1987). *A multi-dimensional approach to clinical research in schizophrenia.* Springfield, IL: Charles C. Thomas.

Harrow, M., Adler, D., & Hanf, E. (1974). Abstract and concrete thinking in schizophrenia during the prechronic phases. *Archives of General Psychiatry, 31,* 27–33.

Harrow, M., Carone, B. J., & Westermeyer, J. F. (1985). The course of psychosis in early

phases of schizophrenia. *American Journal of Psychiatry, 142,* 702–707.

Harrow, M., Grinker, R., Silverstein, M., & Holzman, P. (1978). Is modern day schizophrenic outcome still negative? *American Journal of Psychiatry, 135,* 1156–1162.

Harrow, M., & Marengo, J. T. (1986). Schizophrenic thought disorder at followup: Its persistence and prognostic significance. *Schizophrenia Bulletin, 12,* 373–393.

Harrow, M., Marengo, J., & McDonald, C. (1986). The early course of schizophrenic thought disorder. *Schizophrenia Bulletin, 12,* 208–224.

Harrow, M., Rattenbury, F. R., Marengo, J., & King, G. (1988). A manual to assess positive thought disorder using the object sorting test. Unpublished manuscript.

Harrow, M., Marengo, J., Pogue-Geile, M. F., & Pawelski, T. J. (1987). Schizophrenic deficits in intelligence and abstract thinking: Influence of aging and long-term institutionalization. In N. Miller (Ed.), *Schizophrenia, paranoia and schizophreniform disorders in later life* (pp. 133–144). New York: Guilford Press.

Harrow, M., & Quinlan, D. (1985). *Disordered thinking and schizophrenic psychopathology.* New York: Gardner Press.

Hollingshead, A. B., & Redlich, F. C. (1958). *Social class and mental illness.* New York: John Wiley & Sons.

Huber, G., Gross, G., Schuttler, R., & Linz, M. (1980). Longitudinal studies of psychiatric patients. *Schizophrenia Bulletin, 6,* 595–605.

Kraepelin, E. (1919). *Dementia praecox and paraphrenia* (R. M. Barclay, Trans.), G. M. Robertson, Ed.). Edinburgh: E. S. Livingstone.

Langfeldt, G. (1937). *The schizophrenic states.* Copenhagen: E. Munksgaard.

Marengo, J., Harrow, M., & Rogers, C. (1980). *A manual for scoring abstract and concrete responses to the Proverbs Test* (p. 1–15). ASIA/NAPS #03646. New York: Microfiche Publications.

Marengo, J., Harrow, M., Lanin, I. B., & Wilson, A. (1986). A comprehensive index of positive thought disorder. *Schizophrenia Bulletin, 12,* 497–511.

Pogue-Geile, M. F., & Harrow, M. (1984). Negative and positive symptoms in schizophrenia and depression: A follow-up study. *Schizophrenia Bulletin, 10,* 371–387.

Pogue-Geile, M. F., & Harrow, M. (1985). Negative symptoms in schizophrenia: Their longitudinal course and prognostic importance. *Schizophrenia Bulletin, 11,* 427–439.

Pogue-Geile, M. F., & Zubin, J. (1988). Negative symptomatology and schizophrenia: A conceptual and empirical review. *International Journal of Mental Health, 16,* 3–45.

Rubin, N. S., Harrow, M., & Pogue-Geile, M. F. (1987). *The prognosis of deficit-negative and positive symptoms in post-hospital schizophrenia.* Paper presented at the 95th annual meeting of the American Psychological Association, New York.

Schneider, K. (1959). *Clinical psychopathology* (M. W. Hamilton, Trans.). New York: Grune & Stratton, Inc.

Spitzer, R. L., & Endicott, J. (1978). *Schedule for affective disorders and schizophrenia (SADS)* (3rd ed.). New York: Biometrics Research, New York State Psychiatric Institute.

Strauss, J. S., & Carpenter, W. T. (1972). The prediction of outcome in schizophrenia: I. Characteristics of outcome. *Archives of General Psychiatry, 17,* 739–746.

Strauss, J. S., & Carpenter, W. T. (1974). The prediction of outcome in schizophrenia: II. Relationships between predictor and outcome variables: A report from the WHO International Pilot Study of Schizophrenia. *Archives of General Psychiatry, 31,* 37–42.

Strauss, J. S., & Carpenter, W. T. (1977). The prediction of outcome in schizophrenia: III. Five year outcome and its predictors. *Archives of General Psychiatry, 34,* 159–169.

Strauss, J. S., Carpenter, W. T., & Bartko, J. J. (1974). The diagnosis and understanding of schizophrenia: Part III. Speculations on the processes that underlie schizophrenic symptoms and signs. *Schizophrenia Bulletin, 11,* 161–179.

Vygotsky, L. S. (1962). *Thought and language* (E. Hanfman & G. Vaskar, Eds. & Trans.). New York: John Wiley & Sons.

Wechsler, D. (1939). *Measurement and appraisal of adult intelligence.* Baltimore: Williams & Wilkins.

Wechsler, D. (1955). *Wechsler Adult Intelligence Scale manual.* New York: Psychological Corporation.

Wechsler, D. (1981). Wechsler Adult Intelligence Scale—Revised. San Antonio, The Psychological Corporation.

Wynne, L. C., Cromwell, R. L., & Matthysse, S. (Eds.). (1978). *The nature of schizophrenia: New approaches to research and treatment.* New York: John Wiley & Sons.

Zubin, J., & Spring, B. (1977). Vulnerability—A new view of schizophrenia. *Journal of Abnormal Psychology, 86,* 103–126.

15

The Heterogeneous Prognosis of Schizophrenia: Possible Determinants of the Short-Term and 5-Year Outcomes

ECKART R. STRAUBE

The objective of this prospective study was to investigate characteristics of schizophrenic patients that may determine the short-term (6 weeks') response to neuroleptics and the medium-term (5-year) "natural course of the illness," and whether common factors exist that predict both. Because the prediction of response to a 4-week standard haloperidol treatment and the prediction concerning the 2-year course was described elsewhere (Straube, Wagner, Foerster, & Heimann, 1989), this chapter deals with the new analysis of the results of our comprehensive project. We analyzed the course of the illness after the termination of 4 weeks of standard therapy when the selection of the neuroleptic drug was freely determined by the treating therapist (observation up to 6 weeks after index admission). The interest in this kind of analysis is to find out whether a free choice of medication may cause a change in the response to neuroleptics and in the set of outcome predictors, compared to the predictors of the outcome from standard therapy. Another interest was to compare the prediction of the 5-year course with our previous analysis of the 2-year course.

The following set of predictors was assessed:

1. The response of the autonomic nervous system (ANS; electrodermal and heart rate response) to a set of mild-intensity tones and to reaction time stimuli.
2. Behavioral features, such as attention disorder, stimulus barrier function, reaction time, ward behavior, and attitude toward the treatment. A computerized tomography (CT) study was included in this set of data.
3. Psychopathological symptoms and syndromes—that is, positive symptoms, negative symptoms, and the degree of premorbid adjustment.

The reasons for assessing these three sets of potential predictors are the following. The ANS variables and some of the behavioral measures had already been shown to be related to short-term outcome (see a more detailed description of the expected correlations below). Therefore, replicability of these findings was examined. In contrast to this, the psychopathological set of predictors did not show a clear relationship to *short*-term outcome (and drug response) in previous studies, but with respect to medium- and long-term outcome some investigations show a relationship of outcome with specific symptoms. The most interesting aspect of the analysis presented here is that the predictive power of different features of the schizophrenic disturbance, ranging from electrodermal responses to orienting stimuli, attention disorder, the attitude toward medication and negative symptoms, is analyzed in the same study. This was done only in separate investigations in the past. Furthermore, some of the variables tested here were never examined as predictors. The other unusual feature of the present study is that we examined whether the predictor variables of short-term outcome are the same as those for medium-term outcome. Such a comparison including such a wide variety of schizophrenic features has never been done in previous studies.

METHODS

Sample and Definition of the Sample

We investigated the short- and medium-term course of 45 newly admitted schizophrenic patients. All patients were examined with rating scales and experimental tests before onset of neuroleptic treatment. All of the patients had been off medication for at least 4 weeks. Patient selection was based on the so-called WHO criteria/Carpenter Flexible Checklist (Carpenter, Strauss, & Bartko, 1974) on admission. The diagnosis was then assured a second time by CATEGO, which is a computerized diagnostic system based on the Present State Examination (PSE). Most of the patients (61%) were first-admission patients. The rest of the patients had had two and sometimes more previous admissions.

Our aim was to examine the "therapeutic course" and the medium-term "natural course" of an unbiased sample that was to be representative for the population admitted to a German university psychiatric hospital. The representativeness of our sample was therefore checked by the psychiatric rating of all patients admitted to the two (acute) admission wards of the hospital. A detailed comparison of the psychiatric profile of the sample tested and of the patients admitted, but not examined, revealed that our criteria of representativeness of the sample were fulfilled; that is, the samples

did not differ with respect to the syndrome profile of the Brief Psychiatric Rating Scale (BPRS). The average age of the patients was 26.5 years (standard deviation 5.6 years).

Standardized Treatment

After the first assessment of the patients with a variety of rating scales (by several raters) and examination of the psychophysiological response in the Psychophysiology Laboratory of our clinic, a standardized treatment with the neuroleptic haloperidol started (dosages were allowed within the range of 15 to 45 mg haloperidol per day). After that period, medication and range of dosage was allowed to change. The compliance of the patient was checked by regularly taking and analyzing blood samples.

The rationale of this analysis was to find out whether the outcome prediction of an "optimized" therapy differs from that of a standardized haloperidol treatment. "Optimized" means that those patients who did not respond to haloperidol treatment could receive an alternative drug. Most of the nonresponding patients received clozapine as an alternative.

The short-term outcome was assessed with several rating scales. In this presentation of the data we analyzed the change in the Global Assessment Scale (GAS) from day 1 to the last assessment. The last assessment in most patients was 6 weeks after index admission. Some patients, however, could be discharged earlier. We therefore chose the 6-week follow-up point in some patients and in other patients the last assessment before discharge. (Time in hospital already had been examined in a separate analysis as a possible predictor; Straube et al., 1989). Five years after discharge, the status of all patients who could be reached was assessed again. Most patients were examined personally by the psychiatrist who was a member of the project staff. Thirty-eight of the 45 patients could be examined; 3 patients were deceased and 4 could not be reached. (We also examined the patients 9 months after index admission and 2 years after index discharge. The analyses of these data were described elsewhere [Straube et al., 1989].)

Predictors

Three sets of predictors were tested in each patient.

Psychophysiological predictors. Included in this set of predictors were electrodermal and heart rate response to a series of 15 innocuous and mild (habituation) tones, to reaction time stimuli, and to a high-intensity white noise. The reaction time test consisted of 15 signal tones (high-pitch tones = button press) and 15 no-signal tones (low-pitch tones = no button press). The measurement of the orienting response paradigm was the same as described in Straube, Schied, Rein, and Breyer-Pfaff (1987) and Straube (1979), the exception being that the intensity of the tones was reduced to 75 dB. We measured 31 psychophysiological variables that were reduced to six factors (factors with an eigenvalue higher than 1; see also Table 15.3 below) by means of a factor analysis.

Psychopathological predictors. Four PSE syndromes and symptoms, one BPRS symptom, and the premorbid adjustment formed the psychopathological set of predictors. In addition to this, the early change in psychopathology was assessed in response to the administration of 10 mg haloperidol (two times within 24 hours). This is the so-called test-dose response. The PSE total score and the negative and positive symptoms of the PSE were compiled as described by Andreason (1983, 1984). Because affective flattening was described as an important predictor of medium-term outcome (Carpenter, Bartko, Strauss, & Hawk, 1978), this negative symptom of the PSE was tested separately. Thought disorder as a hypothetical core syndrome of schizophrenia was also tested (BPRS syndrome). Carpenter et al. (1978) showed that the degree of premorbid adjustment is an important predictor; we therefore included this variable into the set of predictors. Several

authors (e.g., Awad & Hogan, 1985; Gaebel, Pietzcker, Ulrich, Schley, & Müller-Oerlinghausen, 1988; May, Van Putten, & Yale, 1980) showed that a favorable response to a so-called test dose predicted the overall 4-week drug response; we therefore were interested in knowing whether we could replicate these findings.

Clinical psychological predictors (and CT). Attention disorder is described as an important feature of schizophrenia in the literature. It has been tested as a predictor of short- and medium-term outcome in an investigation by May and Goldberg (1978). They tested sustained attention with the Continuous Performance Test (CPT). We therefore developed a 7-point scale to assess attention disorder, because it was impossible to test the drug-free acute patients with another lengthy experimental procedure in addition to the experiments already done.

The rating of the disorder of selective attention was operationalized on the basis of the patients' self-description of selective attention disorders as assessed by McGhie and Chapman (1961). The reduced ability to protect oneself against all sorts of external stimulation may be a complementary feature of the schizophrenics' attention disorder. We measured this with the 13-point scale developed by Bellak, Hurvich, and Gediman (1973). Reaction time was measured with the method described above during the measurement of the ANS responses. Zahn, Carpenter, and McGlashen (1981a,b) found a correlation of reaction time with poor short-term outcome.

We additionally hypothesized that the attitude toward medication, the therapist, the staff, and the admission may be a factor influencing the improvement of the patient during the 4 to 6 weeks of therapy. Therefore, we developed a 7-point scale to measure the attitude of the patient in these four areas. Because extreme differences in psychophysiological activity were described to be related to outcome, we measured the behavioral activity of the patients by means of the scale developed by Venables (1957).

Later, Venables and Wing (1962) indeed showed that the level of electrodermal activity was correlated with the activity level of the patients on the ward.

In addition to these measures, a CT brain scan was obtained for each patient. The degree of cortical regional change (cortical ventricles, etc.) and diffuse atrophy in the brains of schizophrenic patients was rated on a 4-point scale by two independent experienced neuroradiologists. The potential predictive power of each variable was evaluated by means of a multiple regression analysis. In order to assess the predictive power of each data set separately, three separate multiple regression analyses were calculated.

RESULTS

Short-Term Outcome

As can be seen from Figure 15.1, the response to 4 to 6 weeks of therapy with neuroleptics is heterogeneous; that is, a consid-

erable number of patients showed no marked improvement. That means that, after a 4-week trial with standard therapy (15 to 45 mg haloperidol) and even after an additional trial with other neuroleptics (in most cases clozapine) for those patients who did not improve under the standardized therapy, there are still a considerable number of patients who showed no or only minimal improvement. A total of 20% ($n = 9$) of the patients showed only a minimal change in GAS scores (10% or less). Twenty-four percent ($n = 11$) of the patients showed a marked change during the observation period (a change of 30% or more in GAS score). This is illustrated in Figure 15.1, showing the development of these two extreme groups, but further calculations were done with the total sample ($n = 45$).

Prediction of Short-Term Outcome

As can be seen from Table 15.1, there is no prediction of the 4- to 6-weeks' response

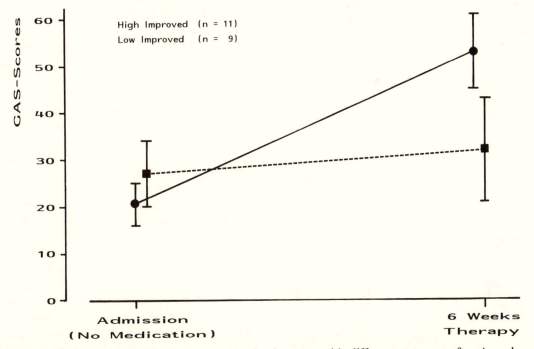

Figure 15.1. Demonstration of the existence of subgroups with different outcome after 4 weeks of standard therapy with haloperidol and an additional period (up to 6 weeks) with a change of the neuroleptic if necessary. The high-improved group ($n = 11$; *solid line*) showed a 30% change in GAS scores; the low-improved group ($n = 9$; *dashed line*) showed only a 10% change or less on the GAS.

Table 15.1. Psychopathological Status, Premorbid Adjustment, and Test-Dose Response at Admission (without Medication) as Potential Predictors of Outcome of 6 Weeks of Neuroleptic Therapy[a]

	Beta[b]	r
PSE total score	.32	.08
PSE negative symptoms	.65	.19
PSE positive symptoms	−.20	.01
PSE affective flattening	−.49	−.16
BPRS thought disorder	−.00	−.18
Premorbid adjustment (Strauss–Carpenter scale)	−.12	.09
Test-dose response (24 hr)	−.23	.14

[a] Outcome criterion: relative difference in GAS rating between admission and follow-up. Overall R^2 = .13 (not significant).
[b] Beta values of the multiple regression analysis.

possible from psychopathology characteristics, including the degree of premorbid adjustment and the 24-hour test-dose response. Interestingly, and in contrast to this, the behavioral scales (clinical psychological scales) do predict outcome. A significant amount of the variance is explained by this data set (R^2 adjusted = .33; see Table 15.2). The stimulus barrier function scale provided the highest predictive power (beta = −.55). The attention disorders are also correlated with the outcome (r = .39), although the beta value for attention disorder is low. Because stimulus barrier function and attention disorder are negatively correlated, the multiple regression analysis selects the variable with the highest correlation with the outcome criterion. This finding therefore means that a low stimulus barrier function and a high degree of attention dis-

Table 15.2. Clinical Psychological Status and CT Rating at Admission (without Medication) as Potential Predictors of Outcome of 6 Weeks of Neuroleptic Therapy[a]

	Beta[b]	r
Attention disorder	.12	.39**
Stimulus barrier function	−.55**	−.54**
Reaction time	−.01	.05
Attitude toward treatment	.18	.27[(*)]
Ward activity scale	.03	.22[(*)]
CT rating	.15	−.14

[a] Outcome criterion: relative difference in GAS rating between admission and follow-up. Overall R^2 = .33 ($p < .01$).
[b] Beta values of the multiple regression analysis.
**, $p < .01$; *, $p < .05$; (*), $p < .10$.

order is correlated with the *better response* to neuroleptic treatment. That is, low tolerance toward external stimulation, and problems in directing attention selectively to relevant stimuli in the environment seem to predict a favorable response to neuroleptic treatment.

One may further suggest that this pattern of features (more distraction and higher vulnerability toward stimulation) may define a certain subgroup of patients who are primarily positive symptom patients. Interestingly, however, this pattern is *not* correlated with the global rating of positive symptoms, although attention disorder is highly correlated with the single positive symptom of thought disorder (r = .76). Stimulus barrier function correlates negatively with thought disorder (r = −.58; see Figure 15.2). In contrast to this, thought disorder itself does not play a role in the prediction of drug response, as can be seen from Table 15.1. The significance of this finding is discussed in more detail below.

There is also a slight tendency (r = .22, $p < .10$) for ward activity (less withdrawn, less mute, and less retarded) and, surprisingly, for the negative attitude of patients toward treatment (r = .27, $p < .10$) to predict a favorable result from drug treatment (see Table 15.2). However, both beta values are low and insignificant.

As for psychophysiology, there is no global predictive power (R^2 is low and not significant), but a single variable—heart rate at rest—turns out to be significantly (and negatively) correlated with outcome, as can be seen from its highly significant beta value (Table 15.3). That means that patients who have a *lower* heart rate in phases of the experiment that are without stimuli (i.e., phases before the occurrence of tones in the habituation [orienting stimuli] experiment, during the reaction time task, and at rest before starting the experiment) are those who have a *better* short-term outcome. In other words, patients who are less activated in a specific component of cardiovascular arousal tend to respond more favorably to neuroleptic treatment. Again, there is a significant correlation between heart rate (factor 1) and stimulus barrier function ($r = .36$; see also Figure 15.2A), which means that low heart rate arousal and low tolerance for stimulation is a related pattern in patients who tend to improve during medication with neuroleptics.

Medium-Term Outcome (5 Years after Index Admission)

Thirty-eight of the 45 patients were examined 5 years after the index admission. Of the remainder, 3 patients died during the follow-up period and 4 patients could not be reached for a follow-up examination for various reasons (i.e., they moved away, refused participation, or could not be traced). Fifty percent ($n = 19$) of the patients had two to seven relapses (with a median of three relapses) during the follow-up observation period. Thirty-two percent ($n = 12$) of the patients had only one relapse and 18% ($n = 7$) had no relapse. A relapse was defined as a readmission to a psychiatric hospital or as a worsening of symptoms that normally would have caused a readmission.

As for psychiatric status, 6% of the patients reached a GAS rating of 81 points or more at the follow-up assessment, which means no symptoms or rarely occurring symptoms and good social adaptability. Thirty-three percent of the patients had only minimal symptoms and less severe problems in daily life (GAS ratings of 61 to 80 points). Forty-two percent of the patients were in the medium range of psychiatric problems (GAS ratings of 41 to 60 points). Nineteen percent of the patients were more

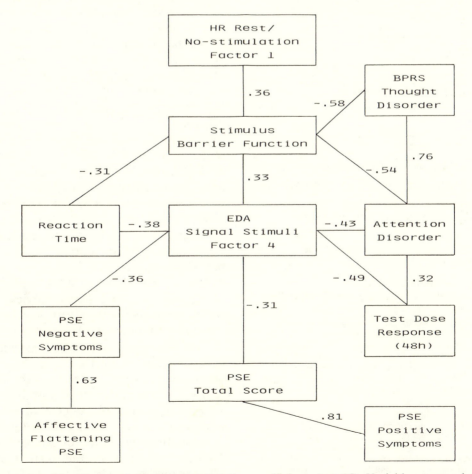

Figure 15.2A. First cluster of significant correlation coefficients ($p<.05$). Variables assessed at admission. $N = 45$ schizophrenic patients not on neuroleptic medication. *Figure continued on following page.*

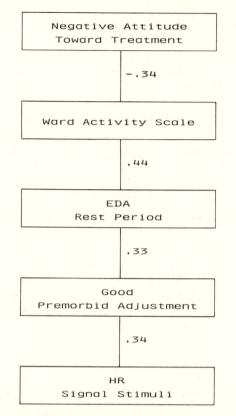

Figure 15.2B. Second cluster of significant correlation coefficients (*p*<.05). Variables assessed at admission. *N* = 45 schizophrenic patients not on neuroleptic medication.

Table 15.4. Results of the GAS Rating 5 Years After Index Admission

GAS rating		*n*	Percentage of patients
81 and above	No symptoms or rarely occurring symptoms	2	6
61–80	Minimal symptoms and minor social problems	12	33
41–60	Psychiatric problems in the medium range	15	42
40 and below	More or less severely ill	7	19

or less severely ill at the follow-up evaluation (GAS ratings of less than 41 points; see also Table 15.4).

In the data analysis presented here, we chose the following outcome criterion: the psychiatric status of the patient at follow-

Table 15.3. Psychological Activity, Electrodermal Activity (EDA), and Heart Rate (HR) Response at Admission (without Medication) as Potential Predictors of Outcome of 6 Weeks of Neuroleptic Therapy[a]

	Beta[b]	*r*
Factor 1 (HR, rest/no stimulation)	− .50**	− .43**
Factor 2 (EDA, orienting stimuli)	− .09	− .07
Factor 3 (EDA, rest period)	− .15	− .11
Factor 4 (EDA, signal stimuli)	− .05	− .03
Factor 5 (HR, signal stimuli)	.23	.16
Factor 6 (HR—Lability, white noise)	− .16	− .12

[a] Outcome criterion: relative difference in GAS rating between admission and follow-up. Overall R^2 = .12 (not significant).
[b] Beta values of the multiple regression analysis.
**, $p < .01$.

up, including the course of the illness. That means that we integrated the number of relapses, the psychiatric and psychosocial adaptability during the 5-year period, and the GAS rating at the follow-up assessment into a 5-point scale. High scores mean poor course and outcome. This scale of global psychopathological and social development correlated with the number of relapses (r = .52) and with the GAS score at the follow-up assessment (r = − .67). We were able to compare the results of this analysis with previous analyses that dealt with (a) the number of relapses and (b) the GAS rating at the follow-up assessment as outcome criteria. Results of these assessments for 2- and 5-year outcomes are described elsewhere (Straube, Wagner, & Ackermann, 1990; Straube et al., 1989). It is important to note that no patient took neuroleptic medication regularly during the follow-up period.

As can be seen from Tables 15.5 through 15.7, only the psychopathological data show a tendency (*p*<.07) to be related to medium-term outcome. Positive symptoms and the PSE total score reached a significant beta value, although the multiple correlation failed to predict outcome (Table 15.5). A *combination* of the severity of the illness at admission and the degree of positive symptoms may be a better predictor of the outcome than one of these variables alone. As expected, and in confirmation of the original finding of Carpenter et al. (1978), the Strauss–Carpenter Scale, which mea-

Table 15.5. Psychopathological Status, Premorbid Adjustment, and Test-Dose Response at Admission (without Medication) as Potential Predictors of the 5-Year Outcome[a]

	Beta[b]	r
PSE total score	.80*	.08
PSE negative symptoms	.44	−.15
PSE positive symptoms	.91*	.25
PSE affective flattening	−.31	.04
BPRS thought disorder	.21	.24
Premorbid adjustment (Strauss–Carpenter scale)	−.52*	.38*
Test-dose response (24 hr)	.49	.19

[a] Outcome criterion: global psychopathological and social development during the last 5 years, rated on a 5-point scale. Overall R^2 = .24 ($p < .07$).
[b] Beta values of the multiple regression analysis.
*, $p < .05$.

sures the premorbid adjustment, predicts the 5-year global outcome (see Table 15.5).

The data set that comprises the clinical ratings, including the CT rating, does not show an overall relationship with the global 5-year outcome but, interestingly enough, attention disorder is again related to outcome (Table 15.6). Patients with *less* attention disorder tended to have a poor medium-term outcome, whereas attention disorder was related to good short-term outcome. Thus, attention disorder seems to be inversely related to short- and medium-term outcomes, respectively.

The psychophysiological data set also is not related to medium-term outcome, but, again, a single variable showed a significant beta value. At a moderate level of correlation ($p < 10$), patients who responded with more electrodermal activity (EDA) to the

Table 15.6. Clinical Psychological Status and CT rating at Admission (without Medication) as Potential Predictors of the 5-Year Outcome[a]

	Beta[b]	r
Attention disorder	−.55**	−.35*
Stimulus barrier function	−.23	.21
Reaction time	.03	.03
Attitude toward treatment	.19	.12
Ward activity scale	.10	.09
CT rating	−.19	.11

[a] Outcome criterion: global psychopathological and social development during the last 5 years, rated on a 5-point scale. Overall R^2 = −.06 (not significant).
[b] Beta values of the multiple regression analysis.
**, $p < .01$; *, $p < .05$.

Table 15.7. Psychophysiological Activity, Electrodermal Activity (EDA), and Heart Rate (HR) Response at Admission (without Medication) as Potential Predictors of the 5-Year Outcome[a]

	Beta[b]	r
Factor 1 (HR, rest/no stimulation)	.29	.18
Factor 2 (EDA, orienting stimuli)	.40*	.29(*)
Factor 3 (EDA, rest period)	−.08	.07
Factor 4 (EDA, signal stimuli)	−.01	−.02
Factor 5 (HR, signal stimuli)	.30	.22
Factor 6 (HR—Lability, white noise)	−.13	−.13

[a] Outcome criterion: global psychopathological and social development during the last 5 years, rated on a 5-point scale. Overall R^2 = .04 (not significant).
[b] Beta values of the multiple regression analysis.
*, $p < .05$; (*), $p < .10$.

orienting stimuli had a tendency to have a poor outcome (see Table 15.7). Psychophysiological factor 2 consisted of the number of spontaneous EDA fluctuations during the habituation experiment, the number of responses until habituation, and the EDA amplitude to the first orienting stimulus. That is, it expresses the EDA activity in response to the innocuous orienting (habituation) stimuli.

DISCUSSION

Clinical Psychological Predictors

Short-term outcome is best predicted by the response of the patient to external stimulation. Patients who are most irritated and distracted and who cannot cope with external stimulation are those who tend to profit most from neuroleptic therapy. This finding cannot be explained by a putatively higher psychopathology rating of these patients, because there exists no correlation between the PSE total score and short-term outcome. However, because no placebo group exists (such would not have been tolerable for this group of highly acute patients), it is not clear whether the remission in this group is spontaneous or in fact caused by neuroleptic treatment. Nevertheless, there is some indirect evidence for the interaction of neuroleptics with attention disorder from other studies. Oltmanns, Ohayon, and Neale (1978) reported that taking schizophrenic patients off medication increased their distractibility in a special version of the digit span test. Strauss, Law, Coyler, & June (1985) saw a negative correlation between plasma level of neuroleptics (i.e., the supposed bioavailability of the drug) and distractibility in the above-mentioned version of the digit span task. May and Goldberg (1978) reported a highly significant correlation between *poor* performance on the CPT, a test that measures sustained selective attention, and a positive response to 4 weeks' treatment with haloperidol (r = .67). These findings suggest that patients with poor selective attention/low stimulus barrier function are those who profit most from antidopaminergic treatment.

However, as far as medium-term outcome is concerned, the issue seems to be more complicated. As can be seen from Table 15.6, patients with *less* attention disorder have a poor outcome. Because no patient took medication regularly, the 5-year outcome of the illness must be considered as being close to the "natural course" of the illness. Thus, patients with higher attention problems at admission (being still drug free) are those who will be better off at the follow-up assessment. This finding is consistent with the separate analysis wherein the GAS rating at the 5-year follow-up is the outcome criterion (Straube et al., 1990). However, if the number of relapses is the criterion, the picture seems to be reversed. Patients with reported problems in stimulus barrier function are those who have *more* relapses during the 5-year period (Straube et al., 1990). These discrepant findings may signify that patients with attention disorder/low stimulus barrier function are those who tend to have an undulating course (with more relapses but with a higher degree of symptomatic and social remission between relapses, which seems to be demonstrated by a higher (better) GAS rating at the 5-year assessment).

One may speculate that the other type of patient, who is less distractible and has fewer problems with overstimulation, belongs to a group with a less spectacular, more process-type course that may

Table 15.8. Number and Percentage of Patients Having Attention Disorder Problems at Admission[a]

Score	n	%	cum %
1 = no Disorder	6	13	100
2	3	7	87
3	5	11	80
4	3	7	69
5	7	16	62
6	15	33	47
7 = Extremely severe	6	13	13

[a] All patients off medication for at least 4 weeks. $N = 45$; rated on a 7-point scale.

progress toward chronicity in the long run. One may also speculate that the type of patients with attention disorder and undulating course are those who have the highest chance to profit from neuroleptic treatment and thus may have the higher chance of preventing poor outcome if on medication continuously. As can be seen from Table 15.8, 69% of the patients had medium to severe attention disorder problems and, as can be seen from Table 15.9, 84% of the patients had medium to severe problems with stimulus barrier function (i.e., low stimulus barrier function at admission when without medication).

The other measurements and scales in the clinical psychological set of data, such as attitude toward treatment and type of activity on the ward, play only a minor role in determining the short-term outcome and no role in determining the long-term outcome. Contrary to expectation from previous findings (Cancro, Sutton, Kerr, & Sugerman, 1971; Zahn et al., 1981b) reaction time did not play a role as a predictor. Slow reaction

Table 15.9. Number and Percentage of Patients with High or Low Stimulus Barrier Function (SBF) at Admission[a]

Score	n	%	cum %
11–13 = High SBF	—	—	100
9–10	1	2	100
7–8	6	14	98
5–6	18	43	84
2–4	12	29	41
1–2 = Low SBF	12	12	12

[a] All patients off medication for at least 4 weeks. $N = 42$; rated on the 13-point scale of Bellak et al. (1973).

time was found to be correlated with poor short-term outcome in these studies. We have no explanation for this discrepancy. The same is true for the CT rating: no correlation with outcome was found. This contradicts the findings of Weinberger, Bigelow, and Kleinmann (1980) and Pandurangi et al. (1989). It may be that direct metric assessment, instead of a global rating as we used, may disclose a relationship between atrophies of the brain and outcome. Subgroup differences between the studies also may play a role. The authors mentioned above examined a more chronic population that may be more prone to atrophic signs. Nevertheless, in our study the rating by the two experienced neuroradiologists revealed a pronounced to severe alteration, as evidenced by atrophy, in at least 32% of the patients. Reports of CT findings vary considerably in the literature, from 6% (Andreasen, Dennert, Olsen, & Damasio, 1982) to 60% (Golden et al., 1980).

Psychophysiological Predictors

With regard to ANS reactivity, there is a considerable amount of data supporting the idea that early electrodermal habituation to orienting stimuli is predictive of a positive short-term development (Cesarec & Nymann, 1985; Frith, Stevens, Johnstone, & Crow, 1979; Straube et al., 1987; Zahn et al., 1981b). These findings are only indirectly confirmed by our analysis. The EDA to orienting stimuli did not differentiate the groups, but lower heart rate activity at rest and during the no-stimulation phases of the experiment tended to be related with better short-term outcome. Again, it is questionable whether this feature is related to spontaneous remission or to treatment with neuroleptics. Because Frith et al. (1979) found reduced electrodermal activity during the habituation/orienting experiment to be related to the outcome of a placebo trial, one may suggest that spontaneous remission (possibly supported and accelerated by neuroleptics) can be expected in those schizophrenic patients who have a low ANS arousal.

Interestingly, regarding the 5-year outcome, there is again a tendency for the low-activity type of schizophrenics to have a more favorable medium-term outcome. In this case early electrodermal habituation to orienting stimuli is related to better outcome. This finding contradicts that of Öhman and Öhlund (1989), who reported that reduced electrodermal activity was associated with poor social outcome 2 years later. In contrast to our study, however, psychopathological outcome criteria were not tested by Öhman and Öhlund (1989).

Psychopathological Predictors

In contrast to the remarkable absence of a predictive value of psychopathology for the short-term outcome (and drug response?), there is at least a tendency for the psychopathological data set to predict the 5-year outcome. In the past a considerable number of scientists have tried to find the pattern of symptoms that is related to drug response or spontaneous remission, but such a pattern has not been revealed (see review by Csenansky, Kaplan, & Hollister, 1985). Nevertheless, at least there are reports that a relationship between the degree of premorbid psychopathology and social capabilities and *short*-term outcome exists (Carpenter & Heinrich, 1981; Evans, Rodnick, Goldstein, & Judd, 1972; Marder, van Kammen, Docherty, Rayner, & Bunney, 1979). This was not confirmed by our analysis, probably because we expressly selected patients who reached at least 61 GAS points in the preadmission period. One may assume that a group with the worst prognosis had been excluded from participation in our study. Nevertheless, for the 5-year outcome, the level of premorbid adjustment clearly predicts outcome, thus confirming the findings of Carpenter et al. (1978), which thereby signifies that, even in our sample of rather acute patients, a subgroup with a poor premorbid course and a poor medium-term course does in fact exist.

Another finding seemingly contradicts the existing literature. We found no correlation between the global change in symptomatology (measured with the GAS) in response to a test dose of haloperidol and short-term outcome. In the present evaluation of the data we analyzed the response to 10 mg haloperidol given two times in the course of 24 hours. This finding contradicts reports of Awad and Hogan (1985), Gaebel et al. (1988), Hogan, Awad, & Eastwood, (1985), and May et al. (1976, 1980). However, further analysis revealed that, after the fifth test dose of 10 mg haloperidol (third day), a significant correlation with the 4-week outcome appeared, thus confirming the findings discussed above. The absence of a correlation for the first test dose may be due to the fact that sedation factors dominated. Most of the patients slept after the first 10 mg of haloperidol; the change of symptomatology therefore was difficult to assess.

Short-Term Versus Medium Term Predictors

If we compare the set of predictors for the 4-week outcome, as described in our previous analysis of the data (Straube et al., 1989), to the present analysis concerning the 4- to 6-week outcome (which allowed an "optimal drug" therapy approach), we note that no difference exists. The 4-week outcome with standard haloperidol therapy correlates with the outcome with the 6-week therapy ($r = .82$). In principle, the same patients who respond to standard therapy with haloperidol also respond to a change in therapy that includes clozapine. From clinical experience one would have expected haloperidol nonresponders to respond favorably to clozapine. This was not the case. Clozapine may ameliorate symptoms further but does not lead to a reversal of the effect. Bitter, Cooper, Crowner, Volavka, and Jaeger (1990) recently presented similar data.

Concerning the medium-term outcome, our previous analysis of the 2-year outcome (Straube et al., 1989) revealed that the same set of predictors (i.e., the clinical psychological data set and the psychophysiological data) were associated with outcome. The same subfactors—attention disorder and

low ANS activity—were involved. However, 2-year outcome was *not* predicted by psychopathological features, in contrast to the present analysis, wherein 5-year outcome was related to a specific pattern of psychopathology at admission.

The change in the pattern of predictors for the short-term (4 to 6 weeks) as compared to the medium-term (5 years) outcome is interesting. Behavioral measures such as the rating of stimulus barrier function and attention disorder tend to be related to short-term outcome whereas psychopathology seems to play a much more prominent role in determining medium-term outcome. This suggests that different features are related to short- and medium-term outcome (and possibly also to long-term outcome). Some other features, such as attention disorder and ANS activity, may be related to both. This seems to be underlined by the fact that no correlation ($r = -.01$) between the 4- to 6-week change in GAS rating and the global outcome rating at the 5-year follow-up assessment exists. In other words, those patients who are better off in the short term (partly because of drug response) are not necessarily those who are better off in the long term.

A pattern consisting of more severe symptoms and positive symptoms seems to be related to a favorable medium-term outcome, but this was not related to short-term outcome. This finding that positive symptoms (together with more severe symptomatology) have a predictive value may be surprising for those who believe that negative symptoms are an indicator of poor prognosis (e.g., Crow, 1980). However, as a detailed analysis of the European and American long-term studies shows with surprising unanimity, there is a clear tendency for at least one positive symptom, hallucinations (in most cases auditory hallucinations, but sometimes also visual hallucinations), to be associated with *poor* long-term outcome of the illness (Ciompi & Müller, 1976; Huber, Gross, & Schüttler, 1979; Marneros, Diester, Rohde, Steinmeyer, & Jünemann, 1989; McGlashan, 1986; Tsuang, 1986). In these studies the long-term course from 10 to over

20 years was analyzed. We did not analyze auditory hallucations as a predictor, but this type of analysis should be conducted in a further evaluation of our data. It may be assumed that a correlation between hallucinations and 5-year outcome will be revealed in such an analysis. Kay and Lindenmayer (1987) even showed that *negative* symptoms predicted a *favorable* outcome at the 2-year follow-up assessment.

The surprising finding was that clinical psychological rating scales (such as attention disorder and low stimulus barrier function) explained a great deal of the variance of the 6-week outcome (up to 33%). This was not the case for psychopathological "predictors," nor was it the case for the psychophysiological measurements, although one single variable (heart rate at rest) was related to short-term outcome. The measurement of information processing, together with the measurement of ANS activity and test-dose response, may help to provide early information about spontaneous remission or drug response. This possibility of early information about the future poor course of the illness in specific patients may be an important hint that additional therapeutic interventions should be undertaken as a consequence. The other important finding is that at least a partial change occurs in the pattern of predictors with respect to short-term compared to medium-term outcome. This was also true for the 2-year outcome compared to the 5-year outcome. The latter may signify that partially different mechanisms are involved in determining short- and long-term outcome, although attention disorder was related to the result of both follow-up assessments. Here again, the relationship is partially inverse. The patient with attention disorder had a more favorable short-term course (more favorable drug response?) but tended to have more relapses and a higher (better) GAS rating between phases of breakdown.

ACKNOWLEDGMENT

The author expresses his thanks to the DFG (German Funding Agency for Science), the team on the A3, and doctors Wagner and Foerster for considerable help in this study.

REFERENCES

Andreasen, N. C. (1983). *The Scale for the Assessment of Negative Symptoms (SANS)*. Iowa City: The University of Iowa.

Andreasen, N. C. (1984). *The Scale for the Assessment of Positive Symptoms (SAPS)*. Iowa City: The University of Iowa.

Andreasen, N. C., Dennert, J. W., Olsen, S. A., & Damasio, A. R. (1982). Hemispheric asymmetries and schizophrenia. *American Journal of Psychiatry, 139*, 427–430.

Awad, A. G., & Hogan, T. P. (1985). Early treatment events and prediction of response to neuroleptics in schizophrenia. *Progress in Neuro-Psychopharmacology and Biological Psychiatry, 9*, 585–588.

Bellak, L., Hurvich, M., & Gediman, H. K. (1973). *Ego functions in schizophrenics, neurotics, and normals: A systematic study of conceptual, diagnostic, and therapeutic aspects.* New York: John Wiley & Sons.

Bitter, I., Cooper, T. B., Crowner, M. L., Volavka, J., & Jaeger, J. (1990, October). *Benztropine and psychopathology in schizophrenia.* Paper presented at the Fifth Congress of the Association of European Psychiatrists, Strasbourg.

Cancro, R., Sutton, S., Kerr, J., & Sugerman, A. (1971). Reaction time and prognosis in acute schizophrenia. *Journal of Nervous and Mental Disease, 153*, 351–359.

Carpenter, W. T., Bartko, J. J., Strauss, J. S., & Hawk, A. B. (1978). Signs and symptoms as predictors of outcome. A report from the International Pilot Study of Schizophrenia. *American Journal of Psychiatry, 135*, 940–945.

Carpenter, W. T., & Heinrichs, D. W. (1981). Treatment-relevant subtypes of schizophrenia. *Journal of Nervous and Mental Disease, 169*, 113–119.

Carpenter, W. T., Strauss, J. S., & Bartko, J. J. (1974). Use of signs and symptoms for the identification of schizophrenic patients. *Schizophrenia Bulletin, 11*, 37–49.

Cesarec, Z., & Nyman, A. K. (1985). Differential response to amphetamine in schizophrenia. *Acta Psychiatrica Scandinavica, 71*, 523–538.

Ciompi, L., & Müller, C. (1976). *Lebensweg und Alter der Schizophrenen: Eine katamnestische Langzeitstudie bis ins Senium.* Berlin: Springer-Verlag.

Crow, T. J. (1980). Drug treatment of schizophrenia and its relationship to disturbances of dopaminergic transmission. In G. Curzon (Ed.), *The biochemistry of psychiatric disturbances* (pp. 61–73). Chichester, England: John Wiley & Sons.

Csenansky, J. G., Kaplan, J., & Hollister, L. E. (1985). Problems in classifications of schizophrenics as neuroleptic responders and nonresponders. *Journal of Nervous and Mental Disease, 173*, 325–331.

Evans, J. R., Rodnick, E. H., Goldstein, J. J., & Judd, L. L. (1972). Premorbid adjustment, phenothiazine treatment and remission in acute schizophrenics. *Archives of General Psychiatry, 27*, 486–490.

Frith, C. D., Stevens, M., Johnstone, E. C., & Crow, T. J. (1979). Skin conductance responsivity during acute episodes of schizophrenia as a predictor of symptomatic improvement. *Psychological Medicine, 9*, 101–106.

Gaebel, W., Pietzcker, A., Ulrich, G., Schley, J., & Müller-Oerlinghausen, B. (1988). Predictors of neuroleptic treatment response in acute schizophrenia: Results of a treatment study with perazine. *Pharmacopsychiatry, 21*, 384–386.

Golden, C. J., Moses, J. A., Zelazowski, R., Graber, B., Zatz, L. M., Horwath, T. B., & Berger, P. A. (1980). Cerebral ventricular size and neuropsychological impairment in young chronic schizophrenics: Measurement by the standardized Luria-Nebraska Neuropsychological Battery. *Archives of General Psychiatry, 37*, 619–623.

Hogan, T. J., Awad, A. G., & Eastwood, M. R. (1985). Early subjective response and prediction of outcome to neuroleptic drug therapy in schizophrenia. *Canadian Journal of Psychiatry, 30*, 241–248.

Huber, G., Gross, G., Schüttler, R. (1979). *Schizophrenie: Eine verlaufs- und sozialpsychiatrische Langzeitstudie.* Berlin: Springer-Verlag.

Kay, S. R., & Lindenmayer, J.-P. (1987). Outcome predictors in acute schizophrenia. Prospective significance of background and clinical dimensions. *Journal of Nervous and Mental Disease, 175*, 152–160.

Marder, S. R., van Kammen, D. P., Docherty, J. P., Rayner, J., & Bunney, W. E. (1979). Predicting drug-free improvement in schizophrenic psychosis. *Archives of General Psychiatry, 36*, 1080–1085.

Marneros, A., Deister, A., Rohde, A., Steinmeyer, E. M., & Jünemann, H. (1989). Longterm outcome of schizoaffective and schizophrenic disorders: A comparative study. I. Definitions, methods, psychopathological and social outcome. *European Archives of Psychiatry and Neurological Sciences, 238*, 118–125.

May, P. R. A., & Goldberg, S. C. (1978). Prediction of schizophrenic patients' response to pharmacotherapy. In M. A. Lipton, A. DiMascio, & K. F. Killam (Eds.), *Psychopharmacology: A generation of progress.* New York: Raven Press.

May, P. R. A., Van Putten, T., & Yale, C. (1980). Predicting outcome of antipsychotic drug treatment from early response. *American Journal of Psychiatry, 137*, 1088–1089.

May, P. R. A., Van Putten, T., Yale, C., Potegan, P., Jenden, D. J., Fairchild, M. D., Goldstein, M. J., & Dixon, W. J. (1976). Predicting individual responses to drug treatment in schizophrenia. A test dose model. *Journal of Nervous and Mental Disease, 162*, 177–183.

McGhie, A., & Chapman, J. (1961). Disorders of attention and perception in early schizophrenia. *British Journal of Medical Psychology, 34*, 103–116.

McGlashan, T. H. (1986). Predictors of shorter-, medium-, and longer-term outcome in schizophrenia. *American Journal of Psychiatry, 143*, 50–55.

Öhman, A., & Öhlund, L. S. (1989). Electrodermal nonresponding, premorbid adjustment and symptomatology as predictors of longterm social functioning in schizophrenics. *Journal of Abnormal Psychology, 98*, 426–435.

Oltmanns, T. F., Ohayon, J., & Neale, J. M. (1978). The effect of anti-psychotic medication and diagnostic criteria on distractibility in schizophrenia. *Journal of Psychiatric Research, 14*, 81–91.

Pandurangi, A. K., Goldberg, S. C., Brink, D. D., Hill, M. H., Gulati, A. N., & Hamer, R. M. (1989). Amphetamine challenge test, response to treatment and lateral ventrical size in schizophrenia. *Biological Psychiatry, 25*, 207–214.

Straube, E. R. (1979). On the meaning of electrodermal nonresponding in schizophrenia. *Journal of Nervous and Mental Disease, 167*, 601–611.

Straube, E. R., Schied, H.-W., Rein, W., & Breyer-Pfaff, U. (1987). Autonomic nervous system differences as predictors of short-term outcome in schizophrenics. *Pharmacopsychiatry, 20*, 105–110.

Straube, E. R., Wagner, W., & Ackermann, K. (1990, October). *Findings significant with respect to short- and medium-term outcome in schizophrenia.* Paper presented at the Fifth European Congress of the Association of European Psychiatrists, Strasbourg.

Straube, E. R., Wagner, W., Foerster, K., & Heimann, H. (1989). Findings significant with respect to short- and medium-term outcome in schizophrenia—a preliminary report. *Progress in Neuro-Psychopharmacology and Biological Psychiatry, 13,* 185–197.

Strauss, M. E., Law, M. F., Coyle, J. T., & June, M. D. (1985). Psychopharmacologic and clinical correlates of attention in chronic schizophrenia. *American Journal of Psychiatry, 142,* 497–499.

Tsuang, M. T. (1986). Predictors of poor and good outcome in schizophrenia. In L. Erlenmeyer-Kimling & N. E. Miller (Eds.), *Lifespan research on the prediction of psychopathology* (pp. 93–101). Hillsdale, NJ: Lawrence Erlbaum Associates.

Venables, P. H. (1957). A short scale for rating "activity-withdrawal" in schizophrenics. *Journal of Mental Science, 103,* 197–199.

Venables, P. H., & Wing, J. K. (1962). Level of arousal and the subclassification of schizophrenia. *Archives of General Psychiatry, 7,* 62–67.

Weinberger, D. R., Bigelow, L. B., & Kleinmann, J. E. (1980). Cerebral ventricular enlargement in chronic schizophrenia: An association with poor response to treatment. *Archives of General Psychiatry, 17,* 22–23.

Zahn, T. P., Carpenter, W. T., & McGlashan, T. H. (1981a). Autonomic nervous system activity in acute schizophrenia. I. Method and comparison with normal controls. *Archives of General Psychiatry, 38,* 251–258.

Zahn, T. P., Carpenter, W. T., & McGlashan, T. H. (1981b). Autonomic nervous system activity in acute schizophrenia. II. Relationships to short term prognosis and clinical state. *Archives of General Psychiatry, 38,* 260–266.

Part V

TREATMENT

16

Neuroleptics and Attention–Information Processing Trait Markers in Schizophrenia

HERBERT E. SPOHN

PERSONAL RESEARCH HISTORY

For the past 15 years I have been concerned with determining the extent to which, and ways in which, neuroleptic treatment is related to attention and information processing impairment in schizophrenia. In this process I have used a variety of measures developed in experimental psychopathology to access, most broadly speaking, cognitive and psychophysiological dysfunction. Thus, I have employed the Continuous Performance Test (Rosvold, Mirsky, Sarason, Bransome, & Beck, 1956), the Conceptual Breadth Test (Chapman & Taylor, 1957), the Thought Disorder Index (Johnston & Holzman, 1979), the Steffy Reaction Time Paradigm (Belissimo & Steffy, 1972), smooth pursuit eye movement recording (Holzman, Proctor, & Hughes, 1973), phasic and tonic electrodermal activity recording, the Wechsler Adult Intelligence Scale Verbal Subtests, the Gorham Proverbs Tests (Gorham, 1956), a size estimation procedure, and the full report span of apprehension procedure.

Initially the aims of the research program were to determine how much of the performance variance on these multiple measures was accounted for by neuroleptic treatment. In this fashion I sought to perform a service to the field. By providing this kind of information, investigators conducting studies concerned with cognitive and psychophysiological dysfunction with mostly medicated schizophrenics would be in a position to discriminate between dysfunction variance due to psychosis or general deficit functioning and variance due to neuroleptic treatment.

As my work progressed, however, my perceptions about the uses of my research program and data were gradually modified. These modifications are due to three major developments occurring in the 15-year time period within which my work has taken place.

For one thing, I came to recognize that my research was unique from the vantage point of its comprehensiveness. No other experimental psychopathologist had employed the multiple tasks and procedures that I have employed in the assessment of cognitive and psychophysiological functions in two large samples of schizophrenic patients. I have acquired a data base that makes it possible to identify interrelationships, for example, among phasic and tonic skin conductance activity, the reaction time crossover (RTX) effect (Spohn & Coyne, 1988), and eye movement dysfunction (EMD) and to partial out correlations due to neuroleptic treatment and tardive dyskinesia (Spohn, Coyne, & Spray, 1988). I return later to a discussion of how these opportunities to tease our relationships among multiple measures can aid in the elucidation of trait markers.

In addition, in the course of the last 15

years, during which I was pursuing studies of neuroleptic effects, the conceptual perspectives that guided research in schizophrenia have undergone profound transformations. Biological psychiatrists have given primary emphasis to neurological, genetic, and neuroscience conceptual tools and technologies. Experimental psychopathologists have become increasingly enamoured of such concepts as vulnerability, vulnerability or trait markers, and genetic markers. Studies of the RTX effect (Spohn & Coyne, 1988) or the skin conductance orienting response (SCOR; Spohn, Coyne, Wilson, & Hayes, 1989) or vigilance à la the Continuous Performance Test (Nuechterlein & Dawson, 1984), which in the past had been aimed at identification of pathological mechanisms, are now directed toward the identification of vulnerability or trait or genetic markers. This shift in conceptual orientation vis-à-vis the traditional tools of the psychological laboratory has had significant influence on interpretation of results derived from the experimental designs I have developed to determine neuroleptic treatment and cognitive dysfunction interrelationships in schizophrenia. I return to this theme when I discuss the central substantive issues of my research.

Finally, during the last 15 years the prevalence of tardive dyskinesia in neuroleptically treated schizophrenics has steadily risen. In 1981 the prevalence of persistent tardive dyskinesia was estimated at 13% (Jeste & Wyatt, 1981), in 1988 estimates had risen to 44% (Chouinard, Annable, Ross-Chouinard, & Mercier, 1988). Issues pertaining to mechanisms, prevention, risk factors, and treatment have received extensive attention during this time period. The supposition that tardive dyskinesia may be associated with specific cognitive dysfunction is only beginning to gain credibility.

I stumbled on evidence on behalf of this supposition in my data base in 1983. Other investigators did so somewhat earlier. In light of the perspectives that have guided my work, that cognitive dysfunction may be mediated by tardive dyskinesia or may represent a risk factor, I came to recognize separate needs. The specific nature of such dysfunction needed to be identified both (a) for purposes of prevention and (b) to gain clarity about cognitive dysfunction variance due to psychosis versus that due to tardive dyskinesia.

In this chapter I weave together the three themes I have touched on here. I show how studies of the relationship between neuroleptic treatment and attention–information-processing (AIP) impairment may lead to the putative identification of pathogenic trait markers and how correlational analysis of multiple measures of AIP dysfunction may significantly aid in this process. What we are learning about the tardive dyskinesia–cognitive functions relationship will provide a cautionary methodological perspective.

I have examined, among others, the relationship between neuroleptic treatment and tardive dyskinesia in three well-established forms of AIP dysfunctions. These are the RTX effect (Spohn & Coyne, 1988), EMD (Spohn et al., 1988), and SCOR nonresponding (Spohn et al., 1989). It is with respect to these three forms of AIP impairment that my studies throw light on their putative traithood and on inter-relationships among them. In order to make my case I must describe the specialized design context in which neuroleptic treatment–AIP relationships were examined as well as present, in synoptic form, the actual findings. A detailed description of this design may be found in Spohn et al. (1988). In so doing, I do not go into methodological, procedural, or data-analytic detail. Some of the work I describe here is in the literature or in press; some of it is being prepared for publication.

STUDY SAMPLE AND METHODOLOGY

Our studies included 100 Research Diagnostic Criteria–diagnosed schizophrenics, all of whom had shown a positive response to neuroleptic treatment. On a proportional random basis, 64 of the patients were abruptly withdrawn from medication and given facsimile placebos. Thirty-six patients remained on the type and schedule of neuroleptics they were receiving prior to research entry. In the course of a 10-week study period patients were tested on, among other procedures, a reaction time paradigm devised by Steffy and his students (Belissimo & Steffy, 1972) and a smooth pursuit eye movement (SPEM) procedure modeled on Holzman's procedure (Holzman et al., 1973). Also, SCOR response to mild innocuous auditory stimuli, as well as skin conductance level and nonspecific response frequency, were recorded. The patients were tested five times, once prior to randomization or at prewithdrawal of medication for the 64 placebo patients, and then at 2-week intervals four times thereafter. On each occasion of testing the Brief Psychiatric Rating Scale (BPRS) (Overall & Gorham, 1962) was rated, presence and severity of tardive dyskinesia was assessed by the Abnormal Involuntary Movement Scale (AIMS), and general deficit functioning was rated.

Two weeks after drug withdrawal (at or near the second test session), 21 of the drug-withdrawn patients had relapsed; at 4 weeks (at the third test session) an additional 32 patients were considered relapsed. (Relapse was indexed by increases in total pathology on the BPRS and by clinical judgment on the part of project and hospital ward staff.) We considered that the relapsed patients were relatively free of drug control over both symptoms and AIP functions at the test session nearest to which the relapse occurred. (I should add here that their relapses were not allowed to run their full course. On the identification of early relapse signs, patients were remedicated but continued with the test schedule of the project.) We assumed further that changes from prewithdrawal performance to test sessions at or near which relapse occurred were due either to neuroleptic medication or to practice. The 36 patients who remained on medication throughout were considered controls for practice and attention.

The logic of this design can also be viewed from another perspective. Our procedures led to the occurrence of an acute episode, or at least an incipient episode, with significant exacerbation of symptoms.

We were thus able to compare the performance of some 53 patients both in neuroleptically mediated remission at prewithdrawal and during an acute episode—that is, at relapse. In data analyses we always contrasted three groups: on-drug controls, nonrelapsed patients, and relapsed patients.

STUDY FINDINGS

Reaction Time Crossover

The procedure in which the RTX derived score is obtained entails measurement of response latencies in a reaction time paradigm in which a warning or ready signal occurs at varying durations (known as the preparatory interval) prior to the imperative tone signal to respond (also see Belissimo & Steffy, 1972). Preparatory intervals in the paradigm we used were 1, 3, and 7 seconds long. These intervals were presented in two orders: (a) regularly, in which the same preparatory interval was presented for four trials, making possible prediction from one to the next trial, and (b) irregularly—that is, in a quasi-random order obviating predictability. Normal subjects are able to take advantage of regular-order predictability at all preparatory interval durations. Schizophrenics are unable to do so at long intervals (in our case 7 seconds), with the result that irregular-order preparatory interval response latencies are shorter than regular-order response latencies. This is the RTX, which has been replicated in numerous studies beginning with that by Huston, Shakow, and Riggs in 1937 (Belissimo & Steffy, 1972) and which has been variously interpreted as an inability to maintain a major set or as reflecting redundancy-associated deficit.

In our data, when we contrasted reaction time performance in two quasi-independent comparisons of on-drug controls, nonrelapsed, and relapsed patients, we did not find differences in patterns of change in RTX from prewithdrawal to postwithdrawal tests. In terms of the logic of our design, we are unable to demonstrate a relation of neuroleptic treatment and the occurrence of the RTX. We found no difference in RTX during remission and during an acute episode in chronic schizophrenics. Parenthetically, let me say that we lacked power to detect anything other than a large effect; however, the RTX in relapsed patients was as stable at prewithdrawal as at postwithdrawal, as was the case for the other two groups.

We believe these findings permit us to argue that the RTX may be regarded as a putative trait marker. Indeed, this is consistent with findings reported by De Amicis and Cromwell (1979) that the RTX is found in 17% of first-degree relatives of schizophrenics and in 8% of the general population.

There is, however, a fly in the ointment here and its name is tardive dyskinesia. We found a substantial positive correlation between the magnitude of the RTX and ratings of severity of orofacial tardive dyskinesia, and no such correlation between RTX and severity of tardive dyskinesia in the extremities (Spohn & Coyne, 1988). This led to the supposition that tardive dyskinesia effects on the RTX are not mediated by interference with psychomotor response. Because age, chronicity, and general deficit functioning are known to be positively correlated, we performed a hierarchical, stepwise multiple regression analysis in which the RTX served as criterion and age, chronicity, and general deficit as predictors were forced into the regression equation in that order, with orofacial tardive dyskinesia as the fourth step. We found that age, chronicity, and general deficit cumulatively accounted for about 4% of RTX variance, whereas tardive dyskinesia accounted for 14% of RTX variance. This finding leads to the following inferences: (a) tardive dyskinesia may exacerbate the inability to maintain a major set, and (b) at least in some schizophrenics, RTX may not be a trait but rather is a tardive dyskinesia–dependent state.

Eye Movement Dysfunction

With regard to SPEM impairment or EMD, its current designation, a series of studies

have shown that about 80% of all schizophrenics manifest EMD (e.g., Holzman et al., 1974). That is, in schizophrenics eye tracking of a moving target is interrupted by small catch-up and spontaneous saccades, and phase lag is significantly greater in schizophrenics than in major depressive disorder patients and normal subjects. Attentional focusing (having numbers on the moving target that subjects are instructed to read) reduces saccadic interruptions but does not completely eliminate them.

Holzman et al. (1988), on the basis of extensive data from first-degree relatives and monozygotic twins, have proposed that EMD is the genetically determined phenotypical alternative to schizophrenia. Most of the eye tracking studies have been performed with neuroleptically treated schizophrenics. Hence, there remained a small margin of doubt about the trait status of EMD. We sought to resolve this doubt in our study (Spohn et al., 1988). We employed the classical procedure involving electro-oculographic recording and a pendulum target. Our results indicated that we could not demonstrate an effect of neuroleptics on EMD; that is, all three of our groups, controls, nonrelapsed, and relapsed patients, showed a slight worsening in eye tracking performance on repeated testing. Again, power was sufficient only to detect large effects. However, in eight patients who showed pre-to-post improvement this proved to be due to a failure on the part of these patients to comply with tracking instructions in the first test session but not in the second test session.

Because our findings indicated that EMD in schizophrenics is present both during neuroleptically mediated remission and during the incipient phases of an acute episode, we concluded that EMD was not a state-dependent phenomenon and that, as far as these findings are concerned, Holzman's genetic hypothesis remained intact.

Again, however, a relationship between tardive dyskinesia and EMD requires some qualification of the above conclusion. In 1985 (Spohn, Coyne, Lacoursiere, & Mazur, 1985) we reported that orofacial tardive dyskinesia accounted for about 10% of eye tracking variance (independent of age and sex, which are correlates of the EMD). In order to determine the specific effects of TD on eye tracking, we devised a two-factor scoring system in which every cycle of eye movement is characterized as to the percentage frequency of small saccades and large nontracking saccades. After satisfying ourselves that there were no differences in the frequency of movement artifacts between two groups equated for age and test session, one of which showed orofacial severity scores of 3 or more and the other of which was free of tardive dyskinesia, we found that the tardive dyskinesia patients showed a significantly larger number of large, nontracking saccades. This finding suggested that tardive dyskinesia patients are more likely to substitute saccadic eye movement for SPEM. This tendency was reduced in tardive dyskinesia patients in trials in which attention-focusing aids were employed, but it remained significantly greater than that of nondyskinetic schizophrenics.

Because our scoring system accounted for over 80% of the signal-to-noise ratio scoring system devised and used by Holzman (Lindsey, Holzman, Haberman, & Yasillo, 1978) to establish cutoff points for normal and abnormal eye tracking, we were forced to conclude that, at least in some schizophrenics, abnormal tracking is state dependent. Moreover, we took our findings in tardive dyskinesia patients to imply that substitution of saccadic eye movement for SPEM was centrally mediated and quite possibly reflected inattention or perhaps impairment in the ability to maintain a major set. This interpretation, of course, is similar to our interpretation of tardive dyskinesia effects on the RTX. I return to this issue at a later point.

Skin Conductance Activity

It is currently the consensus in the field that nonresponding (mostly indexed by the SCOR) to mild, innocuous stimulation (typically tones) is found in 40% to 50% of schizophrenics. Bernstein (1987), the leading authority in this field, has speculated that nonresponding reflects an inability or unwillingness to allocate attention to novel stimuli. Nonresponding has been found both during acute episodes and in remission. This finding, along with equivocal evidence that nonresponding is unaffected by neuroleptics and is characteristically associated with a tonic skin conductance activity significantly lower than that displayed by responders, has led to the supposition that nonresponding may be a trait marker.

In our effort to determine neuroleptic treatment relationships with nonresponding, we used state-of-the-art procedures to assess SCOR responding/nonresponding (to mild innocuous tones) as well as recording of skin conductance levels and nonspecific response frequencies (Spohn et al., 1989). We were unable to demonstrate a relationship between responding/nonresponding and neuroleptic treatment. That is, the pattern of change from prewithdrawal to postwithdrawal was essentially the same in the on-drug control, nonrelapsed, and relapsed patients. Cross-session habituation occurred to the same extent in all three groups. Moreover, no patient who had been a nonresponder in the prewithdrawal test became a stable responder in the two following postwithdrawal sessions. Again, another way of stating our results is that nonresponding was present in the same patients both during neuroleptically mediated remission and during the incipient phases of an acute episode.

We also found that patients who had been nonresponders on three occasions of testing showed significantly lower skin conductance levels and nonspecific response frequencies than either (a) responders (on all three occasions) or (b) cross-session habituators. These findings led us to the conclusion that nonresponding merited putative trait marker status at least in some schizophrenics.

Our findings for tonic skin conductance activity, however, were quite different. It was clearly evident in our data that either neuroleptic treatment is associated with a reduction in tonic activity or an episode-related increase in tonic activity (at the psychophysiological response level) parallels symptomatic exacerbation (at the psychopathology level).

Finally, tardive dyskinesia was not related in any extent to phasic activity. Tonic skin conductance activity, however, was moderately correlated with tardive dyskinesia in the extremeties. Because we recorded skin conductance from the phalanges of the middle and index fingers, we interpreted this finding as reflecting movement artifacts.

Relationships Among Study Measures

Our multiple dimensions of assessment enabled us (Spohn & Coyne, unpublished manuscript, 1990), by multiple regression analysis, to determine that both nonresponding and RTX share non-negligible variance in common with EMD, but do not share variance with each other. To state it in terms of direction of relationships, nonresponders are likely to show both larger crossover effects and poorer eye tracking than responders. However, nonresponding is to no extent predictive of the magnitude of the crossover effect. I should add that these relationships obtained after tardive dyskinesia had been partialled out.

DISCUSSION

There are several generalizations that may be derived from the results we obtained for the RTX, EMD, and phasic and tonic electrodermal activity. Let me emphasize that all such generalizations apply only to neuroleptic treatment–susceptible schizophrenics. At the lowest level of inference I believe we have demonstrated that the study of neuroleptic effects on AIP dysfunction can make a contribution to the identification of putative trait markers. Next, our results for the crossover effect, for EMD, and for SCOR nonresponding, when taken in concert with evidence from other pertinent studies, establishes these three forms of AIP dysfunction as trait markers with some

degree of credibility or, at least, nominates them as hypothetical trait markers worthy of empirical pursuit by other means.

Let me expand on this argument a bit. I assert, not only on the evidence I have presented here but also on evidence from other sources both in my data base and in those of others (Spohn & Strauss, 1989), that neuroleptic treatment reduces or normalizes only dysfunctions and symptoms that are exacerbated or arise de novo in the course of an acute psychotic episode. As I have tried to show, there are severely disabling dysfunctions that are not exacerbated in acute episodes. These same dysfunctions are not normalized or reduced (in drug treatment–susceptible patients) when neuroleptic treatment leads to partial remission. My argument is that such AIP impairments merit the hypothesis that they are trait markers, possibly pointing in the direction of pathogenic traits rooted in genetic loadings for schizophrenia. Moreover, they may be promising candidates, as Cromwell has suggested, for research aimed at identifying behavioral phenotypes to be found in unaffected first-degree relatives of schizophrenics. De Amicis and Cromwell (1979) have demonstrated this potential for the RTX and Holzman et al. (1974) have done so for EMD.

The question may well be asked whether the practical, ethical, and financial costs of the designs I have used may not prohibit assays of AIP impairments as potential trait markers. My answer is certainly yes. There are, however, simpler and cheaper procedures that are within the reach of many investigators. In many clinical settings schizophrenics are withdrawn from medication on admission to facilitate diagnosis and treatment planning and then returned to neuroleptic treatment after a 2- to 3-week washout assessment period. Such patients could be tested at the beginning and end of washout and then 2 to 3 weeks after remedication with an equated on-drug group to control for practice. Such studies can provide strong hints as to the neuroleptic treatment resistance of these AIP impairments which are candidates for traithood.

I want to be very clear on the point that I am not by any means excluding from potential traithood those AIP impairments that are exacerbated in acute episodes and reduced in neuroleptically mediated remission. Indeed, my colleague and collaborator, Dr. Lolafaye Coyne (personal communication), was able to show in a paradigmatic study that the BPRS symptom severity profile in a neuroleptically mediated remission predicted with remarkable accuracy which symptoms would show the greatest exacerbation. That is, those symptoms rated as most severe in remission were precisely the symptoms showing the greatest exacerbation at relapse. I am simply saying that AIP dysfunctions not exacerbated in acute episodes and not normalized or reduced by neuroleptic treatment are reasonable and indeed promising candidates for the imputation of trait marker status.

Finally, in the present connection I want to call attention to an interesting and suggestive difference between AIP trait markers that are susceptible to neuroleptic normalization and those that are not. The dopamine-blocking action or reduction of dopaminergic state at the onset of acute episodes is, of course, widely regarded as the primary mechanism of neuroleptic symptom and dysfunction reduction. From this one might infer that neuroleptically non-normalized or nonreduced dysfunction is not directly mediated by anomalies in a single neurotransmitter system nor necessarily directly mediated by neurochemical anomalies at all; rather, it is mediated by neuroanatomical or neurohistological defects. This speculation seems to me to point to the possibility that the identification of neuroleptically resistant trait markers may open up new perspectives concerning pathogenesis and pathophysiology in schizophrenia. Let me emphasize that I am not talking about dysfunctions found primarily in neuroleptic treatment–resistant patients in whom negative symptoms predominate.

Moving from one bold speculation to another, I now deal with the correlational relationships among SCOR, RTX, and EMD reported above. I believe that such relationships may lead to the discovery of underlying traits not accessible to traditional AIP measures and their conceptual infrastructure. By way of illustration, let me speculate on what the trait structure underlying the RTX-SCOR relationship with eye tracking might be like. What the pattern of shared variances makes evident is that EMD is not a unidimensional trait. Rather, it appears to be a component element in a trait structure comprised of two dimensions in a domain of dysfunction in orientation to events before they undergo later stages of information processing. SCOR nonresponding to novel stimuli may be akin to the inability to maintain orientation to the change in direction of a moving target in SPEM. Similarly, inability to maintain a major set to an impending event in the reaction time task, such that it can undergo processing, may be related to impairment in the ability to anticipate the direction of movement of a target changing orientation. Indeed, it is conceivable that this pathogenic trait structure reflecting impairment in orientation to events early in information processing may represent a primary dysfunction in some schizophrenics.

I hold no particular brief for this fanciful intellectual exercise, and, indeed, radically different interpretations are compatible with the correlational relationships we observed. I do believe, however, that it illustrates that our armamentarium of AIP measures, singularly studied, may not be capable of reflecting underlying and largely unknown trait structures. Assessment by multiple AIP measures, correlational analysis, and tests of construct validity are, in my view, the strategy of choice in the elucidation of these trait structures.

I close with some comments on tardive dyskinesia. Tragic as the consequences of this as yet untreatable affliction are in the lives of schizophrenics with persistent tardive dyskinesia, from the vantage point of the issues that we need to address, tardive dyskinesia is a nuisance variable. As such, however, it needs to be treated with respect and caution. Our data suggest that there is a relationship between the presence of severe tardive dyskinesia and cognitive dysfunction such that tardive dyskinesia may simulate trait markers. It is equally conceivable and possibly more likely that tardive dyskinesia–associated attention impairment may represent a risk factor for the occurrence of tardive dyskinesia. Not only our findings but those of several other investigators (e.g., Chouinard et al., 1988) support this contention. What is needed, therefore, is a research program that will make it possible to rule out one of these two alternative hypotheses. Until that is done we cannot, in good conscience, consider the trait markers, putatively identified as such in the data I have presented, to be pure reflections of AIP phenotypes. An alternative would be to exclude patients with tardive dyskinesia from studies seeking to identify traits. Indeed, in the case of eye movement research, this is already being done. It is, however, a tactic that is costly in terms of generalizability.

REFERENCES

Belissimo, A., & Steffy, R. A. (1972). Redundancy associated deficit in schizophrenic reaction time performance. *Journal of Abnormal Psychology, 80*, 299–307.

Bernstein, A. S. (1987). Orienting response research in schizophrenia: Where we have come and where we might go. *Schizophrenia Bulletin, 13*, 623–641.

Chapman, L. J., & Taylor, J. A. (1957). Breadth of deviate concepts used by schizophrenics. *Journal of Abnormal and Social Psychology, 54*, 118–123.

Chouinard, G., Annable, L., Ross-Chouinard, A., & Mercier, P. (1988). A 5-year prospective longitudinal study of tardive dyskinesia: Factors predicting appearance of new cases. *Journal of Clinical Psychopharmacology, 8*, 215–265.

De Amicis, L. A., & Cromwell, R. L. (1979). Reaction time crossover in process schizophrenics, their relatives and control subjects. *Journal of Nervous and Mental Disease, 167*, 593–600.

Gorham, D. R. (1956). Use of the Proverbs Test for differentiating schizophrenics from normals. *Journal of Consulting Psychology, 20*, 435–440.

Holzman, P. S., Kringlen, E., Matthysse, S. W.,

Lipton, R. B., Cramer, G., Levin, S., Lange, K., & Levy, D. (1988). A single dominant gene can account for eye tracking dysfunction and schizophrenia in offspring of discordant twins. *Archives of General Psychiatry, 45*, 641–650.

Holzman, P. S., Proctor, L. R., & Hughes, D. W. (1973). Eye tracking patterns in schizophrenia. *Science, 181*, 179–181.

Holzman, P. S., Proctor, L. R., Levy, D. L., Yasillo, N., Meltzer, H. Y., & Hurt, S. W. (1974). Eye tracking dysfunctions in schizophrenic patients and their relatives. *Archives of General Psychiatry, 31*, 143–151.

Huston, P. E., Shakow, D., & Riggs, L. A. (1937). Studies of motor function in schizophrenia. II. Reaction time. *Journal of General Psychology, 16*, 39.

Jeste, D. V., & Wyatt, R. J. (1981). Changing epidemiology of tardive dyskinesia: An overview. *American Journal of Psychiatry, 138*, 297–309.

Johnston, M. H., & Holzman, P. S. (1979). *Assessing schizophrenic thinking*. San Francisco: Jossey-Bass.

Lindsey, D. T., Holzman, P. S., Haberman, S., & Yasillo, N. J. (1978). Smooth pursuit eye movements: A comparison of two measurement techniques for studying schizophrenia. *Journal of Abnormal Psychology, 87*, 491–496.

Nuechterlein, K. H., & Dawson, M. E. (1984). Information processing and attentional functioning in the developmental course of schizophrenic disorders. *Schizophrenia Bulletin, 10*, 160–203.

Overall, J. E., & Gorham, D. R. (1962). The Brief Psychiatric Rating Scale. *Psychological Reports, 10*, 799–812.

Rosvold, H. E., Mirsky, A. F., Sarason, I., Bransome, E. D., Jr., & Beck, L. H. (1956). A continuous performance test of brain damage. *Journal of Consulting Psychology, 20*, 343–350.

Spohn, H. E., & Coyne, L. (1988, November). *The effect of neuroleptics on reaction time.* Paper presented at the meeting of the Society for Research in Psychopathology, Cambridge, MA.

Spohn, H. E., & Coyne, L. (1990). *Pathogenic traits in schizophrenia: A proposal for their conceptualization, identification and research utilization.* (Unpublished manuscript).

Spohn, H. E., Coyne, L., Lacoursiere, R., & Mazur, D. (1985). Relation of neuroleptic dose and tardive dyskinesia to attention, information processing, and psychophysiology in medicated schizophrenics. *Archives of General Psychiatry, 42*, 849–859.

Spohn, H. E., Coyne, L., & Spray, J. (1988). The effect of neuroleptics and tardive dyskinesia on smooth pursuit eye movement in chronic schizophrenics. *Archives of General Psychiatry, 45,* 833–840.

Spohn, H. E., Coyne, L., Wilson, J., & Hayes, K. (1989). Skin conductance orienting response: The role of neuroleptics. *Journal of Abnormal Psychology, 98,* 478–486.

Spohn, H. E., & Strauss, M. (1989). Relation of neuroleptic and anticholinergic medication to cognitive functions in schizophrenia. *Journal of Abnormal Psychology, 98,* 367–380.

17

Antipsychotic Medications and Schizophrenia: Effects in Acute and Maintenance Treatment of the Illness

NINA R. SCHOOLER

For more than a generation, antipsychotic or neuroleptic medications have had a central role in the treatment armamentarium for schizophrenia. The availability of these drugs is temporally linked to dramatic changes in the setting in which schizophrenia is treated. At the time that chlorpromazine—the prototypic antipsychotic medication—became available in the United States in the mid-1950s, most care of schizophrenic patients took place in hospitals and primarily in large public facilities inconveniently located at some distance from the urban centers that they served. Hospital stays were measured in years. Continued hospitalization was the default option for patients, and discharge had to be justified.

The start of widespread use of antipsychotic drugs parallels the start of a decline in the numbers of hospitalized psychiatric patients in the United States (Brill & Patton, 1959). However, the drop in numbers of hospitalized patients cannot be attributed only to the introduction of medication, because other factors were changing at the same time. Among these were social policies and the implementation of other treatment modalities. Accordingly, early discussions of drug efficacy noted that the greatest drop in hospital census was in hospitals that

had lacked intensive treatment programs in the prechlorpromazine era (e.g., Klerman, 1961). Within 10 years of their introduction, a general consensus had been reached that phenothiazines such as chlorpromazine and related drugs had broad efficacy in the treatment of schizophrenia (Cole & Davis, 1968). At present, both clinicians and researchers ignore the important effects—both clinical benefits and adverse reactions—of these drugs at their peril.

The first section of this chapter describes briefly the drugs that are currently generally available in the United States with a primary indication for the treatment of psychosis. The second section discusses drug efficacy in terms of phase of treatment, examining acute, continued, and maintenance phases. The emphasis here is on specific symptoms rather than on overall improvement, discharge, or prevention of relapse. This section draws heavily on multicenter collaborative studies conducted by the National Institute of Mental Health (NIMH) through its psychopharmacology research program. The final section discusses the only new drug to be approved for use in schizophrenia in over a decade—clozapine—and two other drugs that may be available within the next several years—remoxipride and risperidone.

AVAILABLE ANTIPSYCHOTIC DRUGS

With the exception of clozapine, to be discussed in a subsequent section, antipsychotic drugs are remarkably similar in overall pharmacological action and clinical efficacy. Authors of psychopharmacology texts are consistent in their judgments that the drugs are interchangeable in average efficacy, but generally note that some patients may show better clinical response to one rather than another agent (Mason & Granacher, 1980; Siris & Rifkin, 1983). As shown in Table 17.1, there are about 20 such agents available, representing five different chemical classes. A useful distinction among these agents is that between high- and low-potency agents—those that are used at relatively low milligram doses compared to those for which higher milligram doses are required to achieve similar efficacy. Although milligram potency is not related to therapeutic effect, it is related to the types of side effects that may be seen with these drugs. Lower potency agents are associated with sedation and autonomic side effects, of which orthostatic hypotension may be the most bothersome. These

effects are generally dose related and are more frequently seen early in treatment. Higher potency agents are more likely to cause extrapyramidal side effects such as muscle stiffness, rigidity, tremor, restlessness, or motoric slowing.

The first of these drugs available in the United States was chlorpromazine, a low-potency drug. For many years it remained the most widely prescribed. More recently the trend in prescribing has shifted to higher potency agents such as haloperidol (Reardon, Rifkin, Schwartz, Myerson, & Siris, 1989). With this shift has come a trend toward the use of higher equivalent dosage. This is perhaps due to reduced side effects such as sedation and orthostatic hypotension, which limit dosage escalation with lower potency agents. A number of researchers have developed dose equivalency models. The most widely used in the field is that developed by Davis (1976); dose equivalencies following his scheme are shown in Table 17.1.

For many purposes, strict dose equivalence may provide an illusion of precision that is not warranted. Alberto DiMascio

Table 17.1. Antipsychotic Medications Generally Available in the United States

Drug	Trade name	Relative potency[a]	Dose levels			
			Low	Moderate	Moderately high	High
Phenothiazines						
Chlorpromazine	Thorazine	100	≤300	301–599	600–999	≥1000
Thioridazine	Mellaril	100	≤200	201–400	401–600	≥601
Mesoridazine	Serentil	51	≤100	101–200	201–400	≥401
Piperacetazine	Quide	14	≤30	31–50	51–100	≥101
Acetophenazine	Tindal	19	≤20	21–40	41–60	≥61
Perphenazine	Trilafon	10	≤20	21–40	41–60	≥61
Trifluoperazine	Stelazine	5	≤10	11–20	21–29	≥30
Fluphenazine HCl	Prolixin	2	≤1	2–5	6–19	≥20
Fluphenazine decanoate (q 2 wk)	Prolixin decanoate	—	<25	25–<50	50–62.5	>62.5
Thioanthenes						
Chlorprothixene	Taractan	—	≤50	51–200	201–400	≥401
Thiothixene	Navane	3	≤10	11–25	26–49	≥50
Butyrophenones						
Haloperidol HCl	Haldol	2	≤5	6–20	21–49	≥50
Haloperidol decanoate (q 4 wk)	Haldol decanoate	—	<100	100–<200	200–300	>300
Indoles						
Molindone	Moban	10	≤30	31–75	76–150	≥151
Dibenzoxapines						
Loxapine	Loxitane	—	≤30	31–75	76–150	≥151

[a] *Source:* Data from Davis (1976).

(personal communication, 1978) developed dose ranges for use by researchers in rating hospital charts for medication exposure. These ranges are based on judgments of experienced clinicians and researchers. Dose ranges are defined as "low," "moderate," "moderately high," and "high." The current version of these ranges is presented in the final columns of Table 17.1. One advantage of such ratings is that they do not assume linearity throughout the dose range. Thus, a "moderate" dose of haloperidol spans a 15-mg range, whereas a "moderately high" dose incorporates a 30-mg range. A "high" rating is given to any dose above 50 mg. A second advantage has already been noted—that a ranked scale may be a better mirror of clinical judgment than precise numerical equivalence. Finally, such ratings readily can be made either from patient charts or clinical reports.

Although these antipsychotic medications do not have clear overall differences in terms of efficacy, there are individual differences in response to specific agents, so that some patients who have failed to improve with one drug may do better when shifted to another agent. There is also evidence that clinical deterioration may occur when patients are arbitrarily shifted from one medication to another (Gardos, 1974). Despite these reports, it has not been possible to identify patient symptom patterns (e.g., Goldberg, Frosch, Drossman, Schooler, & Johnson, 1972) or patient characteristics (e.g., Schooler, Boothe, & Goldberg, 1971) that reliably predict differential response to specific antipsychotic drugs.

Antipsychotic medications differ widely in terms of side-effect profile. Often the desire to take advantage of a side effect, such as sedation in the management of the acute phase of the illness, or to minimize one such as tremor or parkinsonian stiffness, may influence the clinical decision regarding which drug to use.

EFFICACY OF ANTIPSYCHOTIC MEDICATION FOR SPECIFIC SYMPTOMS

Antipsychotic drug efficacy encompasses a wide range of actions. The same drugs that serve to treat acute symptom exacerbations during a relatively brief 6-week period (e.g., NIMH-PSC Collaborative Study Group, 1964) allow for continued improvement over a longer period of 6 months (NIMH-PRB, Collaborative Study Group, 1967) and also prevent relapse in relatively asymptomatic patients (Hogarty, Goldberg, Schooler, & Ulrich, 1974). This does not mean that antipsychotic agents represent a "cure" for the illness of schizophrenia. Results of medication discontinuation studies and clinical experience with individual patients provide evidence that symptoms re-emerge when patients stop taking medication. Furthermore, some follow-up studies recently reviewed by Wyatt (1991) suggest that early intervention with antipsychotic medication may improve the long-term course of the illness.

In recent years, characterization of symptoms in terms of whether they reflect positive or negative features of the illness has received a great deal of attention (Carpenter, Heinrichs, & Wagman, 1988). The determination of which symptoms "fit" the negative symptom or syndrome category varies substantially among investigators. DeLeon and his colleagues (deLeon, Wilson, & Simpson, 1989) found that only flattened affect and poverty of speech content were generally included in scales of negative symptoms. Determination of whether negative symptoms respond to antipsychotic medication is also a hotly contested issue (e.g., Crow, 1985; Goldberg, 1985). Other distinctions among the symptoms that characterize schizophrenia have been applied in the effort to determine whether there are symptom-specific effects of antipsychotic medication. These include paranoid versus withdrawal symptoms (Venables & Wing, 1962) and accessory versus fundamental symptoms (Bleuler, 1950/1911).

This section examines efficacy from the perspective of specific symptomatology, and in particular distinguishes between effects of medication in the acute phase of the illness versus the longer term. In general, evidence drawn from studies that involve comparison of medication to placebo or, in the absence of placebo-controlled studies, comparisons of different dosages, is more persuasive regarding efficacy than studies that do not have comparison groups. I rely more heavily on such studies and specifically address whether there are differences in the response to specific symptoms between antipsychotic medication and placebo as well as differences that depend on the phase of the illness.

Short-Term Treatment of Acute Psychotic Exacerbation

Good evidence for efficacy in the acute phase of the illness comes from studies comparing placebo to antipsychotic drugs. A major, early study (NIMH-PSC Collaborative Study Group, 1964) compared three different drugs (chlorpromazine, fluphenazine, and thioridazine) to a placebo. Three hundred forty acutely ill schizophrenic patients at nine hospitals were treated for 6 weeks. There were no differences among the antipsychotic drugs, but significant overall differences were found in ratings of

severity of illness after 6 weeks between drug and placebo. The median rating for placebo-treated patients ($n = 74$) was between markedly and moderately ill; the median score for the 270 drug-treated patients was between mildly and borderline ill. This difference actually represents an underestimate of the magnitude of effect, because only patients who received 6 weeks of treatment were included in analyses. For 29% of patients assigned to placebo, compared to only 2% of those randomized to the three antipsychotic drugs, treatment was discontinued for lack of efficacy before the end of the treatment period.

A detailed analysis of symptom ratings from this study (Goldberg, Klerman, & Cole, 1965) addressed the specificity of the therapeutic effect. Drug-treated patients improved significantly over the 6-week period in all symptoms assessed. Table 17.2 presents the symptoms and indicates whether patients who had the symptoms improved significantly under placebo treatment, whether the difference between drug and placebo was significant, and finally whether patients who did not have the symptom

Table 17.2 Six-Week Outcome of Symtoms[a]

Symptom and behavior	Placebo[b] pre–post improvement	Drug–placebo[b] pre–post difference	Drug–placebo[c] difference in development
Hostility	.05	.01	NS
Disorientation	.01	NS	.05
Guilt	.01	NS	NS
Auditory hallucination	.01	.05	.05
Agitation and tension	.05	.01	NS
Slowed speech and movements	NS	.01	.01
Delusions of grandeur	.01	NS	NS
Indifference to environment	NS	.01	.01
Incoherent speech	.01	.01	.01
Pressure of speech	.01	.01	NS
Ideas of persecution	.01	.01	NS
Hebephrenic symptoms	NS	.01	.01
Nonauditory hallucinations	.01	NS	NS
Memory deficit	.01	NS	NS
Social participation	.01	.01	NS
Irritability	NS	.01	NS
Self-care	NS	.01	.05
Appearance of sadness	.01	NS	NS
Feelings of unreality	.01	NS	NS
Resistiveness	NS	NS	NS
Confusion	.01	.01	NS

[a] Data entries are significance level.
[b] Only patients who had symptoms at pretreatment.
[c] Only patients who did not have symptoms at pretreatment.

were more likely to develop it with placebo treatment. As can be seen from the table, in contrast to the broad efficacy of medication on all symptoms evaluated, improvement from placebo varies among symptoms. Despite a significant difference between drug and placebo in overall improvement, there are indeed some specific symptoms for which medication is not significantly better than placebo. Goldberg and his colleagues suggested that the differences between drug and placebo are greater for symptoms reflecting Bleuler's accessory rather than fundamental symptoms (Bleuler, 1950/1911). This study challenges the notion that negative symptoms in schizophrenia do not respond to antipsychotic drugs (Crow, 1985), because significant drug-related improvement is reported in some of these symptoms.

Three symptoms have been chosen to illustrate different patterns of drug–placebo differences, as shown in Figure 17.1. In hebephrenic symptoms (Figure 17.1*A*), there is no significant placebo improvement and a significant medication–placebo difference. In delusions of grandeur (Figure 17.1*B*), there is significant improvement under placebo treatment and no significant difference between medication and placebo. Finally, in social participation (Figure 17.1*C*), there is significant improvement with placebo but more improvement with medication, so that the medication–placebo difference is significant.

Continuation Treatment

Not many studies have looked at treatment effects beyond 6 to 8 weeks in patients who are acutely symptomatic. In general, overall improvement continues up to 6 months in drug-treated patients, although the increments in improvement are smaller with succeeding weeks (e.g., Casey et al., 1960, NIMH-PRB, Collaborative Study Group, 1967).

The multicenter 24-week study by Casey and his colleagues (1960) included a placebo-treated group and was congruent in results with shorter term studies. Chlorpro-

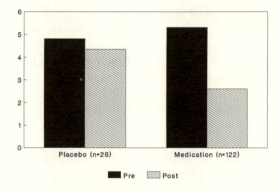

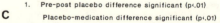

1. Pre-post placebo difference not significant.
A Placebo-medication difference significant (p<.05)

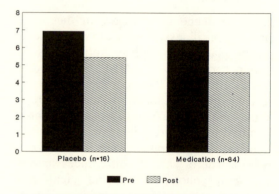

1. Pre-post placebo difference significant (p<.01)
B Placebo-medication difference significant (p<.01)

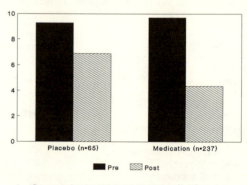

1. Pre-post placebo difference significant (p<.01)
C Placebo-medication difference significant (p<.01)

Figure 17.1. Patterns of drug–placebo differences in short-term symptom reduction. (*A*) Change in hebephrenic symptoms. Pre–post placebo difference not significant; placebo–medication difference significant (*p*<.05). (*B*) Change in delusions of grandeur. Pre–post placebo and placebo–medication differences both significant (*p*<.01). (*C*) Change in social participation. Pre–post placebo and placebo–medication differences both significant (*p*<.01). *Solid bars,* pretreatment; *shaded bars,* post-treatment.

mazine–placebo differences occurred for some but not all specific symptoms. The investigators also found continued improvement in a "total morbidity score" during the first 18 weeks but no change between the 18th and 24th week. However, only one third of the patients were initially described as both "acute and disturbed."

The 6-month multicenter study conducted by the NIMH-PRB Collaborative Study Group (1967), which was restricted to newly hospitalized and acutely ill patients, included three antipsychotic drugs but did not have a placebo-treated group. In agreement with the 6-week study conducted at the same hospitals, all symptoms measured improved significantly over the first 5 weeks (Goldberg, Schooler, & Mattsson, 1967). Ratings of overall severity continued to improve significantly during the subsequent weeks, although, as shown in Figure 17.2A, the rate of improvement slowed. In contrast, only some specific symptoms improved between weeks 5 and 13. No individual symptoms improved significantly after week 13. Paranoid symptoms such as delusions of grandeur and ideas of persecution continued to improve significantly between weeks 5 and 13, as shown in Figure 17.2B. In contrast, as shown in Figure 17.2C, symptoms of withdrawal, such as indifference to environment and slowed speech and movements, showed improvement only during the first 5 weeks. The positive–negative symptom distinction would also be congruent with these findings. Early improvement occurs in both classes of symptoms, but continued improvement is seen only in positive symptoms.

Long-Term Maintenance Treatment

The primary goal of maintenance treatment in schizophrenia has been the prevention of relapse or symptom exacerbation in patients who have achieved either symptom remission or stability. In his review of this literature, Davis (1975) aggregated data from 24 studies and reported that approximately 20% of the 1,858 patients treated with antipsychotic medication relapsed

compared to 52% of the 1,337 patients randomized to placebo. Just as many studies of efficacy have not been restricted to patients who were acutely symptomatic many of the studies included in Davis' review were not limited to patients who were clearly symptomatically stable or in remission. Schooler and Severe (1984) reviewed the same studies in order to evaluate medication effects on specific symptoms, in contrast to relapse. In general, they found that studies conducted with more chronic inpatients were less likely to find medication effects on negative symptoms.

Three placebo-controlled maintenance studies conducted with outpatients assessed symptoms in patients who did not relapse, so that the effects of medication on symptoms can be separated from the decompensation that defines relapse (Engelhardt, Rosen, Freedman, & Margolis, 1963; Hogarty et al., 1974; Rifkin, Quitkin, Kane, Klein, & Ross, 1979). In general, once the symptom exacerbation that defines relapse is eliminated, there are few reliable symptom differences between patients receiving medication versus placebo. Hogarty Goldberg, and Schooler (1974) reported a complex but consistent pattern of results suggesting that gender, medication, and psychosocial treatment all influence symptomatic outcome increasingly over time. In patients who do not relapse, those who received medication and a psychosocial treatment ("major role therapy") showed less symptomatology than those who received medication alone. In contrast, under placebo treatment, patients who received role therapy were more symptomatic than those who did not.

In symptomatically stable schizophrenic patients the primary effect of medication is prevention of relapse or exacerbation. Gains in symptom reduction are won during the first months of treatment. Although these gains can be lost through relapse, continued progress apparently relies on other treatment modalities and is based on prevention of relapse.

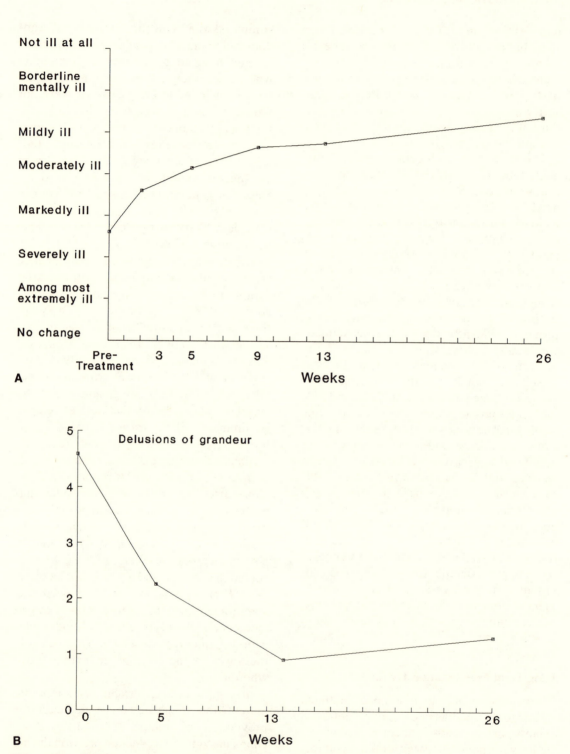

Figure 17.2. Symptom reduction during 26 weeks on medication. (*A*) Global severity. (*B*) Delusions of grandeur. *Figure continued on following page.*

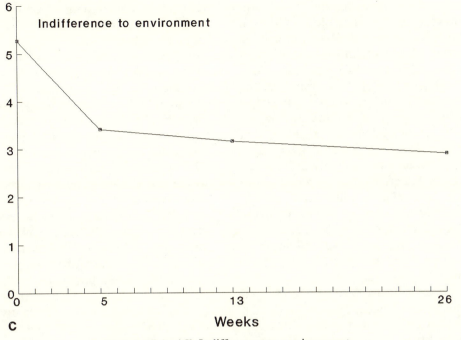

Figure 17.2. (*C*) Indifference to environment.

NEWER MEDICATIONS: ATYPICAL ANTIPSYCHOTIC AGENTS

The tantalizing prospect of new antipsychotic drugs that provide clinical efficacy beyond that of the generally interchangeable drugs discussed earlier in this chapter had been for many years just that—tantalizing, but unrealized. In this section I discuss three drugs that may realize that promise. The first of these, clozapine, appears to be effective for patients who are resistant to treatment with classic antipsychotic drugs. Because of a serious adverse effect it has been available under restrictive conditions and only since mid-1990. The second, remoxipride, is still undergoing investigation in the United States; reports suggest that it does not differ from classic antipsychotic drugs in efficacy, but its side-effect profile in terms of extrapyramidal signs is more favorable (Tamminga & Gerlach, 1987). The third, risperidone, also is still under investigation in the United States. Initial controlled trial results suggest that it too has a more favorable side-effect profile, and it has pharmacological characteristics that are

quite different from the classic antipsychotic agents.

All these drugs are considered to be "atypical" antipsychotic medications, defined by efficacy against psychotic symptoms coupled with a lower propensity to show extrapyramidal side effects. The drugs are diverse both chemically and pharmacologically (Seeman, 1990). Optimally, the hope for these agents is that they will provide a therapeutic advantage as well as a reduced side-effect liability.

Clozapine

In 1990, the Food and Drug Administration approved the marketing of the first new antipsychotic medication in well over a decade. It is the first medication that is substantially different from the medications discussed in earlier sections of this chapter. Clozapine, a dibenzodiazepine, is chemically related to loxapine, but has a very different pharmacological profile and is considered an atypical antipsychotic drug. It also has a checkered history. In 1975, while it was undergoing clinical testing both in the United States and internationally, agranulocytosis—a dramatic lowering of the white blood cell count and protection from infection—occurred in a series of 13 patients in Finland, eight of whom died from secondary infections (Griffith & Saameli, 1975). Research with the drug was halted in the United States and its use was severely restricted worldwide. However, early studies had suggested that clozapine might have specific advantages for patients who were severely ill (Fischer-Cornelssen & Ferner, 1976), and it continued to be available for a limited number of patients who appeared to benefit uniquely from the medication and who received continued monitoring to detect reduction in white blood count before the onset of infection.

Persistent clinical reports of benefit led Kane and his colleagues (Kane, Honigfeld, Singer, & Meltzer, 1988) to conduct a formal clinical trial. They compared clozapine to chlorpromazine in patients who met carefully defined criteria for poor response to at least three other antipsychotic medications and who further failed to respond to a 6-week trial of haloperidol. Results were impressive. After 6 weeks, 30% of the clozapine-treated patients met an improvement criterion compared to only 4% of those treated with chlorpromazine. In the clozapine-treated patients, there was significant pre–post improvement for all specific symptoms with the exception of motor retardation.

Table 17.3 presents findings comparing the efficacy of clozapine and chlorpromazine for specific symptoms. The findings are analogous to the results presented in Table 17.2, comparing antipsychotic medication to placebo during a similar length of treatment exposure for a less restrictive population of schizophrenic patients. As can be seen from Table 17.3, although both clozapine- and chlorpromazine-treated patients improved in a range of symptoms, in this severely ill patient population, chlorpromazine-treated patients did not show significant change in a number of negative symptoms. These are very similar to the symptoms that fail to improve with placebo treatment and develop in the absence of medication for the wider group of schizophrenic patients. It appears that some schizophrenic patients who do not benefit from the classic antipsychotic agents do experience benefit from clozapine, and that improvement is in those symptoms in which

Table 17.3 Six-Week Comparison of Clozapine and Chlorpromazine[a]

Symptom or behavior	Chlorpromazine pre–post improvement	Chlorpromazine–clozapine pre–post difference
BPRS positive symptoms		
Conceptual disorganization	Sig	001
Mannerisms	NS	001
Hostility	Sig	001
Suspiciousness	Sig	001
Hallucinatory behavior	Sig	001
Excitement	Sig	001
Unusual thought	Sig	001
Grandiosity	NS	NS
BPRS negative symptoms		
Emotional withdrawal	NS	001
Uncooperativeness	NS	001
Blunted affect	NS	001
Disorientation	NS	001
Motor retardation	NS	05
BPRS general symptoms		
Somatic concern	NS	01
Anxiety	Sig	NS
Guilt	Sig	NS
Tension	Sig	001
Depressed mood	Sig	NS

[a] Data entries are significance level.

typical antipsychotic drugs differ from placebo for the broader population of schizophrenic patients.

Remoxipride

Remoxipride, like clozapine, is considered an atypical antipsychotic agent. Chemically it is a substituted benzamide (sulpiride is another member of the same chemical class). Remoxipride has been compared to haloperidol, a typical neuroleptic, in a number of short-term (6-week) double-blind studies. In their review of nine such studies, Lewander, Westerburgh, and Morrison (1990) aggregated the data across studies and doses. They reported no differences between remoxipride and haloperidol in short-term efficacy as defined by a number of measures, including global improvement ratings and changes in positive and negative symptoms. About 57% of the 858 patients in the studies were rated as much improved or very much improved. However, none of these studies included a placebo control.

Three further studies that incorporate additional controls provide data regarding short-term efficacy. The first (Chouinard, 1990) compared remoxipride to a standard neuroleptic, chlorpromazine, and to a placebo. In this small study, chlorpromazine was significantly more effective than remoxipride in a wide range of symptoms and marginally more effective than placebo. Remoxipride could not be reliably distinguished from placebo. The second study (Patris, Agassol, Alby, Brion, Burnat, & Castelnau et al., 1990) examined two doses of remoxipride, low and moderate, and haloperidol in a 6-week study. There were no overall differences among the treatment groups, but haloperidol was significantly better for positive symptoms, and the moderate dose of remoxipride was significantly better for negative symptoms. The third study (Lapierre, Nair, Awad, Chouinard, Saxena, & Jones et al., 1990) compared three doses of remoxipride, a very low, a low, and a moderate dose, to haloperidol. The very low dose, which was lower than that administered in other trials, was less effective for a wide range of symptoms than the two higher dose levels of remoxipride and haloperidol.

On balance, remoxipride appears to be an effective antipsychotic, not different from the already available medications in terms of efficacy. It also clearly merits its atypical label. As Lewander and his colleagues reported (1990), it has a significantly lower rate of extrapyramidal symptoms, specifically rigidity, restlessness, and motoric slowing.

Risperidone

Risperidone provides blockade of the D_2 dopamine receptor, like all available antipsychotic agents (Seeman, 1990). In addition, it was specifically formulated to block the S_2 serotonin receptor, based on an observation that ritanserin, a drug that antagonizes the S_2 receptor, was effective against negative symptoms when used in conjunction with haloperidol (Janssen, Niemegeers, Awouters, Schellekens, & Meert, 1988). Its pharmacological profile also predicts that it would be an atypical antipsychotic agent.

Preliminary open studies (Gelders, 1989) appear to support these predictions—symptom levels declined broadly, as did extrapyramidal symptoms. A small, double-blind study comparing risperidone to haloperidol and a placebo also suggests both its efficacy and that it is an atypical antipsychotic (Borison, Pathiraja, Diamond, & Meibach, 1991). Risperidone and haloperidol both reduced psychotic symptoms significantly more than placebo. Risperidone and placebo both showed less severe extrapyramidal symptoms than haloperidol. Results of multicenter studies both in the United States and abroad also suggest that risperidone is an effective antipsychotic drug.

CONCLUSIONS

During most of the past three decades, changes in treatment practice with antipsychotic drugs have been more reflective of style than of differences in available agents. I have reviewed some data that suggest that the effects of these drugs are quite specific in terms of symptoms of psychopathology during periods of active symptom control in relatively symptomatic patients. In patients who have achieved symptom control, these drugs appear to serve to delay or prevent new episodes, but the kind of symptom specificity described for acute treatment is not as clearly shown.

For the first time in over a decade, a new antipsychotic drug is available and the prospect is relatively bright that it will be followed by others. Some of these newer compounds, as described in an earlier section, are hypothesized to have differential effectiveness for specific symptoms. Should this promise be realized, an early hope expressed for antipsychotic drugs—"The right drug for the right patient" (Klett & Mosely, 1963)—may yet be attained.

REFERENCES

Bleuler, E. (1950). *Dementia praecox, or the group of schizophrenias* (J. Zinken, Trans.). New York: International Universities Press. (Original work published 1911).

Borison, R. L., Pathiraja, A. P., Diamond, B. I., & Meibach, R. C. (1991). Risperidone in the treatment of acute exacerbation of chronic schizophrenia. *Schizophrenia Research, 4*, 314–315.

Brill, H., & Patton, R. E. (1959). Analysis of population reduction in New York state mental hospitals during the first four years of large-scale therapy with psychotropic drugs. *American Journal of Psychiatry, 116*, 495–509.

Carpenter, W. T., Jr., Heinrichs, D. W., & Wagman, A. M. I. (1988). Deficit and nondeficit forms of schizophrenia: The concept. *American Journal of Psychiatry, 145*, 578–583.

Casey, J. F., Bennett, I. F., Lindley, C. J., Hollister, L. E., Gordon, M. H., & Springer, M. N. (1960). Drug therapy in schizophrenia: A controlled study of the relative effectiveness of chlorpromazine, promazine, phenobarbital and placebo. *Archives of General Psychiatry, 2*, 210–220.

Chouinard, G. (1990). A placebo-controlled clinical trial of remoxipride and chlorpromazine in newly admitted schizophrenic patients with acute exacerbation. *Acta Psychiatrica Scandinavica Supplementum, 358*, 111–119.

Cole, J. O., & Davis, J. M. (1968). Clinical efficacy of the phenothiazines as anti-psychotic drugs. In D. H. Efron (Ed.), *Psychopharmacology: A review of progress* (pp. 1057–1066). Washington, DC: U. S. Government Printing Office.

Crow, T. J. (1985). The two syndrome concept: Origins and current status. *Schizophrenia Bulletin, 11*, 471–485.

Davis, J. M. (1975). Overview: Maintenance medication in psychiatry: I. Schizophrenia. *American Journal of Psychiatry, 132*, 1237–1245.

Davis, J. M. (1976). Comparative doses and costs of antipsychotic medication. *Archives of General Psychiatry, 33*, 858–861.

deLeon, J., Wilson, W. H., & Simpson, G. M. (1989). Measurement of negative symptoms in schizophrenia. *Psychiatric Developments, 7*, 211–234.

Engelhardt, D. M., Rosen, B., Freedman, D., & Margolis, R. (1963). Long term drug-induced symptom modification in schizophrenic out-patients. *Journal of Nervous and Mental Disease, 137*, 231–241.

Fischer-Cornelssen, K. A., & Ferner, U. J. (1976). An example of European multicenter trials: Multispectral analysis of clozapine. *Psychopharmacology Bulletin, 12*, 34–39.

Gardos, G. (1974). Are antipsychotic drugs interchangeable? *Journal of Nervous and Mental Disease, 159*, 343–348.

Gelders, Y. G. (1989). Thymosthenic agents, a novel approach in the treatment of schizophrenia. *British Journal of Psychiatry, 155*(suppl. 5), 33–36.

Goldberg, S. G. (1985). Negative and deficit symptoms in schizophrenia do respond to neuroleptics. *Schizophrenia Bulletin, 11*, 453–456.

Goldberg, S. C., Frosch, W. A., Drossman, A. K., Schooler, N. R., & Johnson, G. F. S. (1972). Prediction of response to phenothiazines in schizophrenia. *Archives of General Psychiatry, 26*, 367–373.

Goldberg, S. C., Klerman, G. L., & Cole, J. O. (1965). Changes in schizophrenic psychopathology and ward behaviour as a function of phenothiazine treatment. *British Journal of Psychiatry, 111*, 120–133.

Goldberg, S. C., Schooler, N. R., & Mattsson, N. (1967). Paranoid and withdrawal symptoms in schizophrenia: Differential symptom reduction over time. *Journal of Nervous and Mental Disease, 145*, 158–162.

Griffith, R. W., & Saameli, K. (1975). Clozapine and agranulocytosis. *Lancet, 2*, 657.

Hogarty, G. E., Goldberg, S. C., Schooler, N. R., & Ulrich, R. F. (1974). Drug and sociotherapy in the aftercare of schizophrenic patients: II. Two-year relapse rates. *Archives of General Psychiatry, 31,* 603–608.

Janssen, P. A. J., Niemegeers, D. J. E., Awouters, F., Schellekens, A. A. H. P., & Meert, T. F. (1988). Pharmacology of *Risperidone (R64 766),* a new antipsychotic with Serotonin-S_2 and Dopamine-D_2 antagonistic properties. *Journal of Pharmacology and Experimental Therapeutics, 244,* 685–693.

Kane, J. M., Honigfeld, G., Singer, J., & Meltzer, H. (1988). Clozapine for treatment resistant schizophrenia. *Archives of General Psychiatry, 45,* 789–796.

Klerman, G. L. (1961). Historical baselines for the evaluation of maintenance drug therapy of discharged psychiatric patients. In M. Greenblatt, D. J. Levinson, & G. L. Klerman (Eds.), *Mental patients in transition:* steps in hospital community rehabilitation. (pp. 287–301). Springfield, IL: Charles C Thomas.

Klett, C. J., & Moseley, E. C. (1965). The right drug for the right patient. *Journal of Consulting Psychology, 29,* 546–551.

Lapierre, Y. D., Nair, N. P. V., Chouinard, G., Saxena, B., Jones, B., McClure, D. J., Bakish, D., Max, P., Manchanda, R., Beaudry, D., Bloom, D., Rostein, E., Ancill, R., Sandor, P., Sladen-Dew, N., Durand, C., Chandrasena, R., Horn, E., Elliot, D., Das, M., Ravindran, A., & Matsos, G. (1990). A controlled dose-ranging study of remoxipride and haloperidol in schizophrenia—a Canadian multicentre trial. *Acta Psychiatrica Scandinavica Supplementum, 358,* 72–76.

Lewander, T., Westerburgh, S-E., & Morrison, D. (1990). Clinical profile of remoxipride—a combined analysis of a comparative double-blind multicentre trial programme. *Acta Psychiatrica Scandinavica Supplementum, 358,* 92–98.

Mason, A. S., & Granacher, R. P. (1980). *Clinical handbook of anti-psychotic drug therapy.* New York: Brunner/Mazel.

NIMH-PRB Collaborative Study Group. (1967). Clinical effects of three phenothiazines in "acute" schizophrenia. *Diseases of the Nervous System, 28,* 369–383.

NIMH-PSC Collaborative Study Group. (1964). Phenothiazine treatment in acute schizophrenia. *Archives of General Psychiatry, 10,* 246–261.

Patris, M., Agussol, P., Alby, J. M., Brion, S., Burnat, G., Castelnau, D., Duluermoz, S., Dufour, H., Ferreri, M., Goudemand, M., Leguay, D., Lamperiere, T., Martin, A., Morin, D., Tignol, J., Vincent, T., & Albaret, C. (1990). A double-blind multicentre comparison of remoxipride, at two dose levels, and haloperidol. *Acta Psychiatrica Scandinavica Supplementum 358,* 78–82.

Reardon, G. T., Rifkin, A., Schwartz, A., Myerson, A., & Siris, S. G. (1989). Changing patterns of neuroleptic dosage over a decade. *American Journal of Psychiatry, 146,* 726–729.

Rifkin, A., Quitkin, F., Kane, J. M., Klein, D. F., & Ross, D. (1979). The effect of fluphenazine upon social and vocational functioning in remitted schizophrenics. *Biological Psychiatry, 14,* 499–508.

Schooler, N. R., Boothe, H., & Goldberg, S. C. (1971). Life history and symptoms in schizophrenia. *Archives of General Psychiatry, 25,* 138–147.

Schooler, N. R., & Severe, J. B. (1984). Efficacy of drug treatment for chronic schizophrenic patients. In M. Mirabi (Ed.), *The chronically mentally ill: Research and services* (pp. 125–141). New York: Spectrum Publications.

Seeman, P. (1990). Atypical neuroleptics: Role of multiple receptors, endogenous dopamine, and receptor linkage. *Acta Psychiatrica Scandinavica Supplementum, 358,* 14–20.

Siris, S. G., & Rifkin, A. (1983). Drug treatment of acute schizophrenia. In A. Rifkin (Ed.), *Schizophrenia and affective disorders: Biology and drug treatment* (pp. 237–280). Boston: John Wright/PSG Inc.

Tamminga, C. A., & Gerlach, J. (1987). New neuroleptics and experimental antipsychotics in schizophrenia. In H. Y. Meltzer (Ed.), *Psychopharmacology: The third generation of progress* (pp. 1129–1140). New York: Raven Press.

Venables, P. H., & Wing, J. K. (1962). Level of arousal and the subclassification of schizophrenia. *Archives of General Psychiatry, 7,* 114–119.

Wyatt, R. J. (1991). Neuroleptics and the natural course of schizophrenia. *Schizophrenia Bulletin, 17,* 325–351.

Part VI

CONCEPTUAL STRUCTURE AND FAMILY INTERVENTION

18

Spontaneous and Induced Cognitive Changes in Rehabilitation of Chronic Schizophrenia

WILL D. SPAULDING

There can no longer be any doubt that cognitive vulnerabilities and impairments play an important role in schizophrenia, as many of the contributions in this volume make clear. So far, our accumulating knowledge of these vulnerabilities and impairments has been applied primarily toward better understanding the etiology and the natural history of the disorder. As a result, we now believe with a reasonable degree of confidence that abnormalities in attention and other aspects of cognition often appear in childhood, that these are either indicators of a psychobiological predisposition to schizophrenia or a cause of impaired development or both, and that these and other abnormalities worsen in severity with the onset of the disorder (Nuechterlein & Dawson, 1984). More recently, we have learned that some cognitive impairments improve with recovery and worsen with relapse throughout the disorder's course, whereas others remain fairly constant (Nuechterlein, Edel, Norris, & Dawson, 1986; Spohn et al., 1986).

More direct application of cognitive psychopathology to clinical assessment and treatment has had a fitful and convoluted history. In the 1950s, as psychiatry emerged from domination by classical psychoanalytical theory, the new "ego psychology" renewed interest in the cognitive hypotheses about schizophrenia proposed by Bleuler. Some well-known writers (e.g., Arieti, 1955; Cameron & Magaret, 1951) developed models of schizophrenic cognition that were complementary to treatment, but the models were not based on verifiable laboratory findings in the cognitive domain, and the treatment techniques to which they contributed never developed beyond traditional analytical–interpretative psychotherapy.

Widespread use of antipsychotic drugs in the 1960s competed with further interest in cognitive models in psychiatry. In retrospect, this seems rather ironic. The efficacy of the drugs was established through measurement of their dramatic effects in the behavioral domain. Nobody ever questioned the tacit assumption that behavioral effects are mediated by effects on cognition and related brain functions, yet almost all research on the "mechanisms" of antipsychotic drug effects addressed histochemical and neurophysiological phenomena. Probably, this was partly because research in nonpsychiatric pharmacology had enjoyed plenty of success with those foci of interest and partly a result of the rise of the "neo-Kraepelinians" in the 1970s.

The neo-Kraepelinians successfully urged psychiatry toward nosologies based on nonoverlapping categories defined by presence or absence of signs and symptoms observable in a case history or interview. The *Diagnostic and Statistical Manual of Mental Disorders,* third edition (American Psychiatric Association, 1980) is the chief result. This preoccupation with sign- and symptom-based classification directed psychiatric research away from analysis of the cognitive mediators of drug effects. The latter research was carried on by only a few experimental psychopathologists (e.g., Spohn, Lacoursiere, Thompson, & Coyne, 1977), and only recently has an integrated picture begun to emerge (Spohn & Strauss, 1989).

Meanwhile, clinical psychology had preoccupations of its own. A radical behaviorism eschewing cognitive models of any kind was the chief competitor with psychodynamic and humanistic approaches to treatment throughout the 1960s and early 1970s. The dramatic success of token economies and related treatments with chronic psychiatric populations (see Curran, Monti, & Corriveau, 1982) seemed to obviate consideration of the cognitive aspects of schizophrenia.

A variety of factors converged in the late 1970s and 1980s to return cognitive psychopathology of schizophrenia to the clinical arena. Antipsychotic drugs came to be seen as less than a panacea, and their inability to normalize key aspects of personal and social functioning suggested lingering deficits in the cognitive domain. Clinical psychology moved away from radical behaviorism as evidence accumulated that many behavior therapy effects are cognitively mediated. The success of the token economy was reevaluated as it became apparent that its effects often do not generalize beyond the institutional treatment setting. Social learning theory helped add social skills training to the behavior therapists' schizophrenia armamentarium, and this in turn pointed to the need for a more sophisticated understanding of schizophrenic social cognition (see Bellak, Morrison, & Mueser, 1989; Liberman, Nuechterlein, & Wallace, 1982; Wallace & Boone, 1984). Clinical neuropsychology began to reach beyond its origins in the neurosurgery wards to explore brain–behavior relationships in functional disorders, especially schizophrenia (e.g., Levin, Yurgelin-Todd, & Craft, 1989). Also, neuropsychologists began to challenge the doctrine that an impaired brain

must remain impaired, introducing the possibility of *cognitive rehabilitation* (e.g., Brodsky, Brodsky, Sever & Sever, 1986; Gianutsos, 1980). It thus became inevitable that clinicians would begin to wonder whether there are ways to identify and correct the cognitive vulnerabilities and impairments of schizophrenia.

Modification of cognitive abnormalities actually has a history within the experimental psychopathology of schizophrenia. Since the 1960s researchers have used specific manipulations to improve or suppress schizophrenic subjects' performance on laboratory tasks (e.g., Kaplan, 1975; Karras, 1962, 1968; Koh, Kayton, & Peterson, 1976; McAllister, 1970). The purpose has been to understand better the nature of the deficits rather than to develop clinically useful techniques. Nevertheless, as a result it has long been known that deficits can be reduced by increasing stimulus intensity or clarity, providing training and/or practice of task-critical cognitive operations, and teaching prosthetic tactics to bolster performance.

In the early 1970s Meichenbaum and Cameron (1973) reported successful use of self-instructional training (SIT), a cognitive–behavior modification technique, to improve schizophrenic subjects' performance in psychiatric interview, social behavior, and even the Rorschach test. Subsequent attempts to replicate their findings yielded mixed results. A recent review and series of new studies (Bentall, Higson, & Lowe, 1987) concluded that SIT can indeed improve cognitively demanding performance, provided the training is sufficiently individualized and suited to the patient's particular cognitive problems.

More than 10 years after the first SIT studies, Spaulding, Storms, Goodrich, and Sullivan (1986) published a review of SIT and other cognitive interventions in schizophrenia. They concluded that, although most of the evidence comes from quasi-experimental and case studies, there is considerable potential for direct modification of cognitive impairments in schizophrenia. Large-scale experimental trials have not yet been completed, but clinical programs for assessing and treating schizophrenic cognitive impairments are beginning to appear.

The remainder of this paper reports on studies completed since the Spaulding et al. (1986) report, and concludes with a description of a large-scale, highly controlled experimental trial of cognitive therapy for schizophrenic patients now in progress at the University of Nebraska–Lincoln. First, however, it should be helpful to review some of the contextual factors that must be considered in designing research and interpreting results in this area.

CONSIDERATIONS IN RESEARCH DESIGN AND INTERPRETATION

Course of the Disorder

Schizophrenia generally proceeds through relatively distinct phases in its course. Different phases have different implications for cognitive assessment and treatment. The first is the *vulnerability phase*. For some patients there are identifiable cognitive abnormalities, possibly as early as the first year of life, that are thought to be linked to vulnerability for eventual onset of schizophrenia. To the degree that these abnormalities produce the vulnerability by interfering with normal development, amelioration should be expected to reduce probability of eventual onset. If they are simply markers of some other biopsychological impairment, amelioration is of course irrelevant. It has not yet been demonstrated that vulnerability-linked cognitive abnormalities exert a direct causal effect on onset. Indeed, experimental reduction of these abnormalities in a high-risk population could usefully be part of a research strategy for addressing the causality issue.

Following vulnerability is the *prodromal* phase. The prodromal phase may be protracted (up to several years) and characterized mainly by gradual and nonspecific deterioration in personal and social functioning. Alternatively, it may be brief (a few days or less) and characterized by distinct perceptual, emotional, and behavioral

anomalies. There is a long-standing hypothesis that these two types of prodrome represent different subtypes of schizophrenia, and there is considerable evidence for different symptomatology, treatment response, and prognosis. Accordingly, their cognitive characteristics should be expected to be quite different. In either case, there may be cognitive abnormalities that appear in the prodrome whose amelioration could abort an impending onset.

The *acute* phase is typically characterized by behavioral agitation, neuro- and psychophysiological hyperarousal, and gross disruption of cognitive functioning. Cognitive abnormalities evident in the vulnerability and prodromal phases become more severe and new ones appear. It is fairly clear that some cognitive impairments respond to treatment in the acute phase, but this is thought to be almost exclusively secondary to normalization of neurophysiological hyperarousal through antipsychotic drugs or psychophysiological interventions.

The *residual* phase gradually emerges as the acute phase abates. In some patients (especially those with a short, intense prodrome), cognitive impairments may almost entirely normalize or return to vulnerability levels. In others, severe cognitive impairments may remain even after all other symptoms of the acute phase are gone. Impairments in the residual stage have two types of clinical implication. They are *obstacles to rehabilitation* to the degree that they prohibit reacquisition of skills for daily living, and they are *new vulnerabilities* to the degree that they increase the probability of relapse.

It is easiest to study cognitive modification in the residual stage, for several obvious reasons. However, simply limiting our conclusions to residual-stage phenomena has its own complications. Although antipsychotic drugs make the length of the acute phase shorter, it can still be quite protracted, and the transition to the residual stage is still gradual in many patients. As many as 20% of schizophrenic patients do not respond to antipsychotic drugs at all. For them, and for many more with minimal drug response, the residual phase is not much different from the acute phase. There is no universally accepted criterion for discriminating between the two phases for research purposes. Therefore, investigators studying cognitive treatment must either adopt conservative criteria for including "residual-phase" subjects, thereby sacrificing some clinical generalizability, or they must adopt liberal criteria and be prepared to deal with the clinical heterogeneity that this produces.

General Versus Specific Cognitive Deficits

Experimental psychopathologists have known for a long time that it is very difficult to demonstrate that any measured cognitive deficit represents a truly specific impairment, rather than the effects of globally impaired cognitive functioning (Chapman & Chapman, 1978, 1989). Accordingly, it is difficult to establish that a specific intervention produces a specific rather than global cognitive change. It is important to distinguish between theoretical and clinical implications when generality and specificity are at issue. Cognitive improvement is desirable, whether it is specific or global, and whether the treatment that produced it is specific or nonspecific. However, to understand the mechanisms of treatment effects, and to optimize the cost-effectiveness of treatment, we must know all about the specificity of the effects and the specificity of the cognitive functions affected.

General Versus Specific Treatment Effects

Most psychosocial treatment approaches exert effects that are common to all approaches. Such nonspecific treatment effects are produced by the empathetic responses of the therapist, the interpersonal warmth generated during treatment, descriptive feedback from the therapist to the patient, and the like. Evaluation of these common factors, and their interactions with factors thought to be specific to certain treatment approaches, is a current concern in psychotherapy outcome research (e.g.,

Jones, Cumming, & Horowitz, 1988). Cognitive changes induced in chronic schizophrenic patients may also be the result of both common and specific therapy factors, so this must also be addressed in research designs.

Generalization of Cognitive Change

Conceptually related to the specificity problem is the problem of generalization. Improvement of performance in circumscribed areas of cognitive functioning does not necessarily produce meaningful change in personal or social functioning.

Context of Psychiatric Rehabilitation

In recent years a number of psychosocial and psychobiological treatment modalities have been woven together into an integrated approach called *psychiatric rehabilitation* (Liberman, 1992; Liberman and Anthony, 1986). Among its special advantages are adoption of functional criteria of success, as alternatives to the "cure" criterion of traditional allopathic medicine, and emphasis on *skill acquisition* as the mechanism for reaching these criteria. These advantages make psychiatric rehabilitation a useful context in which to test cognitive change techniques. Facilitation of progress in rehabilitation can be operationalized as increasing the rate of skill acquisition in its various modalities. So conceived, cognitive improvement can be expected to facilitate rehabilitation progress before more absolute benefits become apparent. Thus, facilitation of rehabilitation represents an intermediate domain of therapeutic outcome in which to measure cognitive treatment effects.

COGNITIVE CHANGES DURING PSYCHIATRIC REHABILITATION

Spontaneous Changes in a 4- to 6-Month Time Frame

If cognitive functioning is at all relevant to progress in psychiatric rehabilitation, one would expect that improvement on cognitive tasks should accompany improvement on other measures of personal and social functioning. Previous studies (e.g., Nuechterlein et al., 1986; Spohn et al., 1986) have evaluated cognitive changes accompanying dramatic changes in clinical status, associated with drug withdrawal and/or psychotic relapse. Such studies generally suggest that some cognitive impairments fluctuate with gross psychiatric status whereas others do not. It is a different question whether longer term changes within the remitted (residual) phase are related to more subtle changes in personal and social functioning.

In our laboratory we have measured the cognitive functioning of a large number of chronic schizophrenic patients as they progress through an inpatient psychiatric rehabilitation program. The cognitive measures are a collection borrowed from the experimental psychopathology of schizophrenia, integrated in a microcomputer-administered battery called COGLAB. The individual tasks of the battery are selected to represent a continuum of cognitive functions, from preattentional (visual feature analysis measured by a backward masking task and a span of apprehension task) to attentional (vigilance and reaction time tasks) to conceptual (a version of the Wisconsin Card Sorting Task). Ten separate measures of cognitive performance are derived from the tasks. The parameters and factor structure of the COGLAB battery are fairly well known (Spaulding, Garbin, & Crinean, 1989; Spaulding, Garbin, & Dras, 1989). It distinguishes between chronic psychiatric patients and normal subjects with high accuracy. Within chronic psychiatric subjects, about 30% of the total variance in performance is common across almost all the individual performance measures; the rest is unique to the individual measures. Thus, in a schizophrenic population the COGLAB battery measures both global and specific aspects of cognitive functioning.

The subjects were tested and retested with COGLAB at an interval of 3 to 8 months, as they progressed through the psychiatric rehabilitation program. The subjects all had been in the program for at least

several months, in some cases several years, when the first testing was done. This means they were all at least 1 year past hospital admission, and at least several months past the point when their acute psychosis was judged to be stabilized (patients are not transferred from the acute ward to the rehabilitation ward until the acute psychosis is judged to be stabilized). Their personal and social functioning was measured weekly with the Nurses Observational Scale for Inpatient Evaluation (NOSIE-30; Honigfeld, Gillis, & Klett, 1966), an observational measure that is known to be sensitive to treatment effects in schizophrenic inpatients. The NOSIE-30 has six subscales, three of which measure behavioral assets (Social Competence, Social Interest, and Neatness), and three of which measure deficits (Irritability, Psychoticism, and Psychomotor Retardation). In addition, there is a Total Assets scale that integrates the six subscales.

For each subject, an average NOSIE score was computed for the month of the first COGLAB testing and the month of the second COGLAB testing, by simply averaging all the weekly NOSIE scores for those months. This was done for each of the seven NOSIE scales. A NOSIE change score was then computed by subtracting the first from the second average score. Similarly, a change score was computed for each of the various performance measures of the COGLAB battery. To evaluate the relationship of COGLAB changes to NOSIE changes, a multiple regression equation was constructed for each NOSIE scale change score, with the NOSIE score as the dependent (target) variable and the ten COGLAB measure change scores as the independent (predictor) variables.

A summary of the results of the regression analyses is shown in Table 18.1. For purposes of comparison, Table 18.1 also shows regression data for concurrent COGLAB prediction of NOSIE scores during the time of testing, and prediction of future NOSIE changes by the initial COGLAB scores.

Table 18.1 shows that: (a) COGLAB vari-

Table 18.1. Prediction of NOSIE-30 Scores and NOSIE-30 Changes by COGLAB Scores and COGLAB Changes: Summary Regression Statistics[a]

NOSIE-30 subscale	COGLAB measure[b]	R	adj R^2	p
I: Prediction of NOSIE-30 subscales by concurrent COGLAB scores				
Social competence	RT trials >1 s	.48	.14	<.022
	Vigilance false alarms			
	Backward masking function			
	RT anticipatory errors			
	Vigilance hits			
	Simple apprehension			
	RT latency			
Neatness	RT trials >1 s	.52	.19	<.006
	Vigilance false alarms			
	Backward masking function			
	RT anticipatory errors			
	Vigilance hits			
	Simple apprehension			
	RT latency			
Irritibility	RT trials >1 s (−)	.39	.12	<.007
	Vigilance hits (−)			
	RT latency (−)			
Psychoticism	WCST consolidation	.56	.26	<.000
	RT redundancy deficit			
	Vigilance hits (−)			
	RT trials >1 s (−)			
	RT latency (−)			
II. Prediction of future NOSIE-30 change by initial COGLAB scores				
Social competence	WCST modulation	.58	.28	<.001
	RT redundancy deficit			
	Vigilance false alarms			
	WCST consolidation			
Social interest	WCST consolidation (−)	.48	.20	<.001
	Size estimation (*)			
Irritibility	RT trials >1 s (−)	.47	.15	<.016
	Vigilance false alarms (−)			
	Vigilance hits (−)			
	RT latency (−)			
Psychoticism	RT anticipatory errors	.48	.12	<.037
	Vigilance false alarms			
	Backward masking function			
III: Predicting longitudinal NOSIE-30 change with longitudinal COGLAB changes				
Social competence	RT redundancy deficit	.69	.44	<.000
	Vigilance false alarms			
	Vigilance hits			
Social interest	WCST consolidation	.66	.36	<.001
	Vigilance false alarms			
	Backward masking function			
	Size estimation (*)			
	RT redundancy deficit			
	Simple apprehension			
Neatness	RT anticipatory errors (−)	.53	.26	<.001
	Vigilance false alarms			
Irritibility	Vigilance false alarms	.46	.16	<.014
	Vigilance hits			
	Simple apprehension			
	Backward masking function			
Psychomotor retardation	WCST consolidation	.36	.09	<.031
	Vigilance false alarms			

[a] Cases of counterintuitive direction of the bivariate correlation (i.e., worse COGLAB performance associated with better NOSIE-30 and vice versa) are indicated by (−) following the COGLAB measure. Size estimation is a bipolar variable not monotonically related to performance efficacy; this is noted by (*).
[b] Key to abbreviations: RT, reaction time; WCST, Wisconsin Card Sorting Task.

ables account for 12% to 26% of the variance in concurrent NOSIE scores, (b) an initial COGLAB predicts 12% to 28% of the change in NOSIE over the next 3 to 8 months, and (c) change in COGLAB performance accounts for 9% to 44% of the change in NOSIE scores over a 3- to 8-month period. These results are evidence for the hypothesis that the gradual improvements in personal and social functioning in the residual phase are accompanied by improvement in cognitive functioning. Interestingly, the strongest relationship, between NOSIE Social Competence change and COGLAB performance change, involves one cognitive task known to be sensitive to psychotic remission associated with drug effects (hits and false alarms on a continuous performance or vigilance task; Spohn & Strauss, 1989), and another that is thought to be a vulnerability-linked variable insensitive to changes in mental status (reaction time redundancy deficit; see Steffy and Waldman, Chapter 8, this volume).

It is also noteworthy that the patterns of COGLAB measures are different with regard to different predictive relationships. The concurrent relationship with the NOSIE Social Competence and Neatness subscales involves many COGLAB measures, suggesting a relatively monotonic global effect of cognitive impairment, whereas the concurrent relationships with Irritibility and Psychoticism suggest a more complicated picture. In the latter cases, greater symptomatology is predicted by *better* COGLAB functioning, at least for some of the COGLAB variables. This may reflect the well-known difference between a predominantly positive-symptom psychotic state, wherein behavioral impairment is produced by the intrusion of disruptive psychotic symptoms, and a negative-symptom state, wherein behavior is impaired by a lack of normal behavioral characteristics. The present data suggest that a negative-symptom clinical picture (low scores on NOSIE-30 Social Competence and Neatness) is characterized by global cognitive impairment, whereas a more positive-symptom picture is characterized by better global

cognitive functioning but with more specific and isolated cognitive impairments.

Also, it is noteworthy that, although many COGLAB measures together produce a relatively weak relationship to concurrent NOSIE Social Competence and Neatness, *changes* in only three COGLAB measures have a strong relationship to changes on those NOSIE subscales. This suggests that only a subset of the cognitive deficits that impair patients' personal and social functioning undergo beneficial spontaneous change in the course of long-term treatment.

Taken together, the results of this rather naturalistic descriptive analysis suggest that there are complex relationships between cognitive and behavioral functioning in chronic psychiatric populations, especially as the patients change over time. Of course, correlation does not imply cause, so it cannot be inferred from these data that improved cognitive functioning causes improved behavioral functioning. Nevertheless, the very complexity of the results is hard to explain with a simple, monotonic model wherein behavioral impairment produces deficient performance on laboratory tasks. In that sense, the results stimulate the hypothesis that improvement in cognition can lead to improvement in behavior. However, the results also suggest a caveat, that cognitive impairment and cognitive change may have quite different implications in different patients.

Further multivariate analyses of this type should be expected gradually to articulate the relationships between neurophysiological, neuropsychological, and behavioral levels of organismic functioning as they are affected by the course of schizophrenia and rehabilitation efforts. A fully articulated picture, achieved through structural modeling with multivariate data, is required to understand fully the mechanisms of any treatment.

There are problems, however, with the multivariate modeling approach. Many subjects are needed to produce reliable correlational pictures of relationships between variables, and the need for longitudinal data compounds this problem. Eventually, confirmatory analyses will be required to establish which of many competing models best fits the available data. However, experimental studies are not necessarily incompatible with structural analyses, and investigators should build this capacity into their designs whenever possible.

Direct Treatment of Attention and Vigilance

Because the idea of cognitive rehabilitation has become popular in clinical neuropsychology, many software packages of therapeutic "video games" have become commercially available. Although designed for patients with organic neuropathy, the cognitive functions these packages address are generally ones known to be deficient in functionally disordered patients as well. Previous research (reviewed by Spaulding et al., 1986) makes it a worthy hypothesis that systematic practice with these games strengthens key cognitive functions in patients with schizophrenia.

In a recent series of studies in our lab (Stuve, 1988), we tested the potential of a selection of therapeutic video games in a group of severely disordered patients. Each subject was given a preliminary performance assessment with a commercially available package of therapeutic video games (Bracy, 1986). From a set of 10 games, all of which put fairly specific demands on attentional functioning, a subset of games was chosen for each patient. The game selection criteria were that the patient could understand and engage in the game, but could perform only at a deficient level. Thereafter each subject practiced the subset of games in 30-minute sessions two to four times per week, over an 8-week period. Instructions to practice for task improvement and a brief demonstration of each game were provided at the beginning of each session, but coaching and other interactions were otherwise avoided. The subjects were paid $1.00 at the end of each session regardless of their performance level.

The subjects' responses to this procedure were complex and individually unique. In the first series of case studies, involving seven patients, one subject "topped out" (reached an errorless performance level and stayed there) on one task. Six of the subjects showed improvement on various combinations of one to five tasks. There were several instances of no change, with one of the subjects showing no change on four out of five tasks. One subject improved on one task but deteriorated on three. Two subjects showed a "trade-off" change (one aspect of performance improved while another aspect deteriorated, such as a trade-off of speed for accuracy), each on a different task. On only one of the tasks, a simple visual scanning task, was there improvement by every subject who practiced the game. A more complex visual scanning task was too difficult for all but one of the subjects, and he deteriorated with practice.

To construct a different view of the results, task improvement or deterioration was then broken down according to categories of performance: whether the change was in a hit rate, a false alarm rate, a response latency, or an error rate. Both improvement and deterioration occurred in all performance categories, with the exception of false alarm rate, for which no subject deteriorated by showing more false alarms with practice. Interestingly, this is complementary to the well-known laboratory finding that patients with chronic schizophrenia generally have an abnormally conservative response bias—that is, they tend to commit fewer than normal false alarms in signal detection tasks.

These cases permit some evaluation of the specificity issue of treatment effects. If the subjects' improvement (or deterioration) is general, one would expect high correlations between performance changes on paired tasks. If improvement is specific to one attentional process, these correlations are expected to be low. In this study, the subjects are heterogeneous with respect to specificity. Four had very few significantly correlated task pairs, indicating a pattern of task-specific change. In three subjects at least half of the pairings were significantly correlated, indicating a more generalized pattern of change.

Finally, we attempted to identify possible molar-level generalization of attentional performance and response to the video game program. The subjects were rank-ordered for overall performance and for amount of improvement on the games they had practiced. Next they were rank-ordered for their scores on the NOSIE-30. There were large and significant correlations between the NOSIE-30 and overall performance ($r = .82$; $p<.05$) and between the NOSIE-30 and amount of attentional improvement ($r = .86$; $p<.05$).

A second series of case studies essentially replicated these findings, except that the relationship between NOSIE level and cognitive performance was considerably weaker in the second series. This appeared to be due to a more restricted range of NOSIE variance in the second series. Also, in the second series an attempt was made to evaluate generalization of effects. No effect of the cognitive training was found in patients' performance in a work skills–oriented occupational therapy program. However, pre- and post-treatment COGLAB testing did show a significant treatment effect. Interestingly, the specific COGLAB measures affected by the training are vigilance hits and false alarms, two of the three measures associated with spontaneous changes in NOSIE Social Competence.

Taken together, the results of this pilot study suggest two important caveats for attentional treatment. First, the well-known heterogeneity of patients' attentional deficits extends to their response to attentional training. Each subject in this study showed a unique pattern of change. Some showed widespread improvement, some improved on some tasks but not others, and one showed widespread deterioration. This complements the previously discussed conclusion about self-instructional training, that individualization of training may be a crucial factor. Second, there appears to be a relationship between severity of attentional impairment, capacity to improve attentional functioning, and social–behavioral func-

tioning. The most socially–behaviorally impaired patients tend to be the ones who have the most severe attentional impairments, and they are the ones who improve the least or even deteriorate in attentional treatment.

Direct Treatment of Social–Conceptual Skills

A more molecular cognitive process known to be deficient in many psychiatric patients is the formation of concepts. Spaulding et al. (1986) reported a case study wherein a series of exercises in conceptual flexibility normalized a patient's performance on the Wisconsin Card Sorting Task (WCST; Lezak, 1983), a task that requires apprehension and manipulation of abstract concepts. Three recent experimental studies (Bellak, Mueser, Morrison, Tierny, & Pedell, 1989; Green, Ganzell, Satz, & Vaclav, 1990; Summerfield, Alphs, Wagman, Funderburk, & Strauss, 1989) confirm that psychological interventions can improve schizophrenic patients' performance on the WCST.

Even patients whose cognitive functioning is grossly intact may have problems with concept *modulation,* the process of discarding a conceptual scheme when it is no longer useful and constructing a new one. This type of deficit appears to be particularly relevant to social cognition, because it is associated with hostility, belligerence, and persecutory beliefs (Spaulding, 1978) (although it also appears in many patients without such characteristics). It may be due to a particular style of processing information, wherein new perceptual data are rejected in favor of memory data (Magaro, 1984). This tendency may in turn be a self-protective reaction to past psychotic experiences or the result of a maladaptively reorganized cognitive response heirarchy. The case study reported by Spaulding et al. (1986) illustrates the clinical potential of modifying a concept modulation deficit in social cognition:

The patient was a 23-year-old man with chronic schizophrenia. After living for about 2 years in a supervised residential setting, he had made no rehabilitative progress, and his life had been punctuated by frequent altercations with service personnel and other patients. He had been denied admission to a residential psychosocial program because of his belligerent behavior and hostile demeanor.

The patient had been on a stable antipsychotic drug regimen for 12 months. His history indicated that drugs were necessary to control more florid psychotic symptoms. He was compliant with his drug regimen and was judged to be optimally medicated. As part of a systematic assessment procedure, the patient was administered the COGLAB battery. The patient was within normal limits in simple reaction time, backward masking performance, span of apprehension, distraction effects and redundancy effects in the reaction time task, vigilance and size estimation. He showed an isolated deficit on the COGLAB version of the Wisconsin Card Sorting Task. His difficulty was a tendency to adopt a particular scheme and perseveratively continue to use it long after the task demands had changed.

The laboratory data suggested that the patient had a specific conceptual deficit that was preventing him from using his reasonably good social repertoire in stressful situations. The nature of the deficit was hypothesized to be a tendency to schematize a situation rapidly, and then perseverate with that schema despite changes in the situation. The quality of the patient's attributional behavior in social situations suggested that he used a stereotypic conceptualization of all interactions—that the other person was trying in some way to take advantage of him. He was able to understand interactions in a better perspective when not in the situation, but this did not help when he was actively engaged.

An exercise was designed to increase his ability to reconceptualize a social situation rapidly, enabling him to reject his stereotype. For 10 therapy sessions, the patient was asked to generate alternative schematizations, first to inkblots and then to Thematic Apperception Test (TAT) cards. That is, he was instructed to generate as many different percepts (to the inkblots) or stories (to the TAT cards) as he could to a single stimulus. He found this extremely difficult, especially with the TAT cards. Gradually, however, he gained an ability to generate three to four stories for each card without bizarre or perseverative elements in subsequent stories. One particular card caused him extraordinary difficulty. He reported that it reminded him of an incident in his past that was still upsetting. Even after responding well to two or three cards, he could only generate one morbid scenario for the problem card. This experience served to demonstrate to the patient that his problem could be exacerbated by stressful situations. The conceptual exercise was accompanied by counseling about the importance of conceptual flexibility, especially in social situations.

After the end of the 10 exercise sessions, he was retested with the initial assessment battery. His previous conceptual deficit was normalized. He continued to receive regular counseling about social interactions, as he had before the exercises. In the following weeks, residential staff reported a positive change in his demeanor and attitudes. This was corroborated by an improvement in weekly NOSIE-30 ratings, particularly on the Irritability subscale. At last followup, he had been accepted to the residential program that had previously rejected him.

In subsequent case studies in our laboratory this social apperception exercise has continued be helpful, especially with partially recompensated paranoid schizophrenia patients whose social rehabilitation progress has stalled. An experimental study of the effects of the exercise (Schlank, 1987) suggests that it may also have more generalized benefits. The subjects were eight chronic schizophrenic patients in an intensive inpatient psychiatric rehabilitation program. Along with other rehabilitation activities, they underwent problem-solving training in a group, similar to that described by Spivak, Platt, and Shure (1976). After every problem-solving training session, each patient was given a rating on an operationalized scale of progress by the group leader. Concomitant with the problem-solving training, each patient was seen individually by a cognitive therapist. For the first 4 weeks, the cognitive therapy was restricted to discussions of the problem-solving group and its application to living situations. In the second 4 weeks, half the patients began doing the apperception exercise in their individual sessions. After 4 more weeks the second half of the patients began the apperception exercise. The problem-solving group leader was blind to which patients had started the exercise.

Figure 18.1 shows the problem-solving progress ratings for the two patient subgroups over the three 4-week epochs of the study. Introduction of the apperception exercise produced a significant change in the progress rate, and by the end of the study the patients who had had 8 weeks of the exercise were doing better in problem-solving training than the patients who had had only 4 weeks. The results of this study suggest that, even when deficits in relatively molecular functions such as concept modulation are not specifically identified, therapeutic strengthening of such functions can benefit more molar rehabilitation-oriented activies such as problem-solving training.

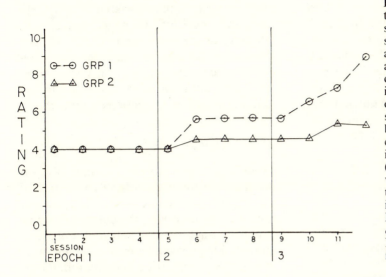

Figure 18.1. Performance of patients in a cognitive problem-solving training group, as measured by therapist's rating. After a baseline period (Epoch 1), an apperception exercise was introduced in Epoch 2 for Group 1 and in Epoch 3 for Group 2. Repeated-measures ANOVA yields a significant interaction for groups by sessions within epochs, indicating the effect of the exercise is detectable within four sessions. (From Spaulding, W., & Sullivan, M. [1992]. From laboratory to clinic: Psychological principles in psychiatric rehabilitation. In R. Lieberman (Ed.), *Handbook of Psychiatric Rehabilitation.* New York: MacMillan. By permission.)

COGNITIVE THERAPY IN REHABILITATION: A PROJECT UNDER WAY

In 1990 a 5-year research project began in our lab to evaluate comprehensively the effects of a group-format cognitive therapy modality on psychiatric rehabilitation of patients with schizophrenia. The project is designed to address the methodological and interpretive complexities discussed above, while, we hope, contributing a new and cost-effective tool to the rehabilitation armamentarium.

Development of Therapy Modality

Development of the modality was begun by Brenner and his colleagues at the University of Bern (Switzerland) psychiatric hospital (Brenner, 1987). Robert Liberman first noticed striking conceptual and technological similarities in the work of the Bern and the Nebraska groups, and through his good offices a collaboration soon flourished. The original Bern modality is a comprehensive package of cognitive therapy and social skills training. The Nebraska group translated the cognitive therapy portions into the American group therapy–skill training idiom and added some specific techniques developed in our lab (most notably the apperception exercise described above).

The modality consists of a number of structured group exercises that target aspects of cognition thought to be crucial for processing social information. The exercises are designed to move quickly from use of simple, nonsocial stimuli to more complex stimuli embedded in a social–interactional context. This movement is thought to be highly desirable for two reasons. First, it produces a broad spectrum of cognitive treatment targets, any one of which may be more relevant to some of the patients in the group than others. Thus, the natural heterogeneity of the group is addressed. Second, systematic integration of social and nonsocial stimuli and responses may facilitate generalization of newly acquired molecular cognitive abilities to useful and important social situations.

Levels of Outcome

The research design identifies three separate domains of outcome in which to evaluate therapy effects. The first is molecular attentional and conceptual functions, such as those measured by COGLAB and similar instruments. It is hypothesized that the therapy will show an immediate or relatively short-term effect in this domain. The second domain is progress in standard psychiatric rehabilitation skill training modalities. It is hypothesized that cognitive therapy will facilitate patients' progress in these modalities, in terms of rate and quality of skill acquisition, over a 3- to 6-month time frame. The third domain is ecologically relevant outcome. It is hypothesized that psychiatric rehabilitation accompanied by the cognitive therapy will produce quicker hospital discharge, lower recidivism rates, and better quality of life over a longer time frame.

Specific and Nonspecific Effects

To discriminate between specific and nonspecific therapy effects, the cognitive therapy will be compared to a supportive therapy modality treated as a control condition. An elaborate Q-sort–based observational measure (Jones et al., 1988) is used to characterize both modalities with respect to the processes and conditions that are thought to produce nonspecific therapy effects. Very little is known about nonspecific group therapy effects with schizophrenic patient populations, or about the therapeutic processes and conditions that characterize cognitive therapy, supportive therapy, and the skill training modalities. In that sense, this part of the project is exploratory and descriptive in nature. It is hypothesized that the cognitive therapy modality will produce both specific effects within the cognitive domain and nonspecific effects in social–behavioral domains (which in this context represent generalization of the specific treatment effects), and that these effects are additive to those that can be produced by a generic therapy modality, which generates only nonspecific therapy effects.

Individual Variation in Treatment Effects

Pilot studies with the cognitive therapy modality suggest that patients vary greatly in their response to the treatment. To articulate further the factors that may predict degree of success or some qualitative aspects of treatment response, multivariate structural models will be constructed at the end of the study. The models will use a large number of subject characteristics, including demographic characteristics, diagnostic subgroup, positive and negative symptomatology, and pretreatment COGLAB performance, to predict outcome with and without cognitive therapy. This will address the important issue of *for whom* group cognitive therapy is a beneficial approach.

CONCLUSION

A number of case studies and partially controlled experimental studies to date strongly suggest that there is considerable potential for directly modifying the cognitive impairments characteristic of schizophrenia. This potential appears to be most relevant in the context of psychiatric rehabilitation, the enterprise of returning patients with residual schizophrenia to the highest possible levels of personal and social functioning and quality of life. Current research in experimental psychopathology and clinical neuropsychology promises to contribute to the development of effective treatment techniques. The question appears to be not so much whether cognitive treatment can work, but for whom, under what circumstances, and with what degree of cost-effectiveness.

REFERENCES

American Psychiatric Association. (1980). *Diagnostic and statistical manual of mental disorders* (3rd ed.). Washington, DC: American Psychiatric Press, Inc.

Arieti, S. (1955). *Interpretation of schizophrenia*. New York: Brunner/Mazel.

Bellak, A., Morrison, R., & Mueser, K. (1989). Social problem solving in schizophrenia. *Schizophrenia Bulletin, 15,* 101–116.

Bellak, A., Mueser, K., Morrison, R., Tierny, A., & Podell, K. (1989). Remediation of cognitive deficits in schizophrenia. Training on the Wisconsin Sorting Test. *American Journal of Psychiatry, 147,* 1650–1655.

Bentall, R., Higson, P., & Lowe, C. (1987). Teaching self-instructions to chronic schizophrenic patients: Efficacy and generalization. *Behavioral Psychotherapy, 15,* 58–76.

Bracy, O. (1986). *Cognitive rehabilitation:* A process approach, *Cognitive Rehabilitation, 4*(2), 10–17.

Brenner, H. (1987). On the importance of cognitive disorders in treatment and rehabilitation. In J. Strauss, W. Baker, & H. Brenner (Eds.), *Psychosocial treatment of schizophrenia* (pp. 136–152). Toronto: Lewistone, Bern, Stuttgart: Huber.

Brodsky, P., Brodsky, M., Sever, H., & Sever, J. (1986). Two evaluation studies of Reitan's REHABIT program for the retraining of brain dysfunction. *Perceptual and Motor Skills, 63,* 501–502.

Cameron, N., & Magaret, A. (1951). *Behavior pathology.* Boston: Houghton Mifflin.

Chapman, L., & Chapman, J. (1978). The measurement of differential deficit. *Journal of Psychiatric Research, 14,* 303–311.

Chapman, L., & Chapman, J. (1989). Strategies for resolving the heterogeneity of schizophrenics and their relatives using cognitive measures. *Journal of Abnormal Psychology, 98,* 357–366.

Curran, J., Monti, P., & Corriveau, D. (1982). Treatment of schizophrenia. In S. Bellak, M. Hersen, & A. Kazdin (Eds.), *International handbook of behavior modification and therapy* (pp. 433–466). New York: Plenum.

Gianutsos, R. (1980). What is cognitive rehabilitation? *Journal of Rehabilitation, 46,* 36–40.

Green, M., Ganzell, S., Satz, P., & Vaclav, J. (1990). Teaching the Wisconsin Card Sort to schizophrenic patients [Letter]. *Archives of General Psychiatry, 47,* 91–92.

Honigfeld, C., Gillis, R., & Klett, J. (1966). NOSIE-30: A treatment-sensitive ward behavior scale. *Psychological Reports, 19,* 180–182.

Jones, E., Cumming, J., & Horowitz, M. (1988). Another look at the nonspecific hypothesis of therapeutic effectiveness. *Journal of Consulting and Clinical Psychology, 56,* 48–55.

Kaplan, R. (1975). *The crossover phenomenon: Three studies of the effect of training and information on process schizophrenic reaction time.* Doctoral dissertation, University of Waterloo.

Karras, A. (1962). The effects of reinforcement and arousal on the psychomotor performance of chronic schizophrenics. *Journal of Abnormal and Social Psychology, 65,* 104–111.

Karras, A. (1968). Choice reaction time of chronic and acute psychiatric patients under primary or secondary aversive stimulation. *British Journal of Social and Clinical Psychology, 7,* 270–279.

Koh, S., Kayton, L., & Peterson, R. (1976). Affective encoding and consequent remembering in schizophrenic young adults. *Journal of Abnormal Psychology, 85,* 156–166.

Levin, S., Yurgelin-Todd, D., Craft, S. (1989).

Contribution of clinical neuropsychology to the study of schizophrenia. *Journal of Abnormal Psychology, 98,* 341–356.

Lezak, M. (1983). *Neuropsychological assessment* (2nd ed.). New York: Oxford University Press.

Liberman, R. (in press). *Handbook of psychiatric rehabilitation.* New York: Pergamon.

Liberman, R., & Anthony, W. (Eds.). (1986). Special issue: Psychiatric rehabilitation. *Schizophrenia Bulletin, 12*(4).

Liberman, R., Nuechterlein, K., & Wallace, C. (1982). Social skills training and the nature of schizophrenia. In J. Curran & P. Monti (Eds.), *Social skills training: A practical handbook for assessment and treatment* (pp. 5–56). New York: Guilford Press.

Magaro, P. (1984). Psychosis and schizophrenia. In W. Spaulding & J. Cole (Eds.), *The Nebraska symposium on motivation, Vol. 31: Theories of psychosis and schizophrenia* (pp. 157–230). Lincoln: University of Nebraska Press.

McAllister, L. (1970). Modification of performance on the rod-and-frame test through token reinforcement procedures. *Journal of Abnormal Psychology, 75,* 124–130.

Meichenbaum, D., & Cameron, R. (1973). Training schizophrenics to talk to themselves: A means of developing self controls. *Behavior Therapy, 4,* 515–534.

Nuechterlein, K., & Dawson, M. (1984). Information processing and attentional functioning in the developmental course of schizophrenia. *Schizophrenia Bulletin, 10,* 160–203.

Nuechterlein, K., Edell, W., Norris, M., & Dawson, M. (1986). Attentional vulnerability indicators, thought disorder and negative symptoms. *Schizophrenia Bulletin, 12,* 408–426.

Schlank, A. (1987). *Facilitation of progress in interpersonal problem-solving training using a cognitive exercise procedure.* Masters degree thesis, University of Nebraska–Lincoln.

Spaulding, W. (1978). The relationships of some information processing factors to severely disturbed behaviors. *Journal of Nervous and Mental Disease, 166,* 417–428.

Spaulding, W., Garbin, C., & Crinean, W. (1989). The logical and psychometric prerequisites for cognitive therapy for schizophrenia. *British Journal of Psychiatry, 155*(Suppl. 5), 69–73.

Spaulding, W., Garbin, C., & Dras, S. (1989). Cognitive abnormalities in psychiatric patients and schizotypal college students. *Journal of Nervous and Mental Disease, 177,* 717–728.

Spaulding, W., Storms, L., Goodrich, V., & Sullivan, M. (1986). Applications of experimental psychopathology in psychiatric rehabilitation. *Schizophrenia Bulletin, 12,* 560–577.

Spohn, H., Coyne, L., Larson, F., Mittelman, J., Spray, J., & Hayes, K. (1986). Episodic and residual thought pathology in chronic schizophrenics. *Schizophrenia Bulletin, 12,* 394–407.

Spohn, H., Lacoursiere, R., Thompson, K., & Coyne, L. (1977). Phenothiazine effects on psychological and psychophysiological dysfunction in chronic schizophrenics. *Archives of General Psychiatry, 34,* 633–644.

Spohn, H., & Strauss, M. (1989). Relation of neuroleptic and anticholinergic medication to cognitive functions in schizophrenia. *Journal of Abnormal Psychology, 98,* 367–380.

Spivak, G., Platt, S., & Shure, M. (1976). *The problem-solving approach to adjustment.* San Francisco: Jossey-Bass.

Stuve, P. (1988). *Computer-assisted cognitive rehabilitation in chronic schizophrenic inpatients.* Masters degree thesis, University of Nebraska–Lincoln.

Summerfeld, A., Alphs, L., Wagman, A., Funderburk, F., & Strauss, M. (1989). *Monetary reinforcement reduces perseverative errors in patients with schizophrenia.* Paper presented at the International Congress on Schizophrenia Research, San Diego, CA.

Wallace, C., & Boone, S. (1984). Cognitive factors in the social skills of schizophrenic patients: Implications for treatment. In W. Spaulding & J. Cole (Eds.), *The Nebraska symposium on motivation, Vol. 31: Theories of schizophrenia and psychosis* (pp. 283–318). Lincoln: University of Nebraska Press.

19

Mapping the Intrafamilial Environment of the Schizophrenic Patient

DAVID J. MIKLOWITZ
MICHAEL J. GOLDSTEIN

Qualities of the family environment that accompany episodes of schizophrenic disorder have long been of interest to clinicians and researchers. Attributes of the family climate may serve as environmental stressors that potentiate genetic vulnerabilities in individuals diagnosed with or at risk for schizophrenia. Identification of family attributes with etiological and/or prognostic significance in schizophrenia has resulted in the development of family psychosocial intervention strategies for modifying these attributes. These interventions, in turn, have been found to affect positively the course of this disorder once it is manifest.

Over the past 25 years, the overriding goal of the research program of the University of California at Los Angeles (UCLA) Family Project (M. Goldstein, Director) has been to map those attributes of the intrafamilial environment that have prognostic significance in schizophrenia. In this chapter, four central questions that have guided the project's most recent research efforts are evaluated:

1. What intrafamilial attributes predict the *onset* of schizophrenia or schizophrenia spectrum disorders?
2. What family attributes contribute to the *course* of schizophrenic disorder once the illness is manifest?
3. What are the origins of these family attributes?

a. Are family variables correlated with attributes of the schizophrenic patient, such as his or her symptomatic profile, emotional attitudes toward parents, or styles of interacting with parents?
b. Are family attributes correlated with attributes of parents, such as a history of diagnosable psychopathology in these parents?
4. Can these family attributes be modified via family psychosocial intervention, and does accomplishing this modification result in a better course of illness for the schizophrenic patient?

WHAT FAMILY ATTRIBUTES ARE IMPORTANT IN THE ONSET AND/OR COURSE OF SCHIZOPHRENIA?

Two types of intrafamilial dysfunction consistently emerge as important contributors to the onset and/or course of schizophrenia: *communication deviance,* or lack of communication clarity (Miklowitz & Stackman, 1992; Wynne & Singer, 1963a, 1963b), and negativity in the family's emotional climate. The latter domain has been operationalized in terms of two distinct but partially overlapping constructs: *expressed emotion* attitudes (criticism, hostility, and/or emotional overinvolvement; Vaughn & Leff, 1976) measured from a semistructured, individual interview with key relatives; and *affective style* verbal interactional behaviors in relatives (supportive, critical, guilt-inducing, or intrusive ["mind-reading"] statements; Doane, West, Goldstein, Rodnick, & Jones, 1981) measured from directly observed, family problem-solving discussions that include the patient.

The communication deviance construct, as discussed below, appears to have utility in prospectively identifying individuals who develop schizophrenia spectrum disorders in adulthood (Goldstein, 1987). The affective dimensions of family functioning (expressed emotion, affective style) appear to be most consistently associated with the course of schizophrenia (Doane, Falloon, Goldstein, & Mintz, 1985; Koenigsberg & Handley, 1986), although at least one study suggests that affective style may be important in predicting its onset as well (Goldstein, 1987). More will be said about these constructs, the way they are measured, the patient and parent correlates of these attributes, and their relative prognostic importance, in the sections that follow.

Role of the Patient

The family attributes described above have typically been measured on key relatives of the index patient–offspring (i.e., biological parents or spouse), with little or no examination of the contributions of this offspring to the family's emotional climate. Important shifts in our own thinking about the prognostic role of parental communication deviance, expressed emotion, and affective style came from applying these constructs to offspring as well as parent behavior in individual or family testing situations. This strategy has allowed us to investigate whether symmetries or complementarities exist when comparing parent and offspring attitudes and/or interactional styles. A central argument made in this chapter is that constructs such as communication deviance, expressed emotion, and affective style tap family-wide transactional processes that cannot be "blamed" on any one individual.

Communication Deviance

Communication deviance refers to unclear, unintelligible, or oddly worded communication during family transactions—the inability of a speaker to "share a focus of attention" with a listener when delivering a spoken message (Singer & Wynne, 1965a, 1965b; Wynne & Singer, 1963a, 1963b). The working assumption of communication deviance research has been that unclear parent–child communication interferes with a child's ability to develop logical thought and to perceive and/or process incoming information accurately. In adulthood, these "acquired vulnerabilities" of perception, thinking, and/or attention become manifest in the core symptoms of schizophrenia when life stressors are maximal (Jones, 1977; Woodward & Goldstein, 1977; Wynne, Singer, Bartko, & Toohey, 1977).

Communication deviance has typically been measured in parents or other key relatives of concurrently schizophrenic offspring, usually from transcripts of an individual projective test such as the Rorschach or Thematic Apperception Test (TAT). The communication deviance system applied to the TAT, originally devised by Singer and Wynne (1966) and modified by Jones (1977; Jones & Doane, 1979), consists of 27 codes that can be roughly subdivided according to whether they measure one of two types of disturbance: disorders of linguistic–verbal reasoning (i.e., unclear sentences, idea fragments, peculiar language) or disorders of perceptual–cognitive processes (i.e., inability to construct a story that integrates elements within the cards; distorting or misinterpreting TAT stimuli).

Numerous studies indicate that levels of communication deviance are indeed higher among parents of schizophrenics than among parents of nonpsychotic or normal individuals, particularly those forms of communication deviance that measure perceptual–cognitive disturbance (for review, see Miklowitz & Stackman, 1992). However, several questions have been raised about communication deviance as a marker of risk for schizophrenia:

1. Because projectives provide a standardized testing situation, the majority of research on communication deviance has relied on projective data rather than on spontaneous communication samples from parents. Is communication deviance, as measured during a projective test, really an accurate measure of how parents actually communicate with their offspring (concurrent validity)?
2. Are high levels of communication deviance found among the parents of patients with other forms of psychosis (specificity)? Prior studies of the specificity of intrafamilial communication deviance (e.g., Wynne & Singer, 1963a, 1963b) systematically excluded comparison groups of nonschizophrenic patients with psychoses or high levels of thought disorder (e.g., bipolar affective patients).
3. Is communication deviance a longitudinal risk marker for the onset of schizophrenia in children at risk for this disorder (predictive validity)? Establishing communication deviance as a risk indicator for schizophrenia is essential to validating the theories of parental influence on which the construct is based.

These questions were recently addressed in a series of studies conducted by our UCLA research group, as outlined below.

Concurrent validity. Do projective tests sample the type of communication dysfunction that occurs in the day-to-day transactions between parents and their patient–offspring? In a study of 59 native English-speaking parents of recent-onset schizophrenics ($n = 37$), Velligan, Goldstein, Nuechterlein, Miklowitz, and Ranlett (1990) compared levels of communication devi-

ance obtained from parents during the TAT task (scored using Jones & Doane's [1979] TAT–Communication Deviance [TAT-CD] system) with their corresponding levels of communication deviance during an unstructured, problem-focused interaction task (scored using the Interactional Communication Deviance (ICD) coding system; Velligan, Christensen, Goldstein, & Margolin, 1988).

Total CD scores from the two tasks correlated at a moderate level ($r = .44, p < .0005$). However, only certain types of parental communication deviance—those communication deviance codes most clearly associated with linguistic anomalies or disorders of verbal reasoning (i.e., fragmented sentences, odd word usage)—were consistent across both settings. Those types of communication deviance that appear to measure perceptual distortion and/or information-processing deficits were only evident on the TAT (a task requiring the parent to clarify ambiguous stimuli). Thus, the domain of communication dysfunction sampled by the TAT is not identical to that sampled by direct interaction tasks.[1]

Specificity to schizophrenia. A second study (Miklowitz, Velligan, Goldstein, Nuechterlein, Gitlin, Ranlett, et al., 1991) investigated whether high levels of communication deviance are unique to parents of schizophrenics or whether these occur with equal frequency among parents of patients with another recurrent psychotic disorder. Biological parents of 39 recent-onset schizophrenics were indistinguishable on total levels of TAT-CD and ICD from a matched sample of biological parents of 16 recent-onset bipolar, manic patients. However, certain communication deviance substyles, particularly the tendency to construct sentences oddly or use words in an

---

1. In the Velligan et al. (1988) study, the TAT-CD and ICD measures were independent of two measures of affective communication—expressed emotion and affective style—derived from interviews with parents and direct family interaction tasks, respectively. Thus, despite the variability of communication deviance across tasks and scoring procedures, there was evidence for its construct validity.

unusual way (e.g., "It's gonna be upwards and downwards along the process all the while to go through something like this"), were actually higher among parents of manic patients than among parents of schizophrenic patients on both the TAT-CD and ICD measures. Thus, levels of parental communication deviance, although perhaps highest in families in which an offspring has a psychotic disorder, do not appear to discriminate between offspring with different types or forms of psychosis.

We also investigated whether patients from these two groups showed levels of communication deviance that paralleled those of their parents. As was true of their parents, schizophrenic and manic patients in this sample were indistinguishable on total levels of ICD (TATs were unavailable on patients). However, manic patients, like their parents, were more likely than schizophrenic patients to show instances of odd word usage, whereas schizophrenics were more likely to make ambiguous references during the interaction task (e.g., "Kid stuff that's one thing but *something else* is different too"). Thus, certain symmetries emerged from comparing the speech deviances found among patients from these two diagnostic groups with those found among the biological parents of these patients.[2]

Predictive validity. Are high levels of communication deviance measurable prior to, and are they predictive of, the onset of schizophrenia or other psychotic disorders? Without prospective evidence of the prognostic utility of intrafamilial communication deviance among at-risk individuals, it remains unclear whether communication deviance is an intrafamilial precursor to psychosis or whether it is simply a correlate of severe psychiatric conditions.

This question was addressed in a 15-year

follow-up of 64 disturbed but nonpsychotic adolescents who presented for treatment at a University clinic in the mid- to late 1960s (Goldstein, 1987). Parents were administered a series of psychological assessments at baseline, including evaluations of their communication styles (based on the TAT and a direct interaction task). At 15-year follow-up, a number of the adolescents (28%) had developed "broad" schizophrenia spectrum disorders, defined with *Diagnostic and Statistical Manual of Mental Disorder,* third edition (DSM-III) criteria (American Psychiatric Association, 1980) for schizophrenia or schizotypal, paranoid, schizoid, or borderline personality disorder.

Those children whose parents were initially high in TAT-CD were far more likely to have developed schizophrenia spectrum disorders at 15-year follow-up than were those whose parents had shown intermediate or low levels of baseline TAT-CD. Furthermore, identification of spectrum outcomes was improved when the level of affective negativity demonstrated by the family during the interaction task (negative affective style) was considered: those families with high communication deviance *and* negative affective style (i.e., high criticism and/or intrusiveness) were the most likely to have children who later developed schizophrenia spectrum disorders. These predictive relationships remained significant when the severity and type of the adolescents' initial symptoms were covaried.

Although the results of this study provide evidence for the role of communication deviance as an intrafamilial precursor to severe psychiatric disorders, it is not clear whether they support the view that communication deviance is specifically associated with the onset of schizophrenia. First, prediction of outcome by parental communication deviance was weakened by excluding persons with borderline and schizoid personality disorders from the schizophrenia spectrum grouping. Second, bipolar and psychotic depressive outcomes were underrepresented in this study. Thus, the question of whether communication deviance is a risk factor for the onset of schizophrenia

---

2. It is important to note that the correlations between levels of parent and patient ICD, when evaluated within each diagnostic group and in the sample as a whole, were rather modest, suggesting that communication deviance in parents is not simply a reaction to dysfunctional communication or thought disorder in patient–offspring.

versus the onset of severe psychiatric disorders is unresolved.

Summary. Our results suggest that communication deviance (a) does show a degree of stability across assessment methods, (b) is present in equivalent amounts among biological parents of schizophrenic and bipolar patients, and (c) is predictive of the onset of disorders within the broad schizophrenia spectrum. Several other questions regarding communication deviance are suggested by these findings and those of others: Is there any evidence that communication deviance is a product of a vulnerable genotype, as evidenced by diagnosable psychopathology in the biological parent(s)? Is communication deviance modifiable via psychosocial intervention, or is it a stable attribute of parents that is not easily altered? These questions are addressed in later sections of this chapter. We now turn attention to the role of the intrafamilial affective climate, which has importance in predicting the *course* of schizophrenic disorders among recently hospitalized patients.

Expressed Emotion

Two attributes of key relatives appear to have prognostic significance for the course of schizophrenic disorders: expressed emotion attitudes, and affective style interactional behaviors. Expressed emotion is scored from the 60- to 90-minute semistructured Camberwell Family Interview (CFI; Vaughn & Leff, 1976) administered to key relatives (typically parents) at the time of the patient's hospitalization for an episode of schizophrenia. This interview explores the relative's emotional reactions to the development of the patient's psychosis. One of three emotional attitudes must be evident during the CFI in order for the relative (and the family) to be classified as high in expressed emotion: high criticism, hostility, or emotional overinvolvement (overconcern or overprotectiveness). Otherwise, the family is classified as low in expressed emotion.

There are now at least ten studies that have independently replicated the finding that schizophrenic patients who are discharged to high–expressed emotion families are two to three times more likely to relapse in the 9 months to 1 year following hospital discharge than are those returning to low–expressed emotion families (for review, see Koenigsberg & Handley, 1986; Mintz, Liberman, Miklowitz, & Mintz, 1987). The family expressed emotion–patient relapse association has also been found in samples of nonpsychotic depressive (Hooley, Orley, & Teasdale, 1986; Vaughn & Leff, 1976), bipolar affective (Miklowitz, Goldstein, Nuechterlein, Snyder, & Mintz, 1988), and obese (Fischmann-Havstad & Marston, 1984) patients.

Methodological limitations. A disadvantage of existing expressed emotion methodology has been the rather lengthy CFI procedure, its even more cumbersome scoring procedure, and the fact that the assessment is temporally tied to an acute episode of psychiatric disorder. Furthermore, the CFI is designed exclusively for interviews of key relatives; expressed emotion attitudes held by patients about their relatives cannot be assessed from this interview.

To address these methodological limitations, we recently developed a brief probe for measuring expressed emotion—the 5-minute speech sample (FMSS)—which requires that relatives "talk for five minutes . . . [about] what kind of person [the patient] is and how the two of you get along together" (Magana et al., 1986). Although it is usually administered during the postdischarge period, the FMSS can be administered at any time. Furthermore, each speech sample can be quickly scored for expressed emotion by trained raters using a scoring system that yields high levels of interrater reliability. Finally, the FMSS can be administered to patients as well as relatives.

Table 19.1 surveys the results of several studies of schizophrenic patients that compared ratings of relatives based on the full CFI with those based on the shorter FMSS

Table 19.1. Correspondence between Camberwell Family Interview (CFI) and 5-Minute Speech Sample (FMSS) Ratings of Expressed Emotion

Sample	N	Sensitivity[a]	Specificity[b]	% Agreement[c]
Magana et al. (1986)	40	.65	.88	.75
Jenkins et al. (1986)	84	.50	.93	.77
Glynn et al. (1990)	49	.42	.89	.59
Leeb et al. (1990)	100	.71	.80	.73
Totals	273	.60	.89	.72

[a] The proportion of relatives rated high in expressed emotion by the CFI that were also rated high in expressed emotion by the FMSS.
[b] The proportion of relatives rated low in expressed emotion by the CFI that were also rated low in expressed emotion by the FMSS.
[c] The ratio of the number of agreements between the two measures divided by the sum of the number of agreements and disagreements.

method. The rate of correspondence between the two measures has ranged from 59% to 77%. Although the FMSS generally has high specificity for identifying CFI ratings, sensitivity has been low to moderate: a significant proportion (23% to 53%) of those relatives rated low in expressed emotion by the FMSS are rated high in expressed emotion by the CFI method. However, 79% to 91% of those rated high in expressed emotion by the FMSS are also rated high in expressed emotion by the CFI method.

The lack of correspondence between the two measures may be due to either of two sources of variance: time and method. The discharge of the patient into the community following hospitalization and his or her corresponding improvements in clinical condition over time may reduce negativity in the attitudes of some relatives, leading to a greater proportion of low–expressed emotion ratings based on the FMSS administered during this postdischarge period. Alternatively, the FMSS may not be long or sensitive enough to capture high–expressed emotion attitudes that appear after a degree of rapport has developed between the interviewer and respondent, which may be easier to achieve with the longer, semistructured CFI. However, the CFI procedure may overidentify high–expressed emotion attitudes, as suggested by the frequent finding that only about 50% of schizophrenic patients from high–expressed emotion homes experience a relapse at 9-month follow-up (Koenigsberg & Handley, 1986; Mintz et al., 1987).

Summary. Because of the documented prognostic utility of the CFI–expressed emotion method, the FMSS is perhaps best viewed as a probe for high–expressed emotion attitudes rather than a substitute for the full CFI. The question of which measure is the most valid indicator of a family's emotional climate, and which is a better predictor of patient relapse rates, would be most easily addressed in a longitudinal study in which the two expressed emotion measures are (a) compared to concurrent measures of family interaction (such as affective style), and (b) used as comparative predictors of longitudinal outcome.

Results of such a study are reported below. It is argued that the *pattern* of expressed emotion attitudes observed when one assesses expressed emotion by the CFI procedure (based on an inpatient assessment) *and* by the FMSS method (based on an assessment conducted during the aftercare period) is a stronger predictor of the family's emotional milieu (including the patient's verbal interactional contributions) and the probability of patient relapse than is either measure taken alone. In order to address these issues more fully, our measure of parental interactional behavior—affective style—is introduced next.

Affective Style

A second construct, affective style, refers to the emotional–verbal behavior of key relatives during a family problem-solving task (Doane et al., 1981). In this task, families are asked to discuss and resolve two family conflict issues for 10 minutes each. Statements made by relatives that qualify as specific criticisms (e.g., "You never try hard in school"), harsh criticisms (e.g., "You are a good-for-nothing"), guilt inductions (e.g., "You are really trying to hurt us"), intrusions ("mind-reading"; e.g., "You're not angry, you're depressed"), or statements of support (e.g., "You really do that well") are tabulated from verbatim transcripts of these interactions. Unlike CFI–expressed emotion ratings, affective style is measured after the patient has returned to the family home or community and has achieved some degree of remission.

As mentioned earlier, family affective style (dichotomized as benign versus negative[3]) was predictive in one study (Goldstein, 1987) of the likelihood that vulnerable adolescents would develop broad schizophrenia spectrum disorders at 15-year follow-up. Furthermore, affective style was associated with short-term relapse rates in one study of schizophrenic patients (Doane et al., 1985) and in one of bipolar patients (Miklowitz et al., 1988).

What Do Expressed Emotion and Affective Style Indicate About Families of Schizophrenic Patients?

Do expressed emotion and affective style measure similar processes within the family? Do attitudes among relatives (expressed emotion) measured during an inpatient period predict their corresponding verbal interactional behavior (affective style) once the patient has returned to the community? Are these attitudes and behaviors among relatives reciprocated by the patient–relative? That is, do expressed emotion and affective style reflect reciprocal, disordered transactional processes within the family system that are mutually produced by parents and patients?

3. A family is classified as affective style negative if one or both relatives makes at least one harsh criticism or guilt-inducing statement or six or more intrusive statements during a single 10-minute interaction. Otherwise, the family is classified as affective style benign.

Are expressed emotion and affective style related? In a sample of 42 relatively chronic schizophrenic patients (Miklowitz, Goldstein, Falloon, & Doane, 1984), high–expressed emotion parents were significantly more likely than low–expressed emotion parents to show high levels of affective style criticism and intrusiveness when interacting with their newly discharged patient–offspring. However, patients in this sample were relatively chronic in illness history, and were often quite symptomatic when the outpatient affective style assessment was conducted. Thus, the correspondence between the two measures may have resulted from the fact that both were administered at times when parents could have been reacting to active symptomatology in the offspring.

In a second study of 36 schizophrenic patients (Miklowitz et al., 1989), parents were once again administered the CFI during the inpatient phase and the affective style interaction assessment several weeks after discharge. This time, however, ratings of parental expressed emotion (based on the FMSS) were also made on the day of the outpatient affective style assessment. Patients in this sample (Nuechterlein, Edell, Norris, & Dawson, 1986; Nuechterlein, Snyder, et al., 1986) were of relatively recent onset (i.e., ill less than 2 years) and were largely clinically remitted by the time of this outpatient assessment.

The two measures of expressed emotion did not overlap in 33% of the cases, which, as discussed earlier, may have resulted from a softening of family attitudes over time or to differences in the sensitivity of the two instruments. However, this moderate level of correspondence proved to be fortuitous, because it enabled us to compare the utility of expressed emotion attitudes measured during a period of high family distress (the inpatient CFI) with that of expressed emotion attitudes assessed at a time of moderate distress (the outpatient FMSS) in predicting affective style behavior.

The FMSS–expressed emotion rating proved to be a stronger predictor of parental affective style behavior than was the

CFI–expressed emotion rating. However, prediction of affective style was maximized through construction of an expressed emotion profile score indicating whether families remained consistent in their emotional attitudes across the CFI and FMSS assessments. Families who remained high in expressed emotion across both measures ($n = 13$) made more harsh criticisms and guilt-inducing statements than did families who shifted from high to low expressed emotion ($n = 9$) or who remained low in expressed emotion across the two assessments ($n = 11$). (Families that became more negative in their attitudes across time and measurement method [low CFI–expressed emotion/high FMSS–expressed emotion group] were too small in number [$n = 3$] to evaluate separately.)[4] Thus, families were most likely to behave negatively toward their patient–offspring if their expressed emotion attitudes toward that offspring were consistently high across time and measurement method.

How Do Patients Contribute to This Intrafamilial Milieu?

A shift in our thinking about these family factors came as a result of observing that negative interchanges in families were frequently initiated by patients. In what ways do schizophrenic patients contribute to the family's emotional climate via their emotional attitudes or interactional behaviors?

Expressed emotion in patients. In a pilot study of 20 newly discharged, relatively remitted patients, patients' expressed emotion attitudes toward their mothers were measured using the FMSS, which simply requires that the patient describe his or her relationship with the parent. Corresponding

4. These family expressed emotion profiles were uncorrelated with degree of clinical improvement in patients from the inpatient to the outpatient period as measured by the Brief Psychiatric Rating Scale (BPRS; Lukoff, Nuechterlein, & Ventura, 1986; Overall & Gorham, 1962) or with severity of BPRS symptoms during the postdischarge aftercare period. Likewise, parents' affective style scores were uncorrelated with patients' BPRS scores.

maternal attitudes were also tabulated based on identical FMSS scoring criteria.

A correspondence between patient and maternal expressed emotion attitudes (high versus low) was recorded in 75% of the cases (Table 19.2). Correspondence of expressed emotion attitudinal subtypes (critical versus emotionally overinvolved) was less consistent. Similar findings were reported by Brown, Monck, Carstairs, and Wing (1962), who found a 67% rate of correspondence when comparing the expressed emotion attitudes of relatives and schizophrenic patients. However, the specific high–expressed emotion attitudes expressed by relatives and patients did not always match.

The finding that expressed emotion attitudes are to some degree reciprocated by patients suggests that (a) the attitudes of either member of the parent–patient dyad may in some cases "drive" or elicit the attitudes of the other member, or (b) expressed emotion may be a measure of a dyadic relationship rather than of an individual's attitudes or idiosyncratic responses to a stressful family situation. A more thorough examination of these questions is currently underway, employing a larger sample of schizophrenic patients and a more comprehensive assessment of patient expressed emotion (Tompson, 1990).

Interactional behavior in patients. The issue of parent–patient reciprocity in direct family interaction was addressed in our study of recent-onset schizophrenic patients ($n = 36$) and their (primarily biological) parents (Strachan, Feingold, Goldstein, Miklowitz, & Nuechterlein, 1989). Patient interactional behavior, based on the same interaction transcripts from which parental affective style was derived, was evaluated using the *coping style* coding system, a system that reflects the domain of possible patient responses to parental affective style statements. Coping style codes include statements of autonomy, self-affirmation, support of the parent, and criticisms of the parent, refusals to perform certain behaviors, and self-denigrating statements. Raw

Table 19.2. Expressed Emotion (EE) in Patients and Their Mothers[a]

EE in patients	EE in mothers		
	Low	High–critical	High–overinvolved
Low	9	1	4
High–critical	0	2	0
High–overinvolved	0	2	2

[a] $X^2 = 12.29$, $p < .02$.

numbers of coping style statements from these various categories were tabulated. Furthermore, a dominant coping style profile was constructed for each patient, based on whether the majority of the coping style statements coded for that patient were primarily "autonomous" in nature (e.g., "I'm going to see a job counselor tomorrow"; $n = 5$); primarily "externalizing" or countercritical or refusing (e.g., "You have never been helpful to me"; $n = 12$); or primarily "internalizing" or self-denigrating (e.g., "I just don't deserve any of your help"; $n = 8$). A minority of patients ($n = 11$) made few or no coping style statements at all ("neutral" profile). Patients with these coping style profiles did not differ on severity or type of concurrent symptoms (based on the BPRS) or on measures of illness history.

A comparison was made between families' dominant affective style profiles (negative versus benign) and these four patient coping style profiles. A strong degree of reciprocity was observed. When parents were rated "benign" in affective style, patients were in most cases (10 of 14, or 71%) rated "autonomous" or "neutral" in coping style. However, when parents were rated "negative" in affective style ($n = 22$) —based primarily on their use of harsh criticisms and/or guilt-inducing statements—only a minority of the patient–offspring showed "autonomous" or "neutral" coping style patterns (6 of 22, or 27%). The majority of these patients (73%) showed "negative" coping style profiles: 36% (8 of 22) were "externalizing" and 36% (8 of 22) were "internalizing." Furthermore, this linkage of negative parent affective style and negative patient coping style profiles was most frequently observed (69% of

cases) among families who were consistently high in expressed emotion (high CFI, high FMSS), and less frequently among families with the high–low (33%) and low–low (27%) expressed emotion patterns.

These results suggest that, when a schizophrenic patient is the recipient of a harsh criticism or a guilt-inducing statement, he or she is likely to counter with a criticism of the relative (a "symmetrical" relational pattern) or a self-denigrating statement (a "complementary" relational pattern) (Haley, 1963). In other cases, the patient may begin this interactional chain. For instance, a patient's criticism of a parent may prompt a countercriticism from this parent. Likewise, a patient's self-denigration may elicit guilt induction from a parent. Thus, negative attitudes in parents of schizophrenic patients, when expressed during a hospitalization and again during the outpatient phase, may tap a reciprocal, relational process marked by escalating, stressful interchanges to which parents (via their affective style behavior) and patients (via their coping style behavior) mutually contribute.

Are these relational processes associated with differential risk of relapse? If stable high–expressed emotion attitudes in parents are tapping a negative relational process in families of schizophrenics, one would hypothesize that patients from these families are at greater risk for relapse than are patients from families with stable low–expressed emotion or unstable high–expressed emotion (high CFI, low FMSS) attitudes. Preliminary data from this recent-onset sample support this hypothesis (Goldstein & Nuechterlein, personal communication, January 18, 1991). When patients are from high CFI–high FMSS expressed emotion families, rates of psychotic relapse at 1-year follow-up are highest. Rates for patients from high–low and low–low families are intermediate and low, respectively, suggesting that those parental attitudes expressed during the inpatient *and* outpatient phases are important in predicting (a) the family's transactional patterns, and (b) the associated risk for patient relapse over a short-term follow-up.

It is important to reiterate that the high–high pattern was associated with high rates of criticism in parents *and* in patients. In fact, the number of coping style criticisms made by patients about their parents was a somewhat better predictor of relapse in this sample than was the number of affective style criticisms made by parents about these patients. However, rates of patient coping style criticisms increased as a linear function of the expressed emotion pattern (low–low, high–low, high–high) observed in their parents.

Final conclusions from this longitudinal study (Nuechterlein, Edell, Norris, & Dawson, 1986; Nuechterlein, Snyder, et al., 1986) must await collection of the full study sample. However, preliminary results suggest that a tense intrafamilial milieu, as indexed by the clustering of negative emotional attitudes in parents, negative affective style behavior in parents, and negative coping style behavior in patients, may provide a better index of risk for psychotic relapse over an outpatient follow-up than will any one family attribute taken alone.

Summary of Findings Regarding the Family Affective Climate

Our findings from samples of recently hospitalized schizophrenic patients suggest several conclusions:

1. Expressed emotion attitudes as measured by the CFI administered during the inpatient phase are frequently but not always indicative of the attitudes expressed by parents once the patient has returned to the community (FMSS).

2. When families are consistently high in expressed emotion across both measures, a negative, reciprocal, relational process is often observed in direct interaction.

3. These negative attitudes and transactional processes are associated with an increased risk of psychotic relapse among index patients followed over a 1-year period.

Many questions remain to be addressed about these constructs. The next section deals with an important issue regarding the genesis of these intrafamilial attributes—are they indices of an increased risk for psychopathology in relatives, and, by extension, of a family history of psychopathology?

FAMILY STRESS FACTORS: INDICES OF PSYCHOPATHOLOGY IN PARENTS?

If communication deviance, expressed emotion, and affective style were found to be indirect or subclinical indicies of psychopathology among parents, the question would arise as to whether offspring from families with these attributes are at greater risk for schizophrenic onset or relapse by virtue of an increased familial loading for schizophrenia or other disorders. Alternatively, the presence of diagnosable disorders in parents may create stress in the intrafamilial environment (as indexed by the communication deviance, expressed emotion, and affective style constructs) that contributes to vulnerability to episodes of schizophrenia in offspring.

A recent study by our group (Goldstein, Talovic, Nuechterlein, Fogelson, Subotnik, & Asarnow, 1992) addressed this set of questions within the Nuechterlein, Edell, Norris, and Dawson (1986) recent-onset schizophrenic sample. Biological parents (*n* = 56) were interviewed for lifetime psychiatric diagnoses using the Diagnostic Interview Schedule (DIS; Robins, Helzer, Croughan, & Ratclift, 1981); the Structured Clinical Interview for DSM-III-R (American Psychiatric Association, 1987) personality disorders (SCID-II; Spitzer, Williams, & Gibbon, 1987); the Global Assessment Scale (GAS; Endicott, Spitzer, Fleiss, & Cohen, 1976); and those portions of the Present State Exam (Wing, Cooper, & Sartorius, 1974) relevant to diagnoses within the psychotic spectrum. Diagnoses were grouped into three primary categories:

1. No DSM-III-R diagnosis ($n = 26$).
2. Unipolar depression, anxiety disorders, substance abuse disorders, and nonschizophrenia spectrum personality disorders (i.e., avoidant, dependent, etc.; $n = 23$).
3. Schizophrenia and bipolar spectrum disorders ($n = 7$).

To date, data have been analyzed on the relation of expressed emotion and communication deviance to parental diagnoses.

Communication Deviance

Levels of parental communication deviance on the TAT were not associated with parental diagnostic group, current parent GAS ratings, or worst lifetime GAS ratings. These negative findings were unexpected. Those forms of parental communication deviance that appear to measure perceptual–cognitive disturbance (e.g., misperceptions of the TAT cards) have been found in other studies to correlate with information-processing disturbances in these parents and in their schizophrenic offspring, which in the latter are presumed to be in large part genetically acquired (Nuechterlein & Dawson, 1984; Nuechterlein, Goldstein, Ventura, Dawson, & Doane, 1989; Wagener, Hogarty, Goldstein, Asarnow, & Browne, 1986). However, it is possible that communication deviance and information-processing disturbances in parents are both manifestations of a vulnerable genotype that is not always expressed as a diagnosable disorder.

It is interesting to note that in Goldstein's (1987) longitudinal study of at-risk adolescents, communication deviance scores in parents were unrelated to a history of severe psychopathology in these parents or in other first- or second-degree relatives of the index offspring. However, those offspring from high–communication deviance families who also had a positive family history of severe psychopathology were far more likely to develop broad schizophrenia spectrum disorders at follow-up (86%) than were those from high–communication deviance families without a family history (20%). Thus, communication deviance and family history of psychopathology may not be associated with the same underlying vulnerability mechanisms. However, knowledge of both factors may increase the probability of correctly predicting which of a cohort of at-risk children are most likely to develop disorders within the schizophrenia spectrum in adulthood.

Expressed Emotion

CFI-based expressed emotion ratings were not associated with parental diagnoses, although a trend existed for parents with high–expressed emotion attitudes to have more diagnoses within the schizophrenic/bipolar spectrum grouping. FMSS expressed emotion ratings, however, were predictive of parental diagnoses: 85% of the parents rated high in expressed emotion by the FMSS had diagnoses within categories 2 (depression and nonspectrum personality disorders, 54%) and 3 (schizophrenia/bipolar spectrum disorders, 31%), whereas only 44% of the low FMSS–expressed emotion parents had these diagnoses. Furthermore, when the pattern of expressed emotion attitudes across time (inpatient versus outpatient period) and measurement method (CFI versus FMSS) was considered, the results were even more striking. Those parents with the high CFI–high FMSS expressed emotion pattern all (100%) had category 2 and category 3 diagnoses, compared with those who showed a shifting pattern (high–low or low–high; 50%) or a consistently low expressed emotion pattern (44%). Parents with the high–high pattern also had lower current GAS ratings, indicating lower concurrent psychiatric functioning, than did those with either of the other two expressed emotion patterns. Thus, psychiatric comorbidity may be one factor affecting the likelihood that a parent will express critical and/or emotionally overinvolved attitudes during and following an offspring's episode of schizophrenia.

Summary

The data presented above are open to several interpretations. First, if one views the discrepancy between CFI and FMSS ratings as due to the passage of time, parents with psychiatric diagnoses may be more likely to react negatively to an episode of psychiatric disorder in their offspring and may not have the emotional resources to shift these attitudes once the patient has returned to the community and has partially recovered. Alternatively, if one views the discrepancy as due to method variance, it is possible that parents with psychiatric diagnoses have a lower threshold for expressing high–expressed emotion attitudes, and manifest these attitudes even when probing by an interviewer is held to a minimum (such as in the FMSS).

These findings suggest that data on parents' histories of psychopathology must be considered when mapping the intrafamilial environment of the schizophrenic patient. The associations found between expressed emotion, family transactional patterns, and relapse may be influenced by a parent's diagnostic status, which may reflect an increased genetic and/or psychosocial vulnerability to episodes of psychiatric disorder within the patient's family of origin. An important future direction for this research is to evaluate whether those patients from stable high–expressed emotion families who do and do not relapse are those with parents who do and do not, respectively, manifest psychiatric disorders. When the full data from the Nuechterlein et al. sample are collected, this question will be addressed.

ARE QUALITIES OF THE INTRAFAMILIAL ENVIRONMENT AMENABLE TO CHANGE THROUGH FAMILY INTERVENTION?

Up until this point, two major issues have been addressed: (a) the predictive utility of family environmental factors, and (b) the origins of these attributes. But what can be done about family stress factors? Once an attribute such as communication deviance is identified within a family, can the family be taught new communication styles that are clearer and more easily interpreted by a listener? Can a high–expressed emotion family be taught to be low in expressed emotion? Can negative transactional patterns be restructured so that families no longer show reciprocal, escalating affective style–coping style interchanges? Does achieving these results bring about better short-term outcomes for schizophrenic patients?

Is Expressed Emotion Modifiable?

Several studies have demonstrated that, when schizophrenic patients are maintained on standard neuroleptic regimens, high–expressed emotion attitudes in parents can be altered via family psychosocial treatment (Hogarty et al., 1986; Leff, Kuipers, Berkowitz, Eberlein-Fries, & Sturgeon, 1982; Leff, Kuipers, Berkowitz, & Sturgeon, 1985; Leff et al., 1989; Tarrier et al., 1988). These family programs were all relatively short term, educational, crisis oriented, skill focused, supportive of medication adherence, and centered on helping the family to adjust to the patient's reentry into the home or community after an episode of schizophrenia. Several of these studies suggest that family treatment is most effective in reducing risk of relapse when families show treatment-associated reductions in initial levels of expressed emotion. Furthermore, reductions in family expressed emotion are not easily achieved in comparison treatment conditions that do not involve the family (Hogarty et al., 1986).

It appears that expressed emotion attitudes are modifiable. However, it may be much easier to modify an attitude than a transactional behavior such as affective style. Whereas the former requires that an initially high–expressed emotion relative simply express more benign attitudes to a neutral clinical interviewer on reassessment, the latter requires that the relative act differently when in the room with the patient. Second, a family-focused program may be effective in changing the attitudes held by relatives, but what about patients and their reactions to relatives (coping styles)? Finally, what about communication clarity (communication deviance)? Is family intervention powerful enough to effect changes in a possibly long-standing family attribute whose appearance may have predated the onset of the disorder (Goldstein, 1987)?

Results of a Family Intervention Study

The findings reported in this section are from a controlled study that investigated the efficacy of a family treatment program—behavioral family management (BFM)—in preventing or delaying episodes of schizophrenia among outpatients maintained on neuroleptics (Falloon, Boyd, & McGill, 1984). BFM consists of three primary components: education for the family about schizophrenia, communication skills training, and training in problem-solving skills. The treatment, conducted in 21 sessions spread over 9 months, is home based and includes the patient. Falloon et al. found that, in 36 relatively chronic, initially hospitalized schizophrenic patients, a 9-month trial of BFM administered in conjunction with neuroleptic medication was, over a 2-year follow-up, far more effective than supportive individual therapy and medication for the patient in reducing relapse rates, reducing number of days in hospital, improving social and occupational adjustment, and reducing the need for high doses of neuroleptics.

By what mechanisms did BFM achieve these results? Were family attributes that are associated with a high risk of patient relapse successfully modified by BFM? In this section, data are reviewed on the efficacy of this family treatment in modifying the pretreatment levels of affective style, coping style, and communication deviance of patients and family members in the Falloon et al. sample. Because these findings were all based on the same controlled treatment

study, results deserve replication in future studies.

Parental affective style. In the Falloon et al. study, family interaction assessments were conducted just prior to the beginning of psychosocial (individual or family) treatment (approximately 2 weeks after hospital discharge) and again after 3 months of treatment. The timing of this 3-month reassessment carried certain advantages over conducting a reassessment at the end of the 9-month treatment: it allowed an investigation of whether potential mediating variables (such as affective style) changed prior to the occurrence of the dependent variable of interest, relapse. In fact, most of the relapses in the Falloon et al. study occurred after the 3-month follow-up.

Data from the Falloon study (Doane, Goldstein, Miklowitz, & Falloon, 1986) are presented in Table 19.3. First, initial levels of parental affective style (criticism or intrusiveness) were more likely to decrease in the BFM plus medication condition than in

Table 19.3. Changes in Parental Affective Style (AS) after Psychosocial Treatment and Their Relation to Patient Outcomes

	N^a	Number of relapses (9-month followup)
Family treatment condition	17	1
AS change group[b]		
Dual increase	2	0
Mixed pattern	6	0
Dual decrease	9	1
Individual treatment condition	16	9
AS change group		
Dual increase	8	5
Mixed pattern	4	3
Dual decrease	4	1

[a] Three families from the original Falloon et al. (1984) sample were excluded from these analyses because they lacked 3-month AS data.
[b] Dual increase = number of critical *and* intrusive statements increased from pretreatment to 3-month follow-up; mixed pattern = one attribute increased while the other stayed the same or decreased; dual decrease = number of critical and intrusive statements both decreased from baseline to 3 months.
Reprinted with permission from Doane, J. A., Goldstein, M. J., Miklowitz, D. J., & Falloon, I. R. H. (1986). The impact of individual and family treatment on the affective climate of families of schizophrenics. *British Journal of Psychiatry, 148,* 279–287.

the individual treatment plus medication condition. In parallel to this, relapse rates at 9-month follow-up were lower in the BFM plus medication condition (6% versus 56%). In the individual treatment plus medication condition, rates of relapse varied according to whether increases or decreases in affective style scores were observed by 3-month reassessment (Table 19.3). Thus, there was evidence that treatment-associated reductions in affective style were a factor mediating the success of this family treatment. In all probability, parents had assimilated communication and problem-solving skills by 3 months that enabled them to behave with greater neutrality toward the patient–offspring.

Patient coping style. If the combination of family treatment and medication for the patient is successful in modifying parent interactional styles, can it also modify those styles observable in patients? In order to underline the significance of this question, three models of influence deserve mention. In the first model, only the interactional behaviors of parents are viewed as directly modifiable by family treatment, and the effects of treatment "trickle down" to patients (in terms of their symptoms and, perhaps, their interactional behaviors) as patients become medically stabilized and parents learn to deal more effectively with the illness. In a second, "reciprocal" model, both parent and patient interactional styles are viewed as modifiable by family treatment, resulting in a family milieu that promotes patient improvement. In a third, "individual skills" model, family treatment is seen as primarily affecting patient interactional behaviors and hence, relapse rates.

Within the Falloon et al. sample, patients became less negative (externalizing or internalizing) and more neutral in coping style interactional behavior from pretreatment to 3 months, regardless of treatment condition (Rea, Strachan, Goldstein, Falloon, & Hwang, 1991). Furthermore, coping style behavior at baseline or 3 months bore no relationship to relapse rates at 9-month follow-up. Thus, patient interactional behav-

iors were less clearly influenced by family management than were parent affective style behaviors, the latter of which were predictive of patient outcomes.

If the coping style system is a valid method for assessing patient interactional styles, these results are most consistent with the first model of influence—the "trickle down" model—in which it is primarily parent behaviors that change as a direct result of family treatment, and patients benefit from the resulting reductions in intrafamilial tension in conjunction with the stabilizing effects of their pharmacotherapy regimens. Of course, it is possible that patients who have recently had an episode of psychosis simply take longer than their parents to assimilate social–interpersonal skills, and that patient coping skills behaviors would have been more strongly affected by family treatment had coping skills been reassessed later in the course of treatment. The question of whether changes in parental interactional behavior are a precondition for corresponding changes in patient interactional behavior is a topic worthy of investigation.

Communication deviance. A final question addressed within the Falloon et al. sample was whether levels of intrafamilial communication deviance are modifiable by family treatment. As discussed earlier, Velligan et al. (1988) developed the ICD system for measuring levels of communication deviance among parents and patients participating in an interaction task. Velligan, Goldstein, and Miklowitz (1990) applied the ICD system to the Falloon et al. sample, using interaction transcripts obtained at pretreatment and at 3 months into the treatment phase. Because BFM emphasizes the learning of communication skills that enhance communication clarity, Velligan et al. hypothesized that greater reductions in communication deviance would be observed among families in BFM than among those in which the patient received individual therapy.

When parent and patient communication deviance scores were summed to form family total scores, a Treatment × Time interaction was observed: families in the BFM plus medication condition showed greater reductions in initial levels of communication deviance than did families in the individual therapy plus medication condition. Furthermore, the effects of family treatment on intrafamilial communication deviance were independent of its effects on affective style. In fact, a multiple regression analysis revealed that improvement scores (from baseline to 3 months) in affective style and communication deviance independently accounted for 16% and 13% of the variance in treatment group membership, respectively.

A closer examination of the Falloon et al. data revealed that the effects of family treatment on family communication deviance scores were largely explained by its effects on *patient* communication deviance. Those patients receiving family treatment and medication showed, at 3 months, substantial reductions from their baseline levels of interactional communication deviance. Reductions in patient communication deviance were also observed in the individual therapy plus medication condition, albeit to a lesser extent. Thus, social skills training for the patient, particularly when administered in a family context, is efficacious in reducing patient communication deviance. Of course, changes in patient communication deviance may reflect overall clinical improvement—perhaps due in part to adjunctive treatment with neuroleptic medications—rather than a patients' acquisition of communication skills.

It is notable that baseline levels of parental communication deviance were not strongly influenced by either the individual or family treatment programs, and tended to remain stable over the 3-month treatment period. For some parents, communication deviance may be an enduring attribute that is not strongly influenced by psychosocial intervention or changes in the patient's clinical condition, at least over a short-term follow-up.

Summary

Certain of the family attributes believed to be important contributors to the onset and/

or course of schizophrenia are more easily modified by family intervention than are others. Prior research by other investigators (Hogarty et al., 1986; Leff et al., 1982, 1985, 1989; Tarrier et al., 1988) suggests that pretreatment levels of parent expressed emotion can be systematically reduced by educationally oriented family interventions administered with medication for the patient. A similar finding emerged from our examination of parental affective style behaviors. However, parental communication deviance was found to be less easily modified by family treatment.

Perhaps the most parsimonious interpretation of our findings concerning dimensions of patient interactional behavior—as measured by coping style and patient CD—is that these attributes improve regardless of whether the patient is treated in an individual or a family context. It seems clear that administering a family intervention is necessary in order to observe reductions in those parent attributes that are most closely associated with high rates of patient relapse (expressed emotion and affective style). However, when patients are maintained on neuroleptics, initial levels of patient coping style and communication deviance improve in both individual and family treatment (although reductions in patient communication deviance are most readily achieved in family treatment). Future research should address the question of whether psychosocial intervention is necessary in order to promote changes in patient interactional behavior, or whether these changes can be accomplished via pharmacological interventions alone.

FUTURE RESEARCH DIRECTIONS

Over the past 25 years, the research program of the UCLA Family Project has focused on intrafamilial attributes that predict the onset and/or course of schizophrenic disorders. Our most recent findings suggest that dysfunctional family communication—in the domains of communication clarity and affective tone—is a precurser to the onset of schizophrenia spectrum disorders. Furthermore, attributes of the intrafamilial affective environment as measured during the acute psychotic episode and the aftercare period are predictive of the course of schizophrenic disorders. We have attempted to describe the nature of these environments in terms of the conjoint, reciprocal contributions of the parents and index patient. Finally, we have presented data to suggest that certain aspects of the family environment are amenable to change through psychosocial intervention.

Many questions remain unanswered about these constructs. Recommendations for future studies of family attributes are presented in this section.

Communication Deviance

Although there is now evidence that communication deviance is a precurser to the onset of schizophrenia and related disorders, it is still unclear what underlying processes are measured by this construct. Levels of communication deviance are uncorrelated with diagnosable disorders or with levels of psychosocial impairment in biological parents of schizophrenics. However, data from other studies (Nuechterlein et al., 1989; Wagener et al., 1986) suggest that certain types of parental communication deviance—particularly those types associated with misperceptions of stimuli on projective tests—are correlated with measures of dysfunctional information processing in these parents and in their schizophrenic offspring. There is also substantial data to suggest that measures of dysfunctional information processing are genetically based vulnerability markers for schizophrenia.

Certain types of communication deviance may reflect underlying perceptual–cognitive vulnerabilities among parents that may also be manifested by their patient–offspring. Future longitudinal studies that investigate the association between parental communication deviance and offspring information-processing deficits, particularly in samples of children at risk for schizophrenia by virtue of genetic and/or psychosocial

factors, would help to determine (a) whether parental communication deviance and offspring perceptual–cognitive deficits are related to similar underlying vulnerability mechanisms, and (b) whether these family and offspring attributes are additive or interactive influences on the gradual development of schizophrenic disorders.

The question of whether high levels of intrafamilial communication deviance are specific to schizophrenia is also unresolved. Our data comparing biological parents of schizophrenic and bipolar patients suggest that levels of parental communication deviance may be less useful in distinguishing between different forms of psychosis than they are in distinguishing psychotic from nonpsychotic disorders. If high levels of communication deviance are in fact associated with forms of psychosis other than schizophrenia, what role do they play in these disorders? Do high levels of communication deviance predict the onset of disorders within the psychotic affective as well as the schizophrenia spectrum? Is the linkage between parental communication deviance and offspring perceptual–cognitive dysfunction also found among patients with bipolar disorder or psychotic depression? Investigation of these issues would help to elucidate the origins of communication deviance and clarify its role as a risk factor in the onset of major mental disorders.

Finally, it remains unclear as to whether parental communication deviance is a state or a trait variable. Our limited data from the Falloon et al. (1984) family treatment study suggest that parental communication deviance is difficult to modify with family treatment, at least over a short period of follow-up. However, it is a conceptual leap to conclude that parental communication deviance is therefore a trait attribute. Future research that evaluates the longitudinal stability of parental communication deviance in the face of abrupt changes in the patient's clinical condition would help to resolve this state–trait question. We also see value in future treatment studies that systematically investigate the linkage between certain types of family interventions and improvements in those forms of parental communication deviance that are specifically targeted by these intervention strategies.

Attributes of the Intrafamilial Affective Climate

There is now substantial evidence to suggest that attributes of the intrafamilial emotional climate have prognostic value in schizophrenic disorders. However, studies that simply document a longitudinal relationship between expressed emotion and relapse rates, without any exploration of the patient, parent, and family mechanisms that mediate this association, are not particularly informative or illuminating. We have described one possible mediating mechanism—a reciprocal, negative transactional process among stably high–expressed emotion parents and their newly discharged schizophrenic offspring—that may help to explain the association between expressed emotion and patient outcomes in some samples. But what other mechanisms account for the expressed emotion–relapse relationship? Do long-standing personality attributes of patients feed into this reciprocal, transactional loop? Are parents in some cases reacting to personality traits of patients that they found objectionable even prior to the onset of the illness? What are the differences between families in which patients primarily initiate negative cycles and those in which parents are the initiators? Identification of those factors that predict the appearance of negative transactional patterns in high–expressed emotion families might help to explain some of the variance in relapse-proneness among patients from these families, and might suggest specific family intervention strategies for modifying these family processes.

As was true for communication deviance, there is also a need to clarify the role of family emotional attitudes and behaviors in disorders other than schizophrenia. Family expressed emotion appears to represent a generic stress factor that affects the course of a variety of disorders, including affective disorders and obesity (Fischmann-Havstad

& Marston, 1984; Hooley et al., 1986; Miklowitz et al., 1988; Vaughn & Leff, 1976). However, are the family transactional patterns associated with these disorders similar to those observed in families of schizophrenic patients? For instance, do bipolar, manic patients interact with their high–expressed emotion parents in the same way that schizophrenic patients do? Do parents of affective patients with stable high–expressed emotion attitudes also have a history of severe psychiatric disorders themselves? Is behavioral family treatment equally effective for these disorders, and if so, is it effective by the same mechanisms as were found significant in our study of schizophrenic patients? Investigation of these questions is important not only for clarifying whether certain family patterns are unique to schizophrenia, but also as an avenue for articulating vulnerability–stress models for the course of other severe, recurrent psychiatric disorders.

Implications for Studies of Prevention

Research in the area of psychosocial factors would benefit from an increased focus on factors relevant to the onset and prevention of schizophrenia. As mentioned above, one means of clarifying the possible etiological role of family factors is to study the association or interaction between these factors and genetic vulnerability mechanisms in at-risk children. However, a potentially more powerful method is to investigate whether these family factors are modifiable through early intervention with families of at-risk children. Prevention studies using designs in which, for instance, one group of at-risk children receives a family treatment specifically tailored to the needs of the premorbid family situation and another group receives individual counseling for the at-risk child (or is followed naturalistically), would help to determine whether family factors are indeed mechanisms contributing to the onset of schizophrenia, and whether altering these factors reduces the risk of developing these disorders in the first place. Thus, the technologies now employed for understanding and altering the course of schizophrenia may also be applicable to the onset of this disorder. If successful preventive strategies can be developed using these technologies, the lives of many psychiatrically vulnerable individuals and their family members would be greatly enhanced.

ACKNOWLEDGMENTS

This research was supported by National Institute of Mental Health grants MH30911, MH08744, MH37705, MH14584, MH42556 and MH43931; a grant from the John T. and Catherine MacArthur Network on Risk and Protective Factors in the Major Mental Disorders; a Young Investigator grant from the National Alliance for Research on Schizophrenia and Depression; and a Junior Faculty Development Award from the University of Colorado, Boulder.

REFERENCES

American Psychiatric Association. (1980). *Diagnostic and statistical manual of mental disorders* (3rd ed.). Washington, DC: American Psychiatric Press, Inc.

American Psychiatric Association. (1987). *Diagnostic and statistical manual of mental disorders* (3rd ed., rev.). Washington, DC: American Psychiatric Press, Inc.

Brown, G. W., Monck, E. M., Carstairs, G. M., & Wing, J. K. (1962). Influences of family life on the course of schizophrenic illness. *British Journal of Preventive Social Medicine, 16,* 55–68.

Doane, J. A., Falloon, I. R. H., Goldstein, M. J., & Mintz, J. (1985). Parental affective style and the treatment of schizophrenia: Predicting course of illness and social functioning. *Archives of General Psychiatry, 42,* 34–42.

Doane, J. A., Goldstein, M. J., Miklowitz, D. J., & Falloon, I. R. H. (1986). The impact of individual and family treatment on the affective climate of families of schizophrenics. *British Journal of Psychiatry, 148,* 279–287.

Doane, J. A., West, K. L., Goldstein, M. J., Rodnick, E. H., & Jones, J. E. (1981). Parental communication deviance and affective style: Predictors of subsequent schizophrenia-spectrum disorders in vulnerable adolescents. *Archives of General Psychiatry, 38,* 679–685.

Endicott, J., Spitzer, R. L., Fleiss, J. L., & Cohen, J. (1976). The Global Assessment Scale: A procedure for measuring overall severity of psychiatric disturbance. *Archives of General Psychiatry, 33,* 766–771.

Falloon, I. R. H., Boyd, J., & McGill, C. (1984). *Family care of schizophrenia.* New York: Guilford Press.

Fischmann-Havstad, L., & Marston, A. R. (1984). Weight loss maintenance as an aspect of family emotion and process. *British Journal of Psychiatry, 23,* 265–271.

Glynn, S., Randolph, E., Eth, S., Paz, G., Leong, G., Shaner, A., & Strachan, A. M. (1990). Psychopathology and expressed emotion in schizophrenia. *British Journal of Psychiatry, 157,* 877–880.

Goldstein, M. J. (1987). Family interaction patterns that antedate the onset of schizophrenia and related disorders: A further analysis of data from a longitudinal prospective study. In K. Hahlweg & M. J. Goldstein (Eds.), *Understanding major mental disorder: The contribution of family interaction research* (pp. 11–32). New York: Family Process Press.

Goldstein, M. J., Talovic, S. A., Nuechterlein, K. H., Fogelson, D. L., Subotnik, K. L., Asarnow, R. F. (1992). Family interaction vs. individual psychopathology: Do they indicate the same processes in the families of schizophrenics? *British Journal of Psychiatry, 161* (suppl. 18), 97–102.

Haley, J. (1963). *Strategies of psychotherapy.* New York: Grune & Stratton.

Hogarty, G. E., Anderson, C. M., Reiss, D. J., Kornblith, S. J., Greenwald, D. P., Javna, C. D., Madonia, M. J., & the EPICS Schizophrenia Research Group. (1986). Family psychoeducation, social skills training, and maintenance chemotherapy in the aftercare treatment of schizophrenia: I. One-year effects of a controlled study on relapse and expressed emotion. *Archives of General Psychiatry, 43,* 633–642.

Hooley, J. M., Orley, J., & Teasdale, J. D. (1986). Levels of expressed emotion and relapse in depressed patients. *British Journal of Psychiatry, 148,* 642–647.

Jenkins, J. H., Karno, M., de la Selva, A., Santana, F., Telles, C. Lopez, S., & Mintz, J. (1986). Expressed emotion, maintenance pharmacotherapy, and schizophrenic relapse among Mexican-Americans. *Psychopharmacology Bulletin, 22,* 621–627.

Jones, J. E. (1977). Patterns of transactional style deviance in the TATs of parents of schizophrenics. *Family Process, 16,* 327–337.

Jones, J. E., & Doane, J. A. (1979). *Communica-*

tion deviance scoring manual. Unpublished manuscript.

Koenigsberg, H. W., & Handley, R. (1986). Expressed emotion: From predictive index to clinical construct. *American Journal of Psychiatry, 143,* 1361–1373.

Leeb, B., Hahlweg, K., Goldstein, M. J., Feinstein, E., Mueller, U., Dose, M., & Magana-Amato, A. (1990). *The cross national reliability, concurrent validity, and stability of a brief method for assessing expressed emotion.* Manuscript submitted for publication.

Leff, J. P., Berkowitz, R., Shavit, N., Strachan, A., Glass, I., & Vaughn, C. (1989). A trial of family therapy versus a relatives' group for schizophrenia. *British Journal of Psychiatry, 154,* 58–66.

Leff, J. P., Kuipers, L., Berkowitz, R., Eberlein-Fries, R., & Sturgeon, D. (1982). A controlled trial of social intervention in the families of schizophrenic patients. *British Journal of Psychiatry, 141,* 121–134.

Leff, J. P., Kuipers, L., Berkowitz, R., & Sturgeon, D. (1985). A controlled trial of social intervention in the families of schizophrenic patients: Two year follow-up. *British Journal of Psychiatry, 146,* 594–600.

Lukoff, D., Nuechterlein, K. H., & Ventura, J. (1986). Appendix A: Manual for expanded Brief Psychiatric Rating Scale. *Schizophrenia Bulletin, 12,* 594–602.

Magana, A. B., Goldstein, M. J., Karno, M., Miklowitz, D. J., Jenkins, J., & Falloon, I. R. H. (1986). A brief method for assessing expressed emotion in relatives of psychiatric patients. *Psychiatry Research, 17,* 203–212.

Miklowitz, D. J., Goldstein, M. J., Doane, J. A., Nuechterlein, K. H., Strachan, A. M., Snyder, K. S., & Magana-Amato, A. (1989). Is expressed emotion an index of a transactional process? I. Parents' affective style. *Family Process, 28,* 153–167.

Miklowitz, D. J., Goldstein, M. J., Falloon, I. R. H., & Doane, J. A. (1984). Interactional correlates of expressed emotion in the families of schizophrenics. *British Journal of Psychiatry, 144,* 482–487.

Miklowitz, D. J., Goldstein, M. J., Nuechterlein, K. H., Snyder, K. S., & Mintz, J. (1988). Family factors and the course of bipolar affective disorder. *Archives of General Psychiatry, 45,* 225–231.

Miklowitz, D. J., & Stackman, D. (1992). Communication deviance in families of schizophrenic and other psychiatric patients: Current state of the construct. *Progress in Experimental Personality and Psychopathology Research, 15,* 1–46.

Miklowitz, D. J., Velligan, D. I., Goldstein, M. J., Nuechterlein, K. H., Gitlin, M. J., Ranlett, G., & Doane, J. A. (1991). Communication deviance in families of schizophrenic and manic patients. *Journal of Abnormal Psychology, 100,* 163–173.

Mintz, L. I., Liberman, R. P., Miklowitz, D. J., & Mintz, J. (1987). Expressed emotion: A call for partnership among relatives, patients, and professionals. *Schizophrenia Bulletin, 13,* 227–235.

Nuechterlein, K. H., & Dawson, M. E. (1984). Information processing and attentional functioning in the developmental course of schizophrenic disorders. *Schizophrenia Bulletin, 10,* 160–203.

Nuechterlein, K. H., Edell, W. S., Norris, M., & Dawson, M. E. (1986). Attentional vulnerability indicators, thought disorder, and negative symptoms. *Schizophrenia Bulletin, 12,* 408–426.

Nuechterlein, K. H., Goldstein, M. J., Ventura, J., Dawson, M. E., & Doane, J. A. (1989). Patient-environment relationships in schizophrenia: Information processing, communication deviance, autonomic arousal, and stressful life events. *British Journal of Psychiatry, 155*(suppl. 5), 84–89.

Nuechterlein, K. H., Snyder, K. S., Dawson, M. E., Rappe, S., Gitlin, M., & Fogelson, D. (1986). Expressed emotion, fixed dose fluphenazine decanoate maintenance, and relapse in recent-onset schizophrenia. *Psychopharmacology Bulletin, 22,* 633–639.

Overall, J. E., & Gorham, D. R. (1962). The Brief Psychiatric Rating Scale. *Psychological Reports, 10,* 799–812.

Rea, M. M., Strachan, A. M., Goldstein, M. J., Falloon, I. R. H., & Hwang, S. (1991). Changes in patient coping style following individual and family treatment for schizophrenia. *British Journal of Psychiatry, 158,* 642–647.

Robins, L. N., Helzer, J. E., Croughan, J., & Ratcliff, K. S. (1981). National Institute of Mental Health Diagnostic Interview Schedule. *Archives of General Psychiatry, 38,* 381–389.

Singer, M., & Wynne, L. (1965a). Thought disorder and family relations of schizophrenics. III. Methodology using projective techniques. *Archives of General Psychiatry, 12,* 187–212.

Singer, M., & Wynne, L. (1965b). Thought disorder and family relations of schizophrenics. IV. Results and implications. *Archives of General Psychiatry, 12,* 201–212.

Singer, M., & Wynne, L. (1966). Principles for scoring communication deviances in parents of schizophrenics: Rorschach and TAT scoring manuals. *Psychiatry, 29,* 260–288.

Spitzer, R. L., Williams, J. B. W., & Gibbon, M. (1987). *A structured clinical interview for*

DSM-III-R Personality Disorders (SCID-II, 3/1/87). New York: Biometrics Research Department, New York State Psychiatric Institute.

Strachan, A. M., Feingold, D., Goldstein, M. J., Miklowitz, D. J., & Nuechterlein, K. H. (1989). Is expressed emotion an index of a transactional process? II. Patient's coping style. *Family Process, 28,* 169–181.

Tarrier, N., Barrowclough, C., Vaughn, C., Bamrah, J. S., Porceddu, K., Watts, S., & Freeman, H. (1988). The community management of schizophrenia: A controlled trial of a behavioral intervention with families to reduce relapse. *British Journal of Psychiatry, 153,* 532–542.

Tompson, M. (1990). *Stress and schizophrenia: Relatives' attitudes, patients' perceptions, and coping*. Unpublished doctoral dissertation proposal, University of California, Los Angeles.

Vaughn, C. E., & Leff, J. P. (1976). The influence of family and social factors on the course of psychiatric illness: A comparison of schizophrenic and depressed neurotic patients. *British Journal of Psychiatry, 129,* 125–137.

Velligan, D., Christensen, A., Goldstein, M. J., & Margolin, G. (1988). Parental communication deviance: Its relationship to parent, child, and family system variables. *Psychiatry Research, 26,* 313–325.

Velligan, D. I., Goldstein, M. J., & Miklowitz, D. J. (1990). *The impact of individual and family treatment on communication deviance in the families of schizophrenic patients*. Paper presented at the Society for Research in Psychopathology, Boulder, CO.

Velligan, D. I., Goldstein, M. J., Nuechterlein, K. H., Miklowitz, D. J., & Ranlett, G. (1990). Can communication deviance be measured in a family problem-solving interaction? *Family Process, 29,* 213–226.

Wagener, D. K., Hogarty, G. E., Goldstein, M. J., Asarnow, R. F., & Browne, A. (1986). Information processing and communication deviance in schizophrenic patients and their mothers. *Psychiatry Research, 18,* 365–377.

Wing, J., Cooper, J. E., & Sartorius, N. C. (1974). *The measurement and classification of psychiatric symptoms: An instruction manual for the PSE and CATEGO programs*. London: Cambridge University Press.

Woodward, J. A., & Goldstein, M. J. (1977). Communication deviance in the families of schizophrenics: A comment on the misuse of analysis of covariance. *Science, 197,* 1096–1097.

Wynne, L. C., & Singer, M. T. (1963a). Thought disorder and family relations of schizophrenics. I. A research strategy. *Archives of General Psychiatry, 9,* 191–198.

Wynne, L. C., & Singer, M. (1963b). Thought disorder and family relations of schizophrenics. II. A classification of forms of thinking. *Archives of General Psychiatry, 9,* 199–206.

Wynne, L., Singer, M., Bartko, J., & Toohey, M. (1977). Schizophrenics and their families: Recent research on parental communication. In J. M. Tanner (Ed.), *Developments in psychiatric research* (pp. 254–286). London: Hodder & Stoughton.

Part VII

CONCLUSIONS

20

A Summary View of Schizophrenia

RUE L. CROMWELL

This book has dealt with the origins, processes, treatment, and outcome of schizophrenia. Many advances have been made, but many questions are yet unanswered. This chapter presents a summary of how schizophrenia might now be viewed, as based on the preceding chapters and related literature. New hypothetical inferences are made that incorporate but also go beyond the content of these chapters. Any such view must be selective. If it provokes researchers to ask good questions and thereby advance knowledge, it has served its purpose.

SYNOPTIC OVERVIEW

Schizophrenia is an oligogenic disorder. That is, it originates from not one, nor many, but a small number of factors. Two of these factors, each with genetic and environmental components, are described. One factor arises from the overexcitatory response to the physical intensity of stimuli. The other arises from the overinhibitory response to meaning (information value) of these stimuli. These two factors confront each other for the first time during the acute phase of psychosis. They determine independent courses for negative and positive symptoms. More important, however, the two factors are proposed as interactive, not additive. This interaction characterizes, more than anything else, the essence of schizophrenia that distinguishes it from other disorders. The interaction locks schiz-

ophrenia into becoming an enduring disorder for many who have it. The typical neuroleptic drugs, when effective, treat (a) the first of these factors and (b) the interaction of the two factors. Typical neuroleptics appear not to treat the second factor. Specialized psychological treatment of the family, when used in combination with the neuroleptic drugs, has proven advantageous, and its effectiveness is not specific to schizophrenia.

BASIC PROCESSES, COURSE, TREATMENT, AND ORIGINS

The following sections describe how information presented elsewhere in the book bears on this summary view of schizophrenia. Much of this new formulation has been inspired by the research legacies of David Shakow and Joseph Zubin. These legacies have been selectively summarized and analyzed in Chapter 8 by Steffy and Waldman. Their chapter also describes the Waterloo extension of those legacies. The works of Hemsley (Chapter 9) and Knight (Chapter 10) represent important new extensions of these legacies.

Many of Shakow's and Zubin's oft-repeated findings, which depict the unusual sensitivities and reliably deviant reactions of people with schizophrenia, have escaped the attention of contemporary investigators. Things tend to go out of fashion if (a) they do not appear to be leading anywhere, especially with respect to amelioration or some other practical benefit, or (b) they are complex, apparently contradictory—difficult to put together in a story of what schizophrenia is about. Perhaps both of these reasons were true of their findings at an earlier time, and Steffy and Waldman (Chapter 8) analyze the reasons for this and show how the Waterloo studies reconcile some of the issues.

Also important to the formulation have been the chapters by Rubin and Harrow (Chapter 14), Schooler (Chapter 17), Spohn (Chapter 16), and Straube (Chapter 15) concerning the course and treatment of schizophrenia.

It might be said that one cannot know schizophrenia unless one knows well the research legacies of David Shakow and Joseph Zubin. It might also be said that schizophrenia will not eventually become understood until its course and symptoms can be seen as unfolding naturally from these salient and complex processes.

Basic Processes

Among the various views that appeared contradictory between Shakow and Zubin, as Steffy and Waldman (Chapter 8) have indicated, was that Shakow emphasized the failure of schizophrenics to maintain a focus of attention (more than a few seconds), whereas Zubin emphasized their persistence of attention. He stressed the fact that immediately prior events were brought to bear unduly on the current situation. As another apparent contradiction, schizophrenics were described, at the same time, as overexcitatory (supersensitive) and overinhibitory. Both Shakow and Zubin agreed that schizophrenics are susceptible to interference of even the most subtle sort. One reconciling view is that an imbalance exists between the excitatory and inhibitory functions that allows these extreme reactions. An alternative view is proposed here: that each tendency exists separately and is under its own genetic and environmental control. The "overinhibitory" factor is referred to here as Factor R. It is arbitrarily named with reference to the redundancy

concept developed by Steffy (see Steffy & Waldman, Chapter 8; Bellissimo & Steffy, 1972, 1975). The "overexcitatory" factor will be referred to here as Factor S. It is arbitrarily named with reference to the supersensitivity factor described by Kendler and Eaves (see Cromwell, Chapter 4; Kendler & Eaves, 1986).

Factor R is characterized by an inhibition in either the latency or the amplitude of response. It is hypothesized here to occur primarily in situations in which the individual is engaged in an activated behavioral sequence. (These situations may also be described as goal directed or as ones involving intent.) When an intrusion with informational value (extrinsic stimulus or covert thought) occurs, the patient either delays, inhibits to lower effort, quits, or substitutes another behavior for the ongoing behavior of intent. The inhibition tends to occur without awareness.

It is speculated here that this "bogging down" of the patient's goal-directed reaction results from the exaggerated tendency to "overconceptualize" the meaning and action sequence implication of the input. Thus, competing activating sequences, involving both approach and avoidance, subdue or interrupt the original one. Then, as the schizophrenic patient continues to detect temporal or part–whole regularities (redundancies) in subsequent input, the overconceptualization (and the resultant overinhibition) accrue.

One example, primarily attributable to Factor R, is the redundancy (or reaction time crossover) deficit. In the task measuring this deficit, a constancy in length of preparatory interval in a reaction time task is of sufficient informational value to result in a progressive slowing in successive reaction time trials.

Factor S is characterized by an overexcitatory (overfacilitatory, supersensitive) response to extrinsic physical stimulus input. It varies as a function of the physical intensity of the input and whether it is novel or perceived as novel. The exaggeration of response may be adaptive (e.g., extensive scanning, fast response to an intense reaction time stimulus), but it is often maladaptive (e.g., response to an intense preparatory stimulus that forewarns of an upcoming reaction time stimulus).

The distinction between Factor S and Factor R may be compared with the distinction between early- and late-evoked response components and early and late visual masks. The amplitude of the N100/P200 visual evoked response is affected by physical stimulus intensity. Some individuals (including schizophrenics) have been shown unable to damp out (reduce) the high-intensity input (Buchsbaum & Silverman, 1968). In the later P300 evoked response, normal subjects' amplitudes reflect uniformly the task relevance of the stimuli. By contrast, the P300 amplitudes of schizophrenics are variously influenced by (a) the task relevance of the stimulus, (b) a predictable regularity of the stimulus that is not relevant to the task, and/or (c) a change in the characteristics of the signal (e.g., Steinhauer, 1985; Steinhauer & Zubin, 1982). Note the parallel of these results to the above contention that the stimulus meaning in the later (P300) phase is overconceptualized in schizophrenics.

The distinction between Factors S and R may also be seen in the work of Knight (Chapter 10), which depicts the separate roles of (early) nonmeaningful and (later) meaningful masks on a visual image. The difficulty in taking advantage of the spatial and temporal redundancies of input, as depicted by Hemsley (Chapter 9), may be viewed in reference to Factor R.

Steffy (see Chapter 8) has devised a technique called "probed reaction time," which appears to separate the R and S factors. After a series of routine regular reaction time trials, a new stimulus of minor informational value (e.g., a bordering of Xs around the "get set" signal on a video screen) is presented at the beginning of the forewarning period. Its effect on reaction time is plotted as a function of the length of this forewarning period. In trials with short forewarning periods (1 to 3 seconds), reaction time latency is prolonged if the unexpected stimulus pattern is present. A recovery occurs among trials with 5 to 7 seconds of forewarning; that is, the novel stimulus makes little or no difference as compared to ordinary trials with the same length of forewarning. Then, a "resurgence" of reaction time deficit occurs when the novel pattern is introduced on trials with 9 seconds or greater forewarning. Thus, two different deficits, early and late, may be observed in patients. It is hypothesized here that these early and late deficits, respectively, represent independent phenomena, that the early slowing is associated with Factor S and the later slowing with Factor R. The early slowing is assumed here to result from the physical character of the novel pattern before any meaning attribution is attempted. The later slowing is assumed to occur only after time has permitted the stimulus to be processed for its meaning.

Course

In their respective studies and reviews of the natural course or treatment of schizophrenia, Harrow (see Rubin & Harrow, Chapter 14), Schooler (Chapter 17), Spohn (Chapter 16), and Straube (Chapter 15) have compiled extensive convergent information about the role of negative and positive symptoms. Positive symptoms refer to those manifestations of schizophrenia that emerge anew and do not exist (at least to the same extent) among normal individuals. Negative symptoms refer to aspects of functioning that normal individuals ordinarily have but that have been lost in schizophrenics.

As a preface to the summary of their findings, it should be noted that major problems exist with regard to the scientific status of these two symptom constructs. They are defined differently in different studies. Even when defined the same, their psychometric (i.e., reliability, internal consistency, validity) status is not strong. Whether positive symptoms should be grouped as a whole is questionable, and sometimes some symptoms called positive are at best marginal. Arndt, Alliger, and Andreasen (1991) have factor-analyzed symptoms, and they have found more than a single positive symptom factor. The emphasis in this chapter on two genetically specific factors in schizophrenia does not preclude the possibility that more may exist or that they may be associated, respectively, with more than one kind of positive or negative syndrome.

Negative symptoms are even more fraught with problems. Such symptoms may coexist with depressive symptoms (Kuck, Zisook, Moranville, Heaton, & Braff, 1992). Standard methods used to measure negative symptoms may be confused with symptoms of depression, sedating or motor side effects of medication, premorbid personality trait structures unrelated to schizophrenia, or, as is discussed later, generalized cognitive deficit. Generalized cognitive deficit emerges separately from negative and positive symptoms primarily during the postacute phase of illness. In spite of these shortcomings, the negative–positive symptom distinctions have value as crude constructs that represent the current state of the art.

Summarizing from the aforementioned chapters, the following characterize the course of the schizophrenic disorder:

1. During the premorbid period, negative symptoms may accrue. They are usually characterized as poor premorbid adjustment. These negative symptoms may persist into later phases when the condition becomes labeled as a psychosis.
2. During the acute phase, positive symptoms emerge. Both positive and negative symptoms become prominent and elevated.
3. Although positive symptoms may be reduced after the acute period (or after any succeeding acute relapse episode), they tend not to disappear. Over 50% of schizophrenic patients continue to have positive symptoms.
4. Compared to negative symptoms, which tend to have an enduring course, positive symptoms are relatively unstable. Relapse episodes

are therefore characterized by the recurrence of positive symptoms. Among the positive symptoms, hallucinations tend to be the most stable.
5. Negative symptoms elevate as well during the acute period. They decrease at the end of the period but not completely. Thus, negative symptoms, like mediated vulnerability markers (Nuechterlein & Dawson, 1984), have both trait and state characteristics.
6. Negative symptoms, when assessed outside the period of acute episode, are therefore the most stable index of severity of disorder.
7. Concrete thinking represents the most enduring of the negative symptoms and, if anything, may even increase from the post acute to a 4.5 year follow-up point.

From these preceding findings, positive and negative symptoms may be seen to run separate and independent courses, except during the acute period. Therefore, it is reasonable to hypothesize that they are driven by separate etiological factors. Factor R is proposed here to be associated with negative symptoms (possibly also with those positive symptoms that endure beyond the acute period). Factor S is proposed to be associated with positive symptoms. The two together produce the generalized cognitive deficit as a third feature.

Treatment

Again, abstracting from Chapters 14 through 17, response to treatment with typical neuroleptics is as follows:

1. Little is known about whether neuroleptic treatment during the premorbid period for individuals at risk for schizophrenia can effectively ward off psychosis.
2. Typical neuroleptics appear to have a useful role during the prodromal or very early stages of ill-

ness. This early treatment appears to be beneficial to the disorder in its later phases.

3. However, for about 20% of schizophrenic patients, neuroleptic drugs have no beneficial effect whatever.

4. Neuroleptics are beneficial to both positive and negative symptoms during the acute period (first 5 months following onset of the illness).

5. If one assumes that change with placebo represents spontaneous change, then hebephrenic symptoms (positive thought disorder, inappropriate affect) improve with drugs but not spontaneously during the acute period.

6. Delusions of grandeur remit spontaneously, but not in response to drugs. (Keep in mind that at least some delusions may develop as patients attempt to construe their own acute perceptual disturbances. Then, when the perceptual disturbances remit or are ameliorated by neuroleptics, the delusional constructions may remain and therefore not be closely linked to the drug treatment.)

7. Social participation improves both spontaneously and in response to the drugs.

8. From 5 to 13 months following the onset of illness, neuroleptics have a beneficial effect in reducing the positive (e.g., delusions other than of grandeur) but not the negative symptoms. According to Straube (Chapter 15), a low stimulus barrier score and the presence of distractibility (each interpreted here as Factor S [supersensitivity]) are associated with good short-term treatment response but with an undulating course (i.e., frequent relapses). In between relapses, however, the remission of symptoms and the restoration of social functioning is fairly complete.

9. For those symptoms, positive or negative, that remain after 13 months, neuroleptic drugs have no ameliorative effect.

10. Nevertheless, neuroleptic drugs continue to play an important role during this chronic (post–13-month) period in preventing either exacerbation of symptoms or relapse. For example, 20% of schizophrenic patients relapse on drugs; 52% of them relapse on placebo.

11. A psychosocial family therapy (e.g., major role, social skills) combined with neuroleptics is superior to treatment with neuroleptics alone.

12. The psychosocial therapy alone—that is, without drugs—produces worse outcome than no treatment at all.

From the foregoing it is clear that both the course and response to treatment of the positive and negative symptoms are relatively independent, except for the acute period of illness. Finally, and very importantly, it will be recalled that the interaction of the two factors (R × S) is proposed to constitute the major essence of what we recognize as schizophrenia. This interaction binds the disorder into an enduring illness. It is proposed that this R × S interaction is reflected by (a) the instability and elevation of symptoms during the acute period and (b) the generalized deficit that characterizes the long-term course.

In other words, it is speculated that the hyperresponsivity to the immediate physical stimulus amplitude during early stages of processing confronts the later overinhibitory response to the information value (see Steffy & Waldman, Chapter 8; Knight, Chapter 10). This confrontation occurs for the first time during the acute phase of illness. The instability and elevation of both positive and negative symptoms represent by-products of the efforts to resolve (or yield to) this unique (overexcitatory and overinhibitory) combination of circumstances. Then, as the acute period passes, the same unique combination of circumstances resolves itself into a generalized deficit that is observed on almost all cognitive tasks.

The role of typical neuroleptic drugs is beneficial with Factor S but not with Factor R. Their impact on Factor R comes only when the reducing of S also reduces the R × S interaction. Thus, the benefit of typical neuroleptics for negative symptoms exists only during the unstable elevated acute phase. Thereafter the neuroleptics may be of value in ameliorating the generalized cognitive deficit so that the patient can develop new conceptual structures about individuals and events. These new conceptual structures help lessen stimulus intensity associated with novelty and threat value of each new demand in the life situation. Otherwise, negative symptoms are not affected during the postacute period.

Origins

. . . a small number of factors. The evidence for schizophrenia originating from at least two factors (see Cromwell, Chapter 4) comes from studies such as those by Heston (1966), McNeil (1971), De Amicis, Wagstaff, and Cromwell (1986), and McCarthy (1993). (In these studies a significant number of healthy first-degree relatives of schizophrenics have creativity or socioeconomic functioning above chance expectancy. Following from Kendler and Eaves (1984), this may be interpreted to mean that at least one factor is accountable for a supersensitivity to environmental information. At least one additional factor is then needed to define the direction of the individual family relative—that is, toward superior functioning or toward schizophrenic deterioration. Unlike Kendler and Eaves (1986), who proposed that a single genetic locus governing supersensitivity interacted with a favorable or unfavorable environment, it is proposed here that the second factor, responsible for setting the direction, has genetic as well as environmental constituents. If one of the factors is missing (not inherited and activated), then the individual has either a benign supersensitivity to stimulation (Factor S only) or else a prolific con-

ceptualizing capacity when interpreting stimuli (Factor R only). Either of these may enhance creativity or socioeconomic functioning.

Keeping in mind that 20% of schizophrenics do not respond beneficially to dopamine-blocking drugs (proposed here to be specific for the treatment of Factor S), the possibility of additional factors responsible for schizophrenia must be acknowledged.

. . . each with genetic . . . components. From the many twin, adoptee, and family studies, it is evident that a prebirth factor exists for schizophrenia. Most people assume that this prebirth factor is a genetic one. To affirm this assumption, evidence is needed regarding mode of transmission and chromosomal locus. No such evidence yet exists. In spite of this general lack of evidence, it is nevertheless hypothesized here that two separate and independent genetic contributions (at least) to schizophrenia are expressed by Factors R and S, respectively.

One provocative example of the search for evidence for genetic loci is presented by Iacono (Chapter 6; Bassett, McGillivray, Jones, & Pantzar, 1988). He describes the emergence of schizophrenia in parallel with a dysmorphic chromosome 5. So, this chromosome may be involved in typical cases of schizophrenia as well.

. . . an oligogenic disorder. With the above hypothesis that Factors R and S are separately gene related, it may also be hypothesized that schizophrenia is oligogenic. This means that only a few genes are involved in the genetics of schizophrenia. This view is in opposition to both a monogenic and a polygenic view of the mode of transmission. Although the evidence to refute the monogenic and polygenic models in favor of an oligogenic one is by no means conclusive (see McGuffin & O'Donovan, Chapter 5), some evidence does exist:

1. The diversity in course and symptoms makes schizophrenia somewhat difficult to interpret as origi-

nating from a single genetic contribution.

2. Single autosomal dominant gene disorders are usually very rare, because they tend to select themselves out of the population. Schizophrenia, with a 1% lifetime incidence, has unusually high frequency. Therefore, it is not likely to be single autosomal dominant (Risch, 1992).

3. Going from monozygotic (MZ) twins to siblings to more remote relatives (who share less and less genetic relationship; expected 50% drop with each step), the frequency of schizophrenia has a different dropoff rate from what one would expect with a single dominant gene. Therefore, it likely involves more than one gene (Risch, 1992).

4. One illustration of this dropoff rate is provided by the study by Gottesman and Bertelsen (1989), who compared the schizophrenia risk levels of the offspring of discordant MZ and dizygotic (DZ) twins. For MZ twins, 16.8% of the offspring of the affected twin were schizophrenic; 17.4% of the offspring of the unaffected twin were schizophrenic. (As an aside, these similar rates affirm that the genetic identity between MZ twins is of greater importance than the full expression of the inherited trait in the parent.) Of importance here are the data of the discordant DZ twin offspring. For the DZ twins, 17.4% of the affected twins were schizophrenic; only 2.1% of the unaffected twins were schizophrenic. The drop in risk rate from the offspring of DZ affected to unaffected twins is dramatic. The latter rate is barely above the incidence rate for schizophrenia in the general population. This can hardly be explained by a polygenic model, because a polygenic dispersion of relevant genes would surely allow a greater level of expected residual risk for the unaffected member of a DZ twin pair. A monogenic model with full penetrance would indeed predict a lowered rate also, but this model does not appear tenable when the data of the MZ twins suggest that full penetrance is not likely. A congenial model for the observed 2.1% risk, therefore, could be an interactive oligogenic model wherein all of a small set of genes must be present before schizophrenia becomes manifest.

5. Still another source of evidence is the discontinuity in frequency distribution of a schizophrenia-related variant among the healthy first-degree relatives of schizophrenics (see Cromwell, Chapter 4; also, Freedman et al., Chapter 7). A distribution that suggests a commingling of two subsets of relatives, one that apparently expresses a schizophrenia-related gene and one that does not, augers against the hypothesis of a polygenic model (wherein relatives differ only in gradations rather than bimodally).

Also, partly in accord with the present proposal is the prevailing view at the 1992 American Psychopathological Association meeting on genetic linkage in psychopathology. This meeting emphasized an oligogenic hypothesis for schizophrenia (Gershon, 1992), except that the implication was primarily toward an additive model. The proposal here is of an interactive model, neither contributor of which could be labeled as a schizotypal gene if present without the other.

. . . *two factors each with . . . environmental components.* A traditional view of environmental factors in schizophrenia has been Rosenthal's (1967) stress–diathesis model, in which constitutional factors interact with environmental stress as a basis for schizophrenia. Attendant to this view has been the vulnerability model (Spring & Zubin, 1977), in which genetic vulnerability adds to stress until a hypothetical threshold is reached to precipitate schizophrenic psychosis. The model presented here tends not to view stress as the monolithic environmental contributor. Instead, it considers environmental factors with respect to how they impinge on the respective genetic components in Factors R and S. In this respect, environmental variance may be separated into R_e and S_e. For example, selected stimulants, such as amphetamine, may combine with the genetic supersensitivity to define Factor S. Exogenous pre- and perinatal events may bear on either factor. Taken together, the environmental contribution to schizophrenia would not be subsumed completely under the construct of stress; however, stress would nevertheless be one type of environmental contributor. Finally, much of environmental variance contributing to schizophrenia is viewed not in terms of the physically defined external events, but instead in terms of the personal conceptual structure (construct system) the individual has developed as a way to pursue and anticipate these events (see Patterson, 1987; Rosenberg, Chapter 13). In other words, it is the match or mismatch of input, not with the remembered past but instead with the conception and anticipation of events, that is the major determinant of behavior.

Another example may be useful to illustrate the separate roles of Factor S and Factor R, because each is necessary interactively to create the schizophrenic process. If Factor S were acting alone, the best analogue in real pathology might be an amphetamine psychosis. High levels of this exogenous stimulant lead to a psychotic delusional episode not easily distinguished from schizophrenia except for its quick and complete remission. Lower levels of the stimulant, such as might be analogous to the relatives of schizophrenics, could conceivably produce high levels of stimulus processing and cognitive functioning. Instead of exogenous amphetamine, the endogenous dopamine receptivity is more congenial to current biochemical models of schizophrenia as an explanatory construct. Nevertheless, the effect may be analogous. Treating the schizophrenia merely with dopamine

(i.e., stimulant) blockers would be expected to suppress the supersensitivity but would not be expected to deal with the negative and deficit aspects of the schizophrenia.

It is further speculated that the analogue for Factor R may be the enduring symptoms of post-traumatic stress disorder (PTSD). Two pieces of evidence are offered to support this suspicion. First, the enduring symptoms of PTSD—that is, the numbing; the loss of interest in activities, occupation, and/or sex; the general anhedonia (loss of sense of pleasure); and intrusions of thought (manifestations of dissociation)—are perhaps more similar than any others in functional psychopathology to the negative symptoms of schizophrenia.

Second, the Perceptual Aberration and Magical Ideation scales (Allen, Chapman, Chapman, Vuchetich, & Frost, 1987), commonly used to study schizophrenia and proneness to other psychosis, have item content often closely related to dissociation. In turn, dissociation and its related characteristics have been studied (Bernstein & Putnam, 1986; Carlson, 1991) in relation to the response to trauma (i.e., PTSD).

If the speculation, that the enduring PTSD symptoms are an analogue to Factor R, is useful, two notions are immediately implied. First, people with PTSD do not also have Factor S, or else they would have a reactive psychosis (or schizophrenia?) rather than PTSD. Second, the Factor R component of schizophrenia may require early traumatic events (as well as genetic predisposition) to precipitate its expression.

DIAGNOSIS, FURTHER TREATMENT IMPLICATIONS, AND RESEARCH

In the remainder of this chapter, issues from the foregoing chapters are discussed that did not lead directly to the formulation presented here but that are nevertheless salient to schizophrenia.

Breadth of Diagnostic Definition

How broad or narrow should the definition of schizophrenia be? Compared to definitions in past decades, the criteria in the *Diagnostic and Statistical Manual of Mental Disorder,* third edition, revised (DSM-III-R; American Psychiatric Association, 1987) are relatively narrow. McGuffin and O'Donovan (Chapter 5) present an impressive set of findings that indicate that the more narrow criteria restrict genetic findings. Their data suggest that a more moderate (broader, but not too broad) set of criteria would be more useful in the genetic study of schizophrenia. This implication is true whether one is investigating a polygenic, monogenic, or oligogenic model.

Indirect evidence is brought in support of McGuffin and O'Donovan (Chapter 5) by Iacono (Chapter 6), who reports that smooth pursuit eye tracking deficit, commonly associated with schizophrenia, occurs in depressives with schizoaffective symptoms and individuals with the social (but not cognitive) symptoms of schizotypal personality disorder.

A different kind of support for the relaxing of definitional boundary comes from the work of Spaulding (Chapter 18). When studying and implementing rehabilitative treatment, Spaulding and other colleagues have often disregarded the DSM categories in favor of the broadly defined category of "chronically mentally ill." The common features and rehabilitative needs of the chronically mentally ill often limit the usefulness of diagnostic divisions.

Further Treatment Implications

Neuroleptic treatment. In addition to the review of efficacy of traditional neuroleptics, Schooler (Chapter 17) also reviewed briefly the more recent "atypical neuroleptics." In the efforts to find medications that (a) minimize side effects, (b) are effective when typical dopamine-blocking drugs fail altogether, and (c) do not oversaturate receptors for short-term symptom gain at the expense of long-term benefit (as typical high-potency neuroleptics are sometimes reputed to do), an important focus has been placed on the study of "atypical neuroleptics." Following from the formulation pre-

sented in this summary chapter, one aspect of this search should be on treatments effect for Factor R as well as for Factor S. [In this respect, the findings that clozapine reduces negative as well as positive symptoms is promising (Kane, Honigfeld, Singer, & Meltzer, 1988).] Beyond this, pharmacological research may continue to be useful in narrowing the candidacy of genetic phenotypes where a one-to-one relationship between genes and treatment responsivity exists.

Conceptual structure and family therapy. The beneficial effect of certain family therapies (when combined with pharmacotherapy) on the relapse rate of schizophrenic patients has now been well established (see Miklowitz & Goldstein, Chapter 19; Schooler, Chapter 17). It is reasonable to assume that this benefit occurs at least partly because of changes this therapy has induced in the conceptual structure of the patient. The patient acquires new ways of construction (organizing information about and anticipating encounters with family and other significant individuals). If so, then greater understanding of conceptual structure may have implications for improving family therapy or even providing alternative interventions that are beneficial.

Many recent advances have occurred in assessing how individuals organize this personal information (Rosenberg, Chapter 13). Much of the current methodology originates from Kelly's (1955) personal construct theory and the role construct repertory paradigm (the Rep Grid). In this procedure a list of elements (names of individuals, events, or other items to be construed) is provided, and in a systematic procedure the subjects apply their own concepts (personal constructs) to classify and rate these elements. The finished product is a matrix of numerical data with an element representing each column and a construct dimension of the subject representing each row of the matrix. In analyzing these data, a distinction is made between content and structural analysis. Content analysis depends on knowing the personal definition a subject ascribes to his or her respective constructs. Structural analysis does not require this knowledge. Instead, various mathematical indices can be derived from the matrix that have high reliability and validity but do not deal with the personal lexicon of the subject.

Through a hierarchical analysis (HICLAS) technique based on set theory, Rosenberg (Chapter 13) and his co-workers have developed an index that assesses the extent to which each given element enters into relationships with other elements. In so doing, a hierarchy of element organization is mathematically derived. Rosenberg and his co-workers have studied how the "self," as one of the elements in the matrix, is hierarchized (elaborated) by schizophrenic patients. They report a strong confirmation of their hypothesis that the "self" element of schizophrenics is low in elaboration. That is, the self does not enter into relationships with other constructs as does the self of normal individuals. This finding is not attributable to the complexity level of the hierarchical structure.

The finding may be compared with another finding (Sewell, 1991) that PTSD patients from Vietnam combat cannot construe their major traumatic combat event in an elaborated (hierarchically elevated) way. Thus, it may be hypothesized that PTSD victims dissociate—that is, are unable to bring the traumatic combat event into identifiable relationships with other events before and after Vietnam. Thus, they cannot put the trauma event into a story that has a smooth cause–effect progression.

The same failing may be hypothesized for schizophrenics, except that the "self," rather than a traumatic event, is the element being conceptualized. If schizophrenics are deficient in relating "themselves" in multiple and meaningful ways to other family members and other people in general, family therapy may make its beneficial difference through facilitating an elaboration of conceptual structure. In turn, the elaboration of conceptual structure may suppress the overexcitatory (Factor S) and/or overinhibitory (Factor R) tendencies that precipitate or exacerbate psychotic symptoms.

These comments do not preclude the ben-

eficial effect of stable reconceptualization that occurs among family members as a result of the family therapy. Miklowitz and Goldstein (Chapter 19) have provided an extensive review of how family interactive style bears on this beneficial family therapy–drug therapy intervention. Their review makes clear that, at least in part, the benefit that comes from family therapy is not specific to the disorder of schizophrenia. Similar predictions and outcomes can occur with other pathologies, such as bipolar mood disorder and obesity.

Of special interest theoretically, however, is the note by Schooler (Chapter 17) that such family psychosocial therapy without drugs is less beneficial than no drugs at all. If the dopamine-blocking drugs suppress Factor S, as has been proposed here, then one may speculate that family therapy alone increases the supersensitivity (i.e., S Factor).

As implied by Miklowitz and Goldstein (Chapter 19), the disturbed behavior of the patient can place high stress on the construct systems of family members, and vice versa. Ordinary personal constructs of a family member can be painful to discard when the patient, for example, responds to the family member as a hostile stranger. Such may be the case when the patient cannot retrieve from his or her memory store and acknowledge the history of loving care and commitment a family member has given. Both Neufeld, Vollick, and Highgate (Chapter 11) and Hemsley (Chapter 9) have provided evidence of the particular impairment that paranoid schizophrenic patients have in this retrieval ability. Thus, family therapy can be beneficial to the family as well as to the patient in helping them accommodate to these "social violations," which arise from the patient's illness. In this respect, the study of the family members' conceptual structure and its parameters of change should not be neglected.

Not all schizophrenic patients have families (or else families willing to conjoin in the treatment process). This represents one impetus for the development of rehabilitative treatment programs for the chronically mentally ill, such as has been studied and reported by Spaulding (Chapter 18). Among the various findings reported are the successful results in using as a treatment/training procedure the repeated creation of alternate Thematic Apperception Test (TAT) stories based on the same stimulus card. The positive results reported with this technique may potentially have some bearing on the Factor R component among schizophrenic patients. Through alternate meaning (informational) attributions to a single stimulus, the counterinhibition of one activation sequence over another may be reduced. One may speculate that such exercises may impinge indirectly on the dissociative tendencies and allow a repertory of cause–effect constructs to be produced that allow reality to be viewed and experienced in a continuous, uninterrupted stream.

Implications for Research

For the psychopathology researcher interested in applying attention and information-processing (AIP) concepts to the genetics of schizophrenia, the summary view of schizophrenia presented here is not entirely encouraging. Until now, at least some researchers in psychopathology have envisioned that AIP variables would be demonstrated as useful markers and phenotypes in the study of genetic transmission in schizophrenia. This view now becomes less likely—or, at least more complicated. Most AIP measures are bilithic (or polylithic), rather than monolithically related to Factor R or Factor S. Thus, they are unlikely to be related to a single gene. Mean reaction time, for example, although highly useful in pinpointing the underlying impairment common to all schizophrenia, is inevitably the summative result of both factors. Even reaction time crossover (RTX; redundancy deficit), which ordinarily would be associated with Factor R, would be elevated by the R × S interaction during the acute stage of illness. Spohn (Chapter 16) reports that eye tracking deficit has a significant correlation with RTX and also with skin conductance orienting response (SCOR), yet these latter two variables have an essentially zero correlation with each other. Such a finding would suggest that the eye tracking deficit, shown clearly to be familial (Iacono, Chapter 6), may be componential rather than monolithic.

Although some AIP and psychophysiological measures may be salvaged as having relatively more loading on Factor R than S, or vice versa, a more likely hope may be in measures like the probed reaction time procedure of Steffy (Steffy & Waldman, Chapter 8) that are hypothesized to separate Factor S from Factor R impairment.

The bilithic nature of most traditional AIP and psychophysiological measures may help explain some of the inconsistencies reported in some findings in schizophrenia. Such inconsistencies have been reported here by Bernstein (Chapter 12) using the responder–nonresponder dimension of the orienting response and by Spaulding (Chapter 18) using the COGLAB battery. Depending on the type of schizophrenic patient being examined, the relative balance of Factor R and Factor S during the patients' respective natural courses, and their different responses to treatment, the results may appear contradictory or at least nonreplicable. This may be true even though the responder–nonresponder dimension of SCOR and the COGLAB variables are highly predictive under other circumstances.

Implications also exist for genetic research. McGuffin and O'Donovan (Chapter 5) have pointed out that the new developments in genetic linkage methodology and DNA probes are highly promising even though results are yet to be forthcoming. However, if a restricted set of specific genes, such as may be revealed separately by Factors R and S, are present, successful genetic linkage methodology would require that separate phenotypes be identified for the respective gene.

Similar implications are present for the quest to identify the biochemical and neuroanatomical correlates of schizophrenia. At least two classes of variables, rather than one, should be the object of the quest. In the work reported by Oke, Carver, and Adams (Chapter 3) the findings of high dopamine, as compared to norepinephrine, levels in the thalamus of schizophrenic brains would be viewed as most likely related to Factor S rather than Factor R. The interpretation of the work reported by Early (Chapter 2), however, presents a greater challenge for interpretation. Both positron emission tomography and behavioral (levorotatory turning preference) variables are brought together to argue that schizophrenia results from *decreased* dopaminergic input to the nonmotor parts of the left basal ganglia. It is unclear whether this intriguing formulation should be hypothesized in association with the suppressive and deficit aspects of Factor R or the supersensitivity aspects associated with Factor S.

As well as suggesting new research directions, other evidence in the preceding chapters has discouraged certain other directions. Both Knight (Chapter 10) and Neufeld, Vollick, and Highgate (Chapter 11), from different vantage points, have argued that the "limited-capacity" explanation for basic processes in schizophrenia is not a fruitful one. Knight analyses the hypothetico-deductive logic of the model against the empirical evidence. Neufeld et al. present a mathematical analysis in which capacity is inferred from slope/zero-intercept analysis of target recognition with various sizes of memory sets. They conclude that the "limited-capacity" model does not have explanatory value. In the same vein, Hemsley (Chapter 9), from yet a different vantage point, restricts the explanatory value of the "limited-capacity" model to controlled (as opposed to automatic) processing activities. Strauss, Buchanan, and Hale (in press) find the partial-report span of apprehension task to be related to negative symptoms (interpreted here as Factor R) and the degraded stimulus continuous performance task to be related to positive thought disorder (interpreted here as Factor S). They conclude that constructs beyond high momentary processing load (i.e., capacity limit) must be invoked to explain the perfor-

mance of schizophrenic patients on these tasks.

As for promising directions for investigation, the work by Freedman and his coworkers (Chapter 7) on the failure of schizophrenics (and a subset of their first-degree relatives) to gate (reduce the P50 average evoked potential of a stimulus that is presented 50 ms following an initial identical one) appears to be closely related to the supersensitivity factor (S). Freedman et al. present these data with their neurotransmitter and neuroanatomical, as well as their psychopathological, implications. They indicate how the failure in gating may be advantageous to those relatives who share the trait but who have otherwise healthy brains.

Knight (Chapter 10) has conducted a fascinating exploration and analysis of the interplay of two successive stimuli in a way different from Freedman et al. (Chapter 7). Knight and his co-workers have focused on the qualitative differences between poor premorbid schizophrenics and other (pathological and normal) subjects in backward masking. In normal subjects a meaningless visual pattern, presented approximately 100 ms after a visual stimulus, will mask it (i.e., make the subject unable to affirm that the original stimulus occurred). From 200 to 600 ms after the original visual stimulus, only a "conceptual mask" (a stimulus with meaning [information value]) will accomplish this masking function for normal subjects. Knight and co-workers have shown that at 250 ms either a patterned (meaningless) or conceptual (meaningful) mask is effective for poor premorbid schizophrenics. For other subjects only a meaningful mask at this 250-ms latency is effective in blocking the original stimulus.

Knight reasons that this overlap in meaningless/meaningful mask properties for poor premorbid schizophrenics might be explained in two possible ways: either meaning is attributed to a nonmeaningful mask or else a weakness exists in attributing meaning at a time when it is normally attributed. Knight and his group then proceed to design research that supports the latter alternative. In particular, the poor premorbid schizophrenics are less sensitive and retentive of holistic meaning in a stimulus presentation. This formulation places the deficit of poor premorbid schizophrenics in the realm of visual memory (i.e., after a visual image has been adequately registered). He also explains how the findings are compatible with those of studies such as by Place and Gilmore (1980), wherein the schizophrenic patients are shown to be superior in dealing with dissembled elements of a visual presentation (e.g., counting) while being inferior in comprehending the holistic meaning of the total stimulus field. Knight's choice of poor premorbid schizophrenics as his focus of study has probably been a prudent one. His findings are more likely related to Factor R; the class of variables, prominant in good premorbid schizophrenics, referred to as Factor S, are less likely to contaminate the data. Notably, the formulation in this chapter concerning Factor R involves one assumption beyond that of Knight. His conclusion that poor premorbid schizophrenics fail in timely attribution of meaning, especially holistic meaning, is assumed in Factor R to be an inhibition resulting from overattribution of alternate meanings.

The work reported by Hemsley (Chapter 9) is impressive in that its implications bear on the works of Steffy and Waldman (Chapter 8) and of Knight (Chapter 10), and vice versa. Moreover, his work may present a challenge to a formulation that separates Factor R from Factor S. Finally, more than many other current investigators, Hemsley attempts to identify the bridge between basic processes and the ultimate symptom features (delusion, hallucination, thought disorder) that characterize schizophrenia. All of these issues merit discussion.

Following from Hemsley's (Chapter 9) theoretical perspective, normal individuals take advantage of temporal and spatial redundancies (regularities) in their life experience in order to reduce their information-processing demands. When Event A has ordinarily led to B but not to C, the very appearance of A will evoke both (a) an A-B association and (b) at least some resistance to an A-C association (i.e., the latter being

negative transfer of training). When Pattern X has ordinarily been a part of Whole Y but not of Whole Z, the very appearance of X will evoke the X-Y, but will resist the X-Z, part–whole relationship. Hemsley asserts that schizophrenics fail in this processing and retrieval skill.

Following from this assertion, Hemsley and his co-workers have devised tasks in which redundancy (regularity) acquisition is paradoxically obstructive to performance. In this way, the schizophrenic's failure in redundancy acquisition allows her or him to produce the correct response more readily than the normal subject. One such task is the latent inhibition paradigm. In this paradigm, repeated exposure to a stimulus (with no specific consequences) reduces the capability in normal individuals for that stimulus to be viewed later in association with a subsequent reinforcement. This preexposure does not limit the ability for schizophrenics in an acute episode to acquire the new association with subsequent reinforcement. Such paradigms (also demonstrated by Place & Gilmore, 1980, Knight in Chapter 10) are crucial in that they circumvent the generalized cognitive deficit (R $\times$ S interaction) that usually makes cognitive studies of schizophrenia noninformative.

The research and formulation by Knight (Chapter 10) appears to be highly similar to that by Hemsley (Chapter 9). Knight describes the failure of schizophrenics to process the holistic aspects of visual memory. It would appear that holistic processing would require the perception of the part–whole (spatial), if not also the cause–effect (temporal), regularities to which Hemsley is referring.

An additional factor, however, appears to be introduced in Steffy's (Steffy & Waldman, Chapter 8) redundancy formulation. Steffy observes not only a failure of schizophrenics (primarily poor premorbid [i.e., process type]) to take advantage of the temporal regularities (redundancy) in reaction time trials but also an additional impairment beyond what would occur if no redundancy of experience had occurred. In other words, Steffy indicates that the schizophrenic does not just "fail" to respond to the temporal regularity but instead actively responds counterproductively to it. Such a finding would appear to challenge the completeness of the Hemsley formulation.

Next, however, comes the implicit challenge by Hemsley (Chapter 9) of the formulation presented here, which separates Factor R from Factor S in schizophrenia. He reviews evidence and reports the effect of a stimulant (amphetamine) on the latent inhibition and related phenomena. He describes how the normal tendency toward latent inhibition is reduced or eliminated by the stimulant. In so doing, normal individuals are then able to improve functioning up to the "superior level" observed in the schizophrenics. These data, of course, would appear analogous to what a dopaminergic effect, which is commonly assumed to be endogenous to schizophrenia, would produce. Such findings would suggest that Factor S is the mediating component of that schizophrenic process which is being affected in the latent inhibition paradigm. Yet, the work of Knight (described here to be similar to that of Hemsley) is with poor premorbid schizophrenics, who have been attributed here to be strongly loaded on Factor R. For that matter, the RTX finding, central to Steffy's formulation (see Steffy & Waldman, Chapter 8), has been attributed primarily to Factor R. One alternative explanation is that the proposed separation of Factors R and S is challenged. An alternative possibility is that the R × S interaction is reflected by all these findings. Still another possibility is that all the work—that is, of Hemsley (Chapter 9), of Knight (Chapter 10), and of Steffy and Waldman (Chapter 8)—is indeed interpretable as Factor R, but that the interpretation of the amphetamine results must be changed. Instead of exogenous amphetamine being an analogue of endogenous dopamine, acting on Factor S, it may be that amphetamine is the analogue of some other endogenous substance or mechanism that acts on Factor R.

Regardless of which interpretation is correct, the research enterprise benefits from the insight and clarity of the presentations of these respective authors; the "potential to disconfirm" such alternative various formulations should aid the progress of knowledge about schizophrenia.

REFERENCES

Allen, J. J., Chapman, L. J., Chapman, J. P., Vuchetich, J. P., & Frost, L. A. (1987). Prediction of psychoticlike symptoms in hypothetically psychosis-prone college students. *Journal of Abnormal Psychology, 96,* 83–88.

American Psychiatric Association. (1987). *Diagnostic and statistical manual of mental disorders* (3rd ed., rev.). Washington, DC: American Psychiatric Press, Inc.

Arndt, S., Alliger, R. J., & Andreasen, N. C. (1991). The distinction of positive and negative symptoms: The failure of a two-dimensional model. *British Journal of Psychiatry, 158,* 317–322.

Bassett, A. S., McGillivray, B. C., Jones, B. D., & Pantzar, J. T. (1988). Partial trisomy chromosome 5 cosegregating with schizophrenia. *Lancet, 1,* 799–801.

Bellissimo, A., & Steffy, R. A. (1972). Redundancy-associated deficit in schizophrenic reaction time performance. *Journal of Abnormal Psychology, 80,* 299–307.

Bellissimo, A., & Steffy, R. A. (1975). Contextual influences on crossover in the reaction time performance of schizophrenics. *Journal of Abnormal Psychology, 84,* 210–220.

Bernstein, E. M., & Putnam, F. W. (1986). Development, reliability, and validity of a dissociation scale. *Journal of Nervous and Mental Disease, 174,* 727–735.

Buchsbaum, M. S., & Silverman, J. (1968). Stimulus intensity control and the cortical evoked response. *Psychosomatic Medicine, 30,* 1222.

Carlson, E. B. (1991). Trauma experiences, posttraumatic stress, dissociation, and depression in Cambodian refugees. *American Journal of Psychiatry, 148,* 1548–1551.

De Amicis, D., Wagstaff, D., & Cromwell, R. L. (1986). Reaction time crossover as a marker of schizophrenia and of higher functioning. *Journal of Nervous and Mental Disease, 174,* 177–179.

Gershon, E. (1992). Summary comments. Made at the Meeting of the American Psychological Association, New York, March 7.

Gottesman, I. I., & Bertelsen, A. (1989). Confirming unexpressed genotypes for schizophrenia. Risks in the offspring of Fischer's Danish identical and fraternal discordant twins. *Archives of General Psychiatry, 46,* 867–872.

Heston, L. L. (1966). Psychiatric disorders in foster home reared children of schizophrenic mothers. *British Journal of Psychiatry, 112,* 819–825.

Kane, J. M., Honigfeld, G., Singer, J., & Meltzer, H. (1988). Clozapine for treatment resistant schizophrenia. *Archives of General Psychiatry, 45,* 789–796.

Kelly, G. A. (1955). *The psychology of personal constructs* (2 vols.). New York: W.W. Norton & Company.

Kendler, K. S., & Eaves, L. J. (1986). Models for the joint effect of genotype and environment on liability to psychiatric illness. *American Journal of Psychiatry, 143,* 279–289.

Kuck, J., Zisook, S., Moranville, J. T., Heaton, R. K., & Braff, D. L. (1992). Negative symptomatology in schizophrenic outpatients. *Journal of Nervous and Mental Disease, 180,* 510–515.

McCarthy, M. (1993). Creativity and crossover as shown by relatives of people with schizophrenia. Masters thesis, University of Kansas.

McNeil, T. F. (1971). Prebirth and postbirth influence on the relationship between creative ability and recorded mental illness. *Journal of Personality, 39,* 391–406.

Nuechterlein, K. H., & Dawson, M. (1984). Informational processing and attentional functioning in the developmental course of schizophrenic disorders. *Schizophrenic Bulletin, 10,* 160–203.

Patterson, T. (1987). Studies toward the subcortical pathogenesis of schizophrenia. *Schizophrenia Bulletin, 13,* 555–576.

Place, E. J. S., & Gilmore, G. C. (1980). Perceptual organization in schizophrenia. *Journal of Abnormal Psychology, 89,* 409–418.

Risch, N. J. (1992, March 5). *How do you find single genes in mental disorders?* Paper presented at the American Psychopathological Association, New York.

Rosenthal, D. (1967). An historical and methodological review of genetic studies of schizophrenia. In J. Romano (Ed.), *The origins of schizophrenia: Proceedings of the First Rochester International Conference on Schizophrenia* (pp. 15–26). Amsterdam: Excerpta Medica Foundation.

Sewell, K. W. (1991). *Conceptual structure of Vietnam combat veterans: Relationship between post-traumatic stress disorder and poorly elaborated trauma constructs.* Unpublished doctoral dissertation, University of Kansas.

Spring, B., & Zubin, J. (1977). Vulnerability: A new view of schizophrenia. *Journal of Abnormal Psychology, 86,* 103–126.

Steinhauer, S. R. (1985). Neurophysiological aspects of information processing in schizophrenia. *Psychopharmacology Bulletin, 21,* 513–517.

Steinhauer, S. R., & Zubin, J. (198). Vulnerability to schizophrenia: Information processing in the pupil and event-related potential. In E. Usdin & I Hanin (Eds.), *Biological markers in psychiatry and neurology* (pp. 371–385). Oxford England: Pergamon Press.

Strauss, M. E., Buchanan, R. W., & Hale, J. (in press). Relations among attention deficits and clinical symptoms in schizophrenic outpatients. *Psychiatry Research.*

Author Index

Subject Index